PROGRESS IN SURGERY OF THE LIVER, PANCREAS AND BILIARY SYSTEM

DEVELOPMENTS IN SURGERY

J.M. Greep, H.A.J. Lemmens, D.B. Roos, H.C. Urschel, eds., Pain in Shoulder and Arm: An Integrated View
ISBN 90 247 2146 6

B. Niederle, Surgery of the Biliary Tract
ISBN 90 247 2402 3

J.A. Nakhosteen & W. Maassen, eds., Bronchology: Research, Diagnostic and Therapeutic Aspects
ISBN 90 247 2449 X

R. van Schilfgaarde, J.C. Stanley, P. van Brummelen & E.H. Overbosch, eds., Clinical Aspects of Renovascular Hypertension
ISBN 0 89838 574 1

G.M. Abouna, ed. & A.G. White, ass. ed., Current Status of Clinical Organ Transplantation. With some Recent Developments in Renal Surgery
ISBN 0 89838 635 7

A. Cuschieri & G. Berci, Common Bile Duct Exploration
ISBN 0 89838 639 X

F.M.J. Debruyne & Ph.E.V.A. van Kerrebroeck, Practical Aspects of Urinary Incontinence
ISBN 0 89838 752 3

S. Bengmark, ed., Progress in Surgery of the Liver, Pancreas and Biliary System
ISBN 0 89838 956 9

PROGRESS IN SURGERY OF THE LIVER, PANCREAS AND BILIARY SYSTEM

edited by

S. BENGMARK

Department of Surgery, University of Lund, Lund, Sweden

1988 **MARTINUS NIJHOFF PUBLISHERS**
a member of the KLUWER ACADEMIC PUBLISHERS GROUP
DORDRECHT / BOSTON / LANCASTER

Distributors

for the United States and Canada: Kluwer Academic Publishers, P.O. Box 358, Accord Station, Hingham, MA 02018-0358, USA
for the UK and Ireland: Kluwer Academic Publishers, MTP Press Limited, Falcon House, Queen Square, Lancaster LA1 1RN, UK
for all other countries: Kluwer Academic Publishers Group, Distribution Center, P.O. Box 322, 3300 AH Dordrecht, The Netherlands

Library of Congress Cataloging in Publication Data

```
Progress in surgery of the liver, pancreas, and biliary
  system.

    (Developments in surgery ; 9)
    1. Liver--Surgery.  2. Pancreas--Surgery.  3. Biliary
tract--Surgery.  I. Bengmark, Stig.  II. Series.  [DNLM:
1. Biliary Tract--surgery.  2. Liver--surgery.
3. Pancreas--surgery.  W1 DE998S v.9 / W1 700 P9646]
RD546.P725  1987        617'.556           87-18558
```


ISBN-13: 978-94-010-8004-0   e-ISBN-13: 978-94-009-3349-1
DOI: 10.1007/978-94-009-3349-1

Copyright

Table of contents

Preface   VII
L. BLUMGART
List of contributors   IX
Introduction   XVII
S. BENGMARK
1. Fifty years of surgery of the liver, pancreas and biliary tract   1
K.W. WARREN
2. Radiology in hepato-pancreatico-biliary disease   45
A. LUNDERQUIST
3. Endoscopic approach to management of hepatico-pancreatico-biliary disorders   57
J.H. SIEGEL
4. Bleeding problems in hepato-biliary patients   95
S.I. SCHWARTZ
5. Septic problems in hepato-pancreatico-biliary surgery   103
M.C.A. PUNTIS AND R.L. SIMMONS
6. Abdominal drains in surgery of the liver, pancreas and biliary system   119
O.T. TERPSTRA, M.C.A. PUNTIS, E.I. GALPERIN AND T. HOLMIN
7. Trauma to the liver, pancreas and porta hepatis: aggressive and conservative management   129
J.M. LITTLE
8. Does ultrasound dissector improve the quality of hepato-pancreatico-biliary surgery?   143
W.J.B. HODGSON, M. KEMENY, J. SCHEELE AND K.G. TRANBERG
9. Hepatic arterial infusion chemotherapy: rationale, results and debits   163
C.J.H. VAN DER VELDE, L.M. DE BRAUW, P.H. SUGARBAKER AND K.G. TRANBERG
10. Primary cancer of the liver: considerations about resection   179
M.A. ADSON

11. Liver resection for colorectal metastases: who, when and to what extent? 189
M.J. KORETZ, K.S. HUGHES AND P.H. SUGARBAKER

12. Surgical management in high bile duct tumours 213
S. BENGMARK AND K.G. TRANBERG

13. Continuing problems in management of benign bile duct stricture 229
Å. ANDRÈN-SANDBERG AND S. BENGMARK

14. Pancreatic pseudocysts 241
M.N. VAN DER HEYDE

15. Surgical treatment of chronic pancreatitis 253
E. MORENO GONZÁLEZ

16. Surgical management of pancreatic cancer 283
H. OBERTOP

17. Identification and treatment of common bile duct stones before cholecystectomy 303
B. LANGER

18. Does preoperative trans-hepatic biliary decompression improve surgical results? 313
P.J. FABRI

19. Problems in surgery of cirrhotic patients 319
G.W. JOHNSTON

20. Selective and total shunts in portal hypertension – facts and myths 333
I.S. BENJAMIN

21. Use of BCAA enriched nutritional regimens in hepatic failure and sepsis – facts or fancy 349
P.B. SOETERS AND J.P. VENTE

22. Pancreas transplantation 363
G. TYDÉN AND C.G. GROTH

23. Transplantation of hepatic segments 379
C.E. BROELSCH AND J.C. EMOND

24. Pancreatic islet transplantation 395
I.D.A. JOHNSTON

25. Hepatic dearterialization in hepatic tumours 407
B. JEPPSSON AND S. BENGMARK

26. Developments in HPB nursing 417
K. ULANDER

Preface

This book reflects a broad spectrum of current opinions and progress in the surgical management of liver, pancreatic and biliary disease.

The enormous advances in diagnostic imaging techniques and in interventional, radiological and biliary approaches, the pathophysiological problems and their management manifest often as complications in the post-operative period, new techniques and the results of surgical approaches are all thoroughly documented.

Historical background is commented upon by Dr. Kenneth Warren of Boston in the first chapter. Subsequent chapters deal with a variety of subjects but always emphasizing differences of opinion and approach and maintaining the discussive environment so typical to the present-day approach to the topic.

Professor Bengmark's efforts to introduce a forum for wide discussion for diseases of the liver, pancreas and biliary tract and many recent advances in research and technology to aspects of the clinical management and outcome of patients is well rewarded in this balanced publication. Advances in this field of surgery have been and continue to be so rapid that such documentation is not only necessary but very welcome.

L.H. Blumgart
Bern/Switzerland
1986

List of contributors

Preface   LESLIE BLUMGART
              Inselspital
              CH 3010 Bern
              Switzerland

Introduction STIG BENGMARK
              Department of Surgery
              University of Lund
              S-221 85 Lund
              Sweden

Chapter 1   KENNETH WARREN
              NE Baptist Hospital
              116 Parker Hill Avenue
              Boston, MA 02120
              USA

Chapter 2   ANDERS LUNDERQUIST
              Department of Diagn Radiol
              Lund University
              S-221 85 Lund
              Sweden

Chapter 3   JEROME H. SIEGEL
              230 East 69th Street
              New York, NY 10021
              USA

X

Chapter 4   SEYMOUR I. SCHWARTZ
             University of Rochester Medical Center
             601 Elmwood Avenue
             Rochester, NY 14642
             USA

Chapter 5   MALCOLM PUNTIS
             University Department of Surgery
             University of Wales
             College of Medicine
             Heath Park, Cardiff CF4 4XN
             Great Britain

             RICHARD L. SIMMONS
             Department of Surgery Medical School
             Phillips Wangensteen Building
             516 Delaware Street SE
             Minneapolis, Minnesota 55455
             USA

Chapter 6   ONNO TERPSTRA
             University Hospital Dijkzigt
             Department of Surgery
             3015 GD Rotterdam
             The Netherlands

             MALCOLM PUNTIS
             See Chapter 5

             EDUARD I. GALPERIN
             1st Moscow Medical Institute
             Hospital 7
             Kolomensky Proezd 4
             Moscow
             USSR

             TORSTEN HOLMIN
             Department of Surgery
             University of Lund
             S-221 85 Lund
             Sweden

Chapter 7   MILES LITTLE
Department of Surgery
Westmead Centre
Westmead, NSW 2145
Australia

Chapter 8   JOHN B. HODGSON
New York Medical College
Manchester Medical Center
Munger Pavillion
Valhalla, NY 10595
USA

MARGARET KEMENY
Department of General and Oncology Surgery
City of Hope Hospital
1500 E Duarte Road
Duarte, CL 91010
USA

JOHANNES SCHEELE
University Hospital Erlangen
Maximiliansplatz 1
D-8520 Erlangen
West Germany

KARL-GÖRAN TRANBERG
Department of Surgery
University of Lund
S-221 85 Lund
Sweden

Chapter 9   CORNELIS VAN DE VELDE
Department of Surgery
University Hospital
PO Box 9600
2300 RC Leiden
The Netherlands

MAURITZ DE BRAUW
Department of Surgery
University Hospital
PO Box 9600
2300 RC Leiden
The Netherlands

PAUL SUGARBAKER
The Winship Cancer Center
Emory University School of Medicine
Atlanta, Georgia
USA

KARL-GÖRAN TRANBERG
See Chapter 8

Chapter 10   MARTIN ADSON
Department of Surgery
Mayo Clinic
Rochester, Minnesota 55905
USA

Chapter 11   MICHEAL J. KORETZ
The Winship Cancer Center
Emory University School of Medicine
Atlanta, Georgia
USA

KEVIN HUGHES
Brown University
Roger Williams General Hospital
825 Chalkstone Avenue
Providence, RI 02908
USA

PAUL SUGARBAKER
See Chapter 9

Chapter 12   STIG BENGMARK
See Introduction

KARL-GÖRAN TRANBERG
See Chapter 8

Chapter 13   AKE ANDRÉN-SANDBERG
Department of Surgery
University of Lund
S-221 85 Lund
Sweden

STIG BENGMARK
See Introduction

Chapter 14   M. NIELS VAN DER HEYDE
Academic Medical Center
University of Amsterdam
Meibergdreef 9
1105 AZ Amsterdam
The Netherlands

Chapter 15   ENRIQUE MORENO GONZALEZ
Instituto National de Salud
Carretera de Andalucia
Ciudad Sanitaria de Seguridad Social
10 de Octubre
Madrid
Spain

Chapter 16   HUUG OBERTOP
Department of Surgery
University Hospital Maastricht
PO Box 1918
6201 BX Maastricht
The Netherlands

Chapter 17   PROF. BERNARD LANGER
Toronto General Hospital
200 Elisabeth Street
Toronto, Ontario M5G 1L7
Canada

Chapter 18   PETER J. FABRI
James A Haley Veterans Administration Hospital
13000 Bruce B Downs Blvd
Tampa, FL 33612
USA

Chapter 19   GEORGE W. JOHNSTON
              Royal Victoria Hospital
              Belfast BT12 6BA
              Northern Ireland

Chapter 20   IRVING S. BENJAMIN
              Royal Postgraduate Medical School
              Ducane Road
              London W12 OHS
              Great Britain

Chapter 21   PETER B. SOETERS
              University Hospital Maastricht
              PO Box 1918
              6201 BX Maastricht
              The Netherlands

              JOHANNES P. VENTE
              University Hospital Maastricht
              PO Box 1918
              6201 BX Maastricht
              The Netherlands

Chapter 22   GUNNAR TYDÉN
              Department of Surgery
              Huddinge Hospital
              114 86 Huddinge
              Sweden

              CARL-GUSTAV GROTH
              Department of Surgery
              Huddinge Hospital
              141 86 Huddinge
              Sweden

Chapter 23   CHRISTOPH BROELSCH
              Department of Surgery
              5841 South Maryland Avenue
              Chicago, IL 60637
              USA

JEAN EMOND
The University of Chicago
5841 South Maryland Avenue
Chicago, IL 60637
USA

Chapter 24   IVAN D.A. JOHNSTON
University of Newcastle upon Tyne
Department of Surgery
The Medical School
Newcastle upon Tyne NE2 4HH
Great Britain

Chapter 25   BENGT JEPPSSON
Department of Surgery
University of Lund
S-221 85 Lund
Sweden

STIG BENGMARK
See Introduction

Chapter 26   KERSTIN ULANDER
Department of Surgery
University of Lund
S-221 85 Lund
Sweden

Introduction

This book presents the experience of a group of outstanding specialists in the field of hepato-pancreatico-biliary surgery.

Surgery of the liver, pancreas and biliary system is a rapidly developing subspeciality. Contributing to this is the increasing knowledge of the pathophysiology of these organs as well as the growing variety of methods to manage the patients when they are very sick. The developments within intensive care are of particular importance including the prevention and treatment of severe complications like sepsis and bleeding. Other fundamental contributions in recent years are the better knowledge and understanding of normal anatomy and the healing of the organs and the greater possibilities of making early diagnoses of diseases in these organs by non-invasive methods like endoscopy, CT and NMR.

Not many years ago most of the diseases in the liver, pancreas and biliary system were chiefly detected during exploratory laparotomy. Today this is rarely the case. Even in emergency cases it is often possible to work the patient up before surgery and plan the operation.

Another contributory factor to the advances made within HPB surgery is the fast development of alternative surgical techniques: interventional endoscopy and radiology. Technology has given us tools which make the surgical operation in these organs easier and safer. Today excellent devices like the ultrasonograph apparatus are available for preoperative diagnosis, mapping of the anatomy and thus, better planning of the operation. When I started my career most of the operations were done with surgical instruments, principally designed more than a hundred years ago, or with the fingers (the finger fracture technique). Now we have access to alternatives like the ultrasound dissector, the laser knife, and more recently, the jet-knife.

In addition to all this, new catheters, shunts, ports, pumps etc. have been developed for implantation in the abdomen. Today, modern HPB surgery, much more than in the past, depends on cooperation with the producer of equipment and materials. This requires working closely with companies who produce the necessary equipment.

These rapid strides made within HPB surgery gave rise to a great need for surgeons to discuss their experiences with each other. As a result, a world organization of HPB surgeons was founded and this will have its second meeting in Amsterdam, May 30 – June 4, 1988.

It is my pleasure to thank Martinus Nijhoff for making this book possible. To those leading scientists in the field of HPB surgery who have responded to the invitation to write chapters for this book I extend my grateful thanks.

Lund, January 1987
Stig Bengmark

1. Fifty years of surgery of the liver, pancreas, and biliary tract

K.W. WARREN

In addressing this comprehensive subject, one might elect to record a chronology of major milestones in the evolution of surgery of these diverse but intimately related organ systems. A Herculean task would encompass the detailed development of both major and minor surgical procedures along with the running controversies that attend almost every subject in this arena. I have elected to base this presentation essentially on my personal experience.

It has been my great good fortune to have started my surgical career about the dawn of the modern era of surgery of the liver, pancreas, and biliary system. Likewise, it has been my lot to have been associated with and influenced by some of the surgical giants who have made permanent imprints on the fabric of surgical history.

Cysts of the biliary tract

Cystic dilatation of the common bile duct may be of the fusiform type or it may be saccular in configuration. It is common for the intrahepatic ducts proximal to the cyst to be dilated. The cysts may be diverticular outpouching from the extrahepatic duct, and they may be multiple. When cysts occur in the distal end of the duct, which they frequently do in infants and children, they are usually associated with profound jaundice (Fig. 1).

An uncommon biliary cyst that occurs as the duct enters the duodenum is called a choledochocele (Fig. 2). Because these cysts are frequently associated with distal obstruction of the duct, it is not uncommon for biliary calculi to be present within the cyst. This is particularly true in adults and especially in patients who have had a previous inadequate operation for the correction of the problem (Fig. 3).

Some controversy exists about the origin of these cysts. One theory is that they are congenital developmental abnormalities; another theory insists that they are acquired. Recently, considerable attention has been focused on the

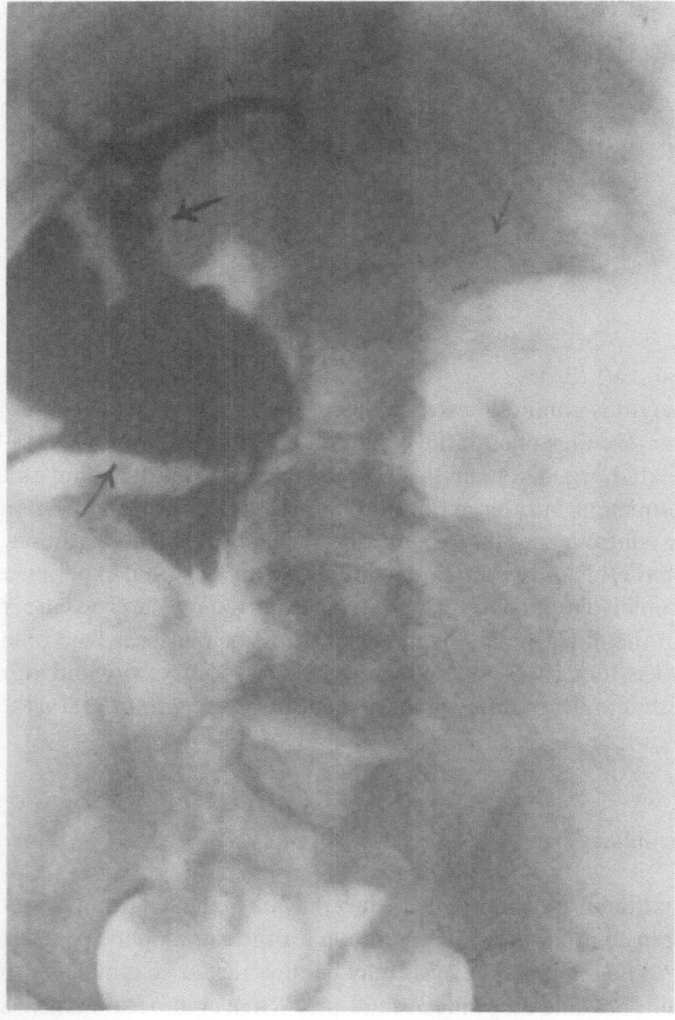

Fig. 1. Large cyst of the distal common bile duct in a 3-year-old boy. Treatment included cystojejunostomy and temporary external drainage with a mushroom catheter.

2% to 5% incidence of malignant tumors in cysts of the biliary tract. The age of
the patient at the onset of symptoms is related to the development of cancer in
cysts. Cancer is more common when the symptoms first appear in adulthood.

A rare form of cystic dilatation of the biliary tract described by Caroli is
characterized by multiple cystic dilatations of the intrahepatic ducts. The degree of dilatation may be extreme; it can occur unilaterally, but unfortunately
its distribution is more commonly bilateral (Figs. 4, 5).

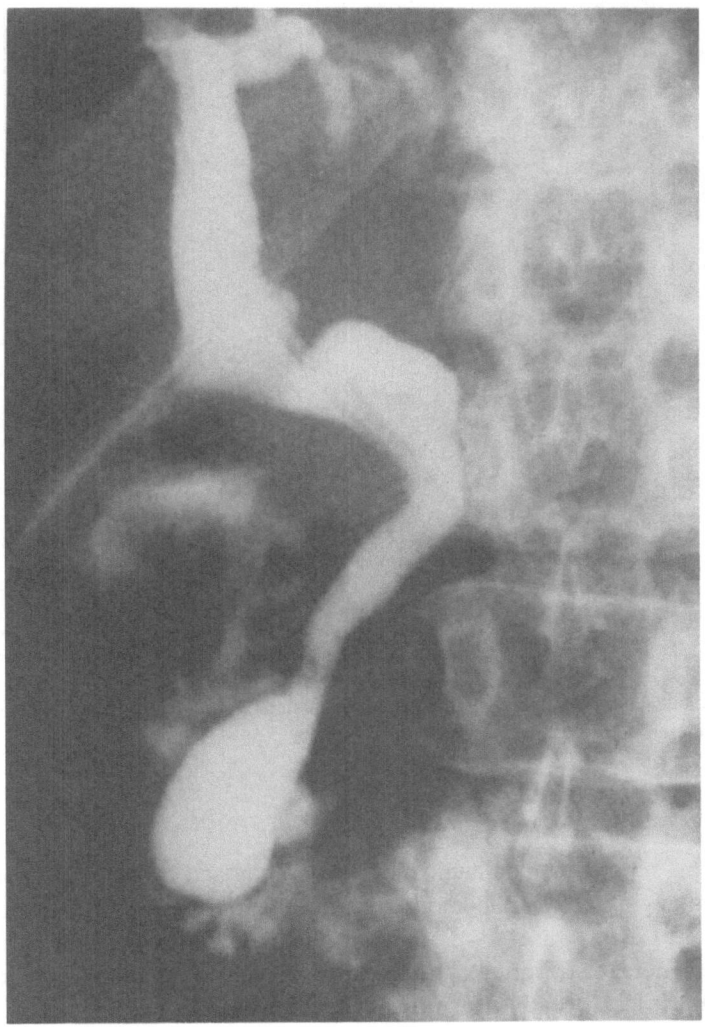

Fig. 2. Choledochocele.

Clinical manifestations

Epigastric or right upper quadrant pain and jaundice are the most frequent complaints. When a palpable tumor is present in the upper part of the abdomen of a child or a young adult with such a history, congenital cystic dilatation of the common bile duct should be considered in the differential diagnosis.

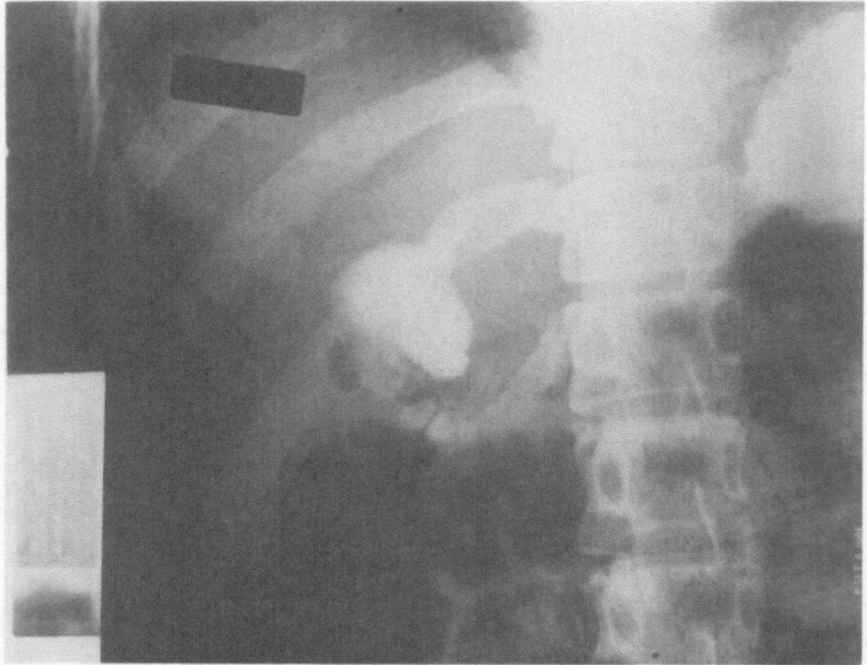

Fig. 3. Choledochal cyst containing multiple calculi treated by subtotal excision and end-to-side choledochojejunostomy.

Current radiologic techniques

Endoscopic retrograde cholangiopancreatography and transhepatic percutaneous cholangiography will demonstrate the essential features in most of these patients. In Caroli's disease, a preliminary computed tomographic scan will show the general distribution of the cystic involvement and the size of the cyst. Ultrasound is less revealing. If sufficient data have not been obtained preoperatively, intraoperative cholangiography will be helpful in assessing the magnitude of the problem.

Treatment

Congenital cystic dilatation of the common bile duct requires surgical treatment. In selecting the surgical procedure, one must realize that in reality the cyst is a tremendously dilated common bile duct with distal obstruction, communications are frequently present between the cystic area and accessory bile ducts, other congenital abnormalities often occur, and the opening between the distal portion of the common bile duct and the duodenum can rarely be found.

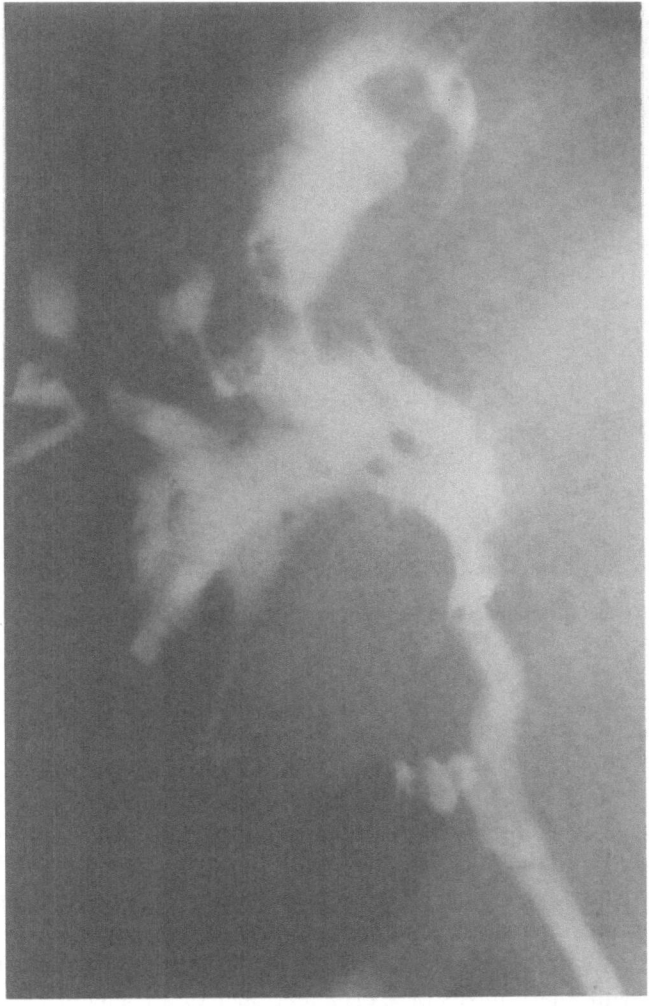

Fig. 4. Cholangiogram showing massive dilatation of intrahepatic ducts (Caroli's disease).

Adequate outflow of bile from the liver into the gastrointestinal tract must be established. A number of surgical procedures have been employed for the treatment of cysts of the bile duct. Choledochoduodenostomy and choledochojejunostomy either in continuity or after the Roux-en-Y procedure have been used according to the bias of the surgeon.

I prefer choledochojejunostomy placing the new stoma at the most dependent portion of the cyst. The opening should be of adequate size to preclude subsequent stricture. Choledochoduodenostomy is simple to execute, but it has a disadvantage – it invites vigorous reflux of food and gastric contents

6

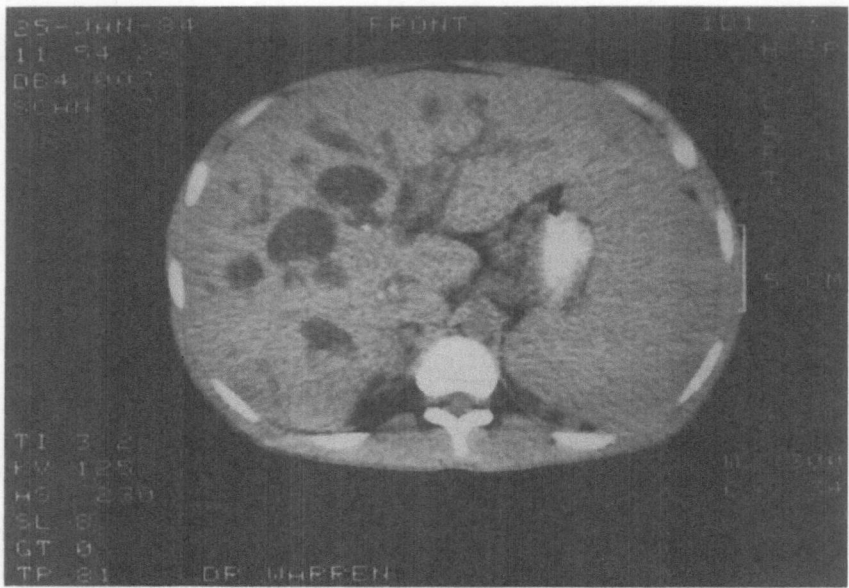

Fig. 5. Computed tomographic scan showing multiple cystic dilatations of intrahepatic ducts (Caroli's disease).

into the biliary ducts. Total excision of the cyst has been advocated recently because of the recognized incidence of cancer in some of these cysts and the failure of cystoenteric bypass to relieve the condition permanently. While I agree it is wise to advocate total excision of the cyst, these cysts are frequently intimately involved with the portal vein and the head of the pancreas, and total removal may not be possible. This is particularly true when multiple operations have been performed and when dense scarring has occurred.

In such a situation, complete removal of the lining of the cyst has been advocated with anastomosis of a proximal duct to a segment of the upper jejunum. This does not appeal to me if the intent is to prevent cancer from arising in the cyst itself. When a large cyst involves the distal segment of the duct that is densely adherent to the portal vein, the hepatic artery, and head of the pancreas, the cyst should be removed completely with anastomosis of the proximal duct to a segment of jejunum preferably by a Roux-en-Y procedure. When a distal portion of the cyst is to be left in place, the pancreatic component, which occurs in an appreciable number of patients, must be controlled properly. Failure to occlude the distal end of the duct by careful suture technique may lead to a persistent fistula that may require further operation.

These cysts must be recognized early to overcome biliary obstruction. This is particularly true in infants and young children in whom prolonged obstruction may lead to an early cirrhosis and ultimately to liver failure.

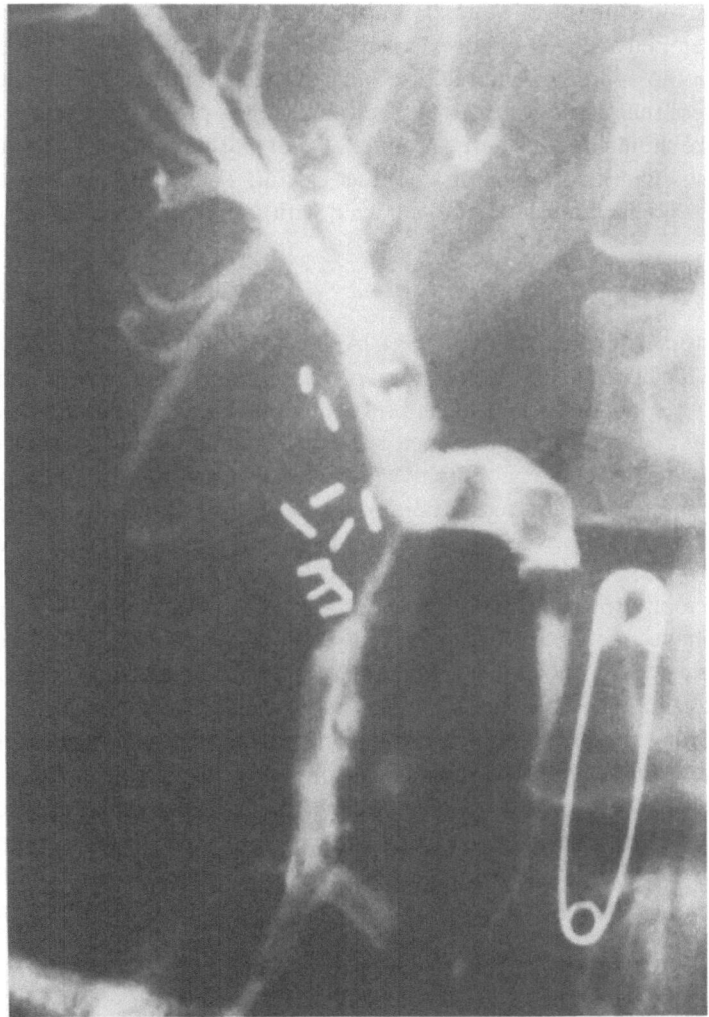

Fig. 6. Multiple common duct calculi above tapered segment of distal common duct.

Choledocholithiasis

Choledocholithiasis may develop de novo (primary) or originate in the gall-bladder (secondary). They may reform after operation (recurrent) or have been overlooked (retained) at cholecystectomy or exploration of the bile ducts (Fig. 6). They may be solitary or so numerous as to fill the entire duct. While some bile duct calculi obviously originate in the duct, most of them migrate from the gallbladder; 10% to 15% of patients with cholelithiasis also have calculi in the common bile duct. It is difficult to determine whether the calculus has developed anew or was overlooked at a previous operation. If the interval between the operation and the discovery of the common bile duct calculus is short (less than a month or two), the calculus was probably overlooked and therefore should be considered retained. Fever and chills followed by jaundice are the hallmarks of common bile duct calculi. Their presence may lead to serious sequelae and should be managed with some urgency and concern.

Diagnosis

The history is extremely important. A presumed diagnosis of choledocholithiasis can be made based on history, physical findings, and simple laboratory data. Ultrasonography may be helpful in demonstrating dilatation of the ductal system and even in the presence of large calculi may reveal the calculus itself. Retrograde cholangiography is much more accurate in the diagnosis of choledocholithiasis and in my opinion is the preferred radiologic diagnostic procedure. Percutaneous cholangiography may show the presence of calculi, but it is a more invasive technique and is associated with some risk. It is customary today to teach that, at the time of cholecystectomy, every patient should have operative cholangiography. While this is an appropriate pronouncement, I do not follow it completely. If the patient has no history of jaundice and has a common bile duct that is smaller than normal and calculi larger than the caliber of the cystic duct, I do not insist on cholangiography. On the other hand, operative cholangiography may reveal calculi that are unsuspected and may reveal no calculi when some relative indication for exploring the duct is present. Consequently, with good judgment, most common bile duct calculi should be detected and removed. No doubt properly performed operative cholangiography may save many unnecessary duct operations.

Treatment

Excellent exposure of the common bile duct at operation is mandatory. This exposure is best obtained by retracting the liver cephalad and duodenum distally, thus placing the common bile duct under slight tension. The duct is aspirated with a fine needle, and the bile is sent to the laboratory for bacteriology, culture, and sensitivity tests. The duct is then opened longitudinally between fine silk guide sutures. If a calculus has been palpated before opening the common bile duct, the position of the calculus should be secured, the duct opened, and the calculus removed without displacing it to a more cephalad position. The duct is thoroughly explored. After all obvious calculi have been removed from the common bile duct and intrahepatic ducts by the use of Randall forceps and appropriate common bile duct scoops, the sphincter of Oddi is calibrated with the gentle passing of Bakes dilators or, if preferred, graduated soft rubber catheters. In the presence of multiple small calculi, the ducts should be irrigated copiously with saline solution. Over the years I have found that use of hydrostatic pressure is an excellent means of removing small calculi from the intrahepatic ducts. Recently, I have employed a Waterpik® with an intermittent jet which I believe, although I cannot prove, is superior to a continuous flow of saline solution.

The use of the choledochoscope by those who have become expert with this instrument claim it is an excellent way of avoiding overlooked calculi.

While choledochoduodenostomy has gained many adherents for the prevention of reoperation for recurrent common bile duct calculi, I have not been impressed with its necessity. When a bypass is indicated, I prefer a Roux-en-Y choledochojejunostomy and have not observed any increased tendency to gastrointestinal hemorrhage after the use of this procedure.

Completion T-tube cholangiography should always be employed to obviate overlooked calculi. Although the tendency among some surgeons today is to avoid the use of a T tube, I have not found that the presence of a T tube for a few weeks has had any ill effect.

Repair of strictures of extrahepatic ducts

The great majority of strictures of the common bile duct are man-made and result from surgical trauma. Injuries to the common bile duct are usually the result of surgical procedures associated with cholecystectomy, but they may be secondary to gastrectomy, choledochostomy, or radical operations on the pancreas.

Table 1. Procedures responsible for biliary stricture in 958 patients (1940–1965).

Procedure	Number of patients	
Surgical trauma		929 (97%)
Biliary tract surgery	918	
Gastric surgery	9	
Pancreatic surgery	2	
Nonsurgical causes		29 (3%)
Inflammatory obstruction	15	
Congenital	5	
Erosion of gallstones	3	
External blunt trauma	2	
Other	4	

From Warren KW, Mountain JC, Midell AI: Management of strictures of the biliary tract. Surg Clin North Am 51: 712, 1971.

10

Anomalies are fequently blamed but rarely are responsible for ductal injuries. In rare instances, a stricture may result from erosion of a gallstone into the common hepatic or right hepatic duct. An analysis of 895 patients with postoperative strictures treated at the Lahey Clinic between 1919 and 1963 showed that 97% could definitely be related to surgical trauma, while 0.4% were the result of the erosion of the bile duct by a gallstone. A total of 3% of these patients had benign biliary strictures not directly the result of previous surgery in this area (Table 1).

Anatomic location of stricture

In a study of 200 consecutive patients with bile duct strictures, the stricture was the result of operative trauma in 190. In 97 patients (51%), the injury definitely involved the common hepatic duct or the right or left hepatic duct. The injury most commonly involved the common hepatic duct where the cystic duct is apposed to its right lateral margin. When the hepatic ducts unite distal to the hilus of the liver, they are particularly prone to surgical injury (Fig. 7 and Table 2).

Pathologic processes that may favor injury

Cholecystitis in two of its pathologic phases predisposes to an injury to the extrahepatic bile ducts during cholecystectomy. In the acute edematous phase of cholecystitis, the gallbladder and surrounding tissue may be so turgid and vascular that obliteration of the cleavage planes in the triangle of Calot makes identification of the cystic artery, the common hepatic duct, and the common bile duct difficult. In the chronic fibrotic phase of cholecystitis with a con-

Table 2. Site of stricture in 958 patients (1940–1965).

Site	Number of patients
Common hepatic ducts	379
Common hepatic and common bile duct	265
Common bile duct, including	
14 in distal common bile duct	217
Bifurcation of hepatic ducts	59
Individual hepatic ducts only	38
Right 27	
Left 11	
Total	958

From Warren KW, Jefferson MF: Prevention and repair of strictures of the extrahepatic bile ducts. Surg Clin North Am 53: 1171, 1973.

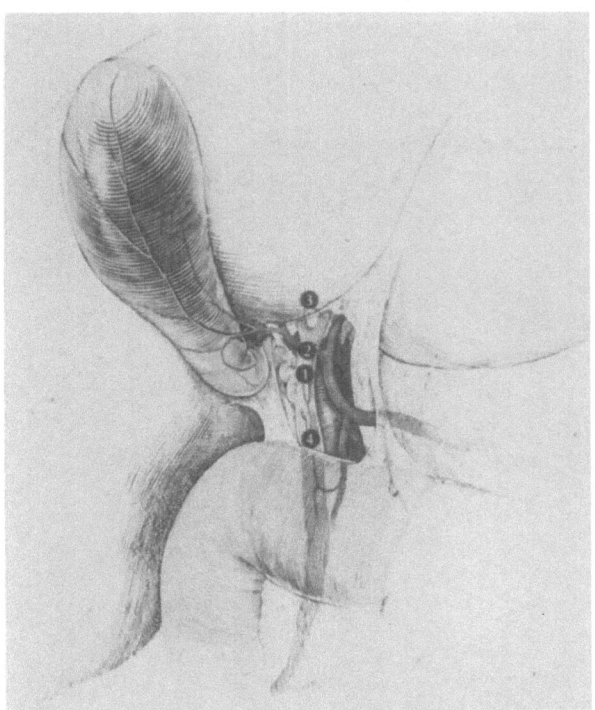

Fig. 7. Incidence of common duct injuries according to anatomic location. 1. Greatest incidence – common hepatic duct; 2. Higher in the common hepatic duct; 3. At the bifurcation; 4. Distal common duct injury usually related to partial gastrectomy.

tracted gallbladder, scarring of the tissues in the triangle of Calot may be so dense that dissection of the individual anatomic structures is extremely difficult.

Diagnosis

The telltale signs of postoperative stricture of the bile duct are jaundice, biliary fistula, or both. The diagnosis of a stricture of the bile duct can usually be made on clinical grounds. The onset of obstructive jaundice possibly associated with biliary drainage from the wound during the immediate postoperative period is indicative of injury to the bile duct.

The radiologic demonstration of a fistulous tract to an obstructed common bile duct is evidence of a stricture. Percutaneous cholangiography gives the best nonoperative visualization of the biliary tree. This should be attempted only if the clotting mechanisms are normal and immediately before exploratory laparotomy. Instead of percutaneous cholangiography, I prefer intraoperative hepatography (Fig. 8).

12

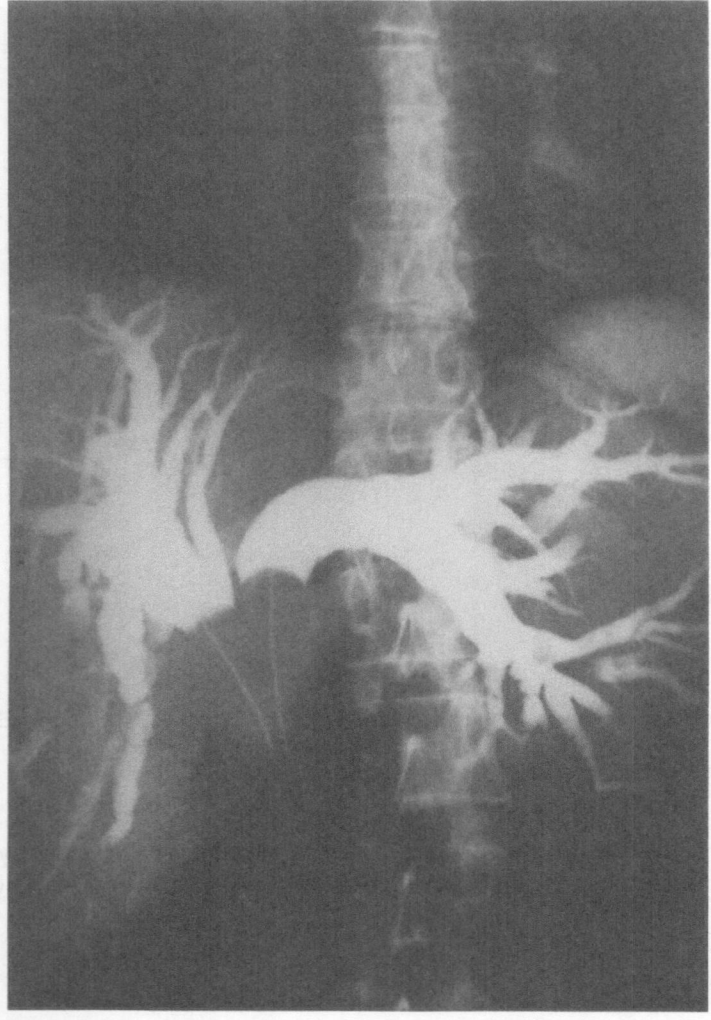

Fig. 8. Hepatogram showing right and left ductal systems when dye has been injected separately through two Foley catheters.

Prevention

The surgeon must have the training and ability to perform safely the surgical procedure undertaken. He or she must have the surgical judgment to know when a procedure will endanger a patient and to perform a less demanding and less hazardous operation if the pathologic process is not favorable for definitive treatment.

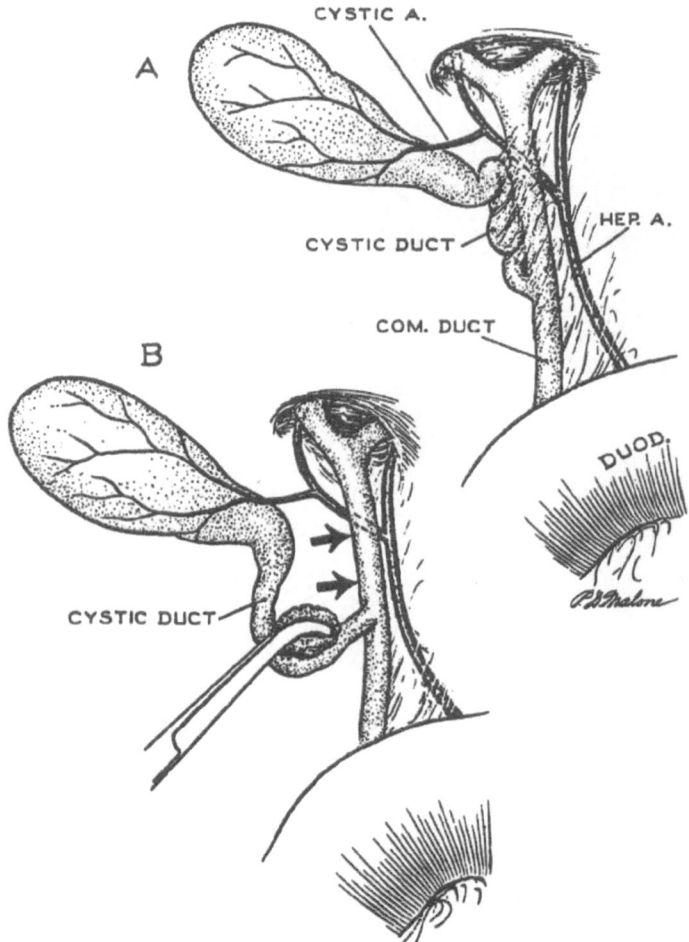

Fig. 9. A. Normal anatomy showing relationship of the cystic duct to the common hepatic duct and the origin of the cystic artery. B. The cystic duct has been mobilized from the right lateral extremity of the common hepatic duct. Note the junction of the cystic duct with the common hepatic duct and the cystic artery.

An incision of adequate length and ideal location that enables faultless exposure and illumination of the operative field is essential if visualization and dissection of the anatomic structures are to be achieved with certainty and confidence. Four structures must be identified before any hemostat is placed. First, the supraduodenal segment of the common duct is exposed; then, the right lateral extremity of the common hepatic duct or the right hepatic duct is visualized. The origin of the cystic artery must be identified, and the approximate junction of the cystic duct with the common hepatic duct to form the

14

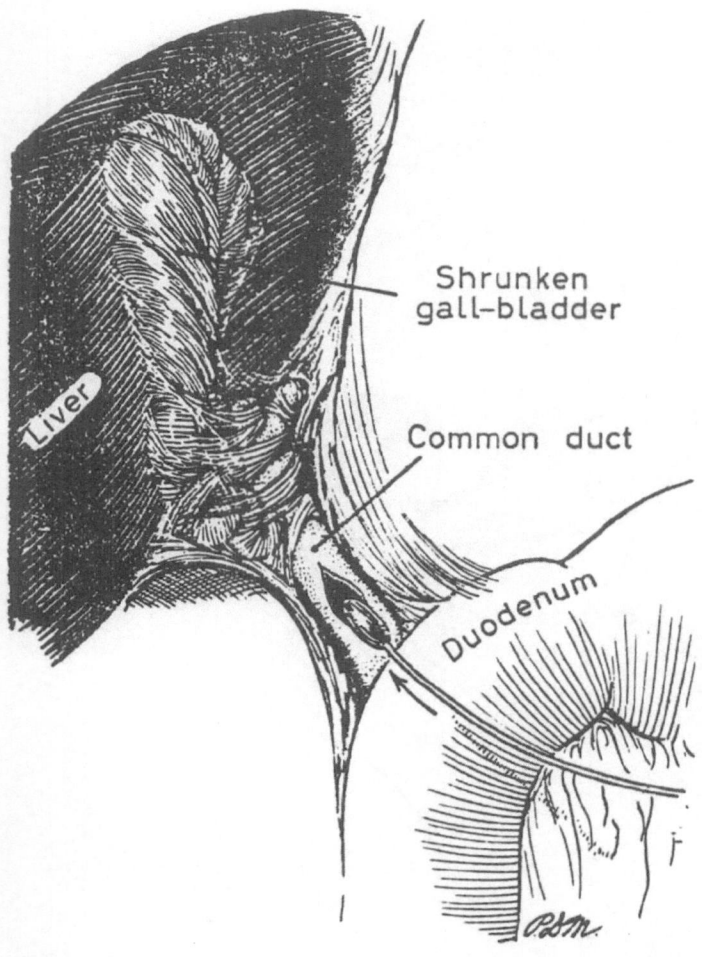

Fig. 10. With the cystic duct and the cystic artery obscured by dense fibrosis, the supraduodenal segment of the common bile duct is opened, and a Bakes dilator is advanced to the region of the cystic duct and the cystic artery to protect the bile duct during dissection of Calot's triangle.

common duct must be demonstrated. These structures are shown in Fig. 9. Each step in the procedure must be deliberate and unhurried. If the turgidity of the gallbladder and the tissues in Calot's triangle prevent visualization of the anatomic structures, the common bile duct should be opened and a Bakes dilator inserted into the common hepatic duct and advanced to the general region of the origin of the cystic artery and the junction of the cystic and common hepatic ducts (Fig. 10).

Treatment

Progressive attrition of the duct occurs with each succeeding operation, and the initial repair is a golden chance for success. The eventual success depends on location of the stricture, caliber of the proximal duct, degree of cholangitis and scarring or local abscess formation, time interval between injury and correction, degree of damage to the hepatic parenchyma, and experience of the surgeon in assessing, selecting, and executing the procedure of choice.

Experience gained from operating on many patients who have this type of injury has taught me that it is not the presence of a defect in the duct that is the problem but the quality and accessibility of the proximal duct that govern the practicality of all corrective procedures. Although a primary end-to-end ductal anastomosis is the ideal treatment, it is doubtful whether the choice of an end-to-end ductal anastomosis or choledochoduodenostomy or choledochojejunostomy with or without Roux-en-Y anastomosis plays a decisive role in the ultimate result. If the proximal duct has been severed high in the transverse fissure of the liver, it is frequently difficult to achieve an ideal anastomosis. Thus, the qualities of the proximal duct will determine the eventual result.

End-to-end anastomosis
Certain conditions must be met to perform a proper end-to-end anastomosis. The relative caliber of the proximal duct has to approximate the caliber of the distal duct. The head of the pancreas and duodenum must be mobilized sufficiently to perform end-to-end anastomosis without tension. The external limb of the T tube, which is used to splint the anastomosis, has to be brought out through a stab wound either in the proximal or distal segment of the duct and never through the anastomotic site. End-to-end anastomosis is reserved for patients who have a short segment of the duct involved in the stricutre where the caliber of the proximal and distal ducts is similar (Fig. 11).

Hepaticoenteric anastomosis
The commonest type of repair today involves some type of anastomosis of the proximal duct to a segment of the upper gastrointestinal tract.

Hepaticoduodenostomy. Hepaticoduodenostomy has the appeal of being less complicated than a Roux-en-Y anastomosis to the jejunum. Despite this advantage, I rarely perform choledochoduodenostomy because it permits the greatest degree of reflux of food and gastric contents into the ductal system; a duodenal fistula is much more difficult to deal with than a biliary jejunal fistula. Despite this obvious bias, series of choledochoduodenostomies with good long-term results are well documented in the literature.

16

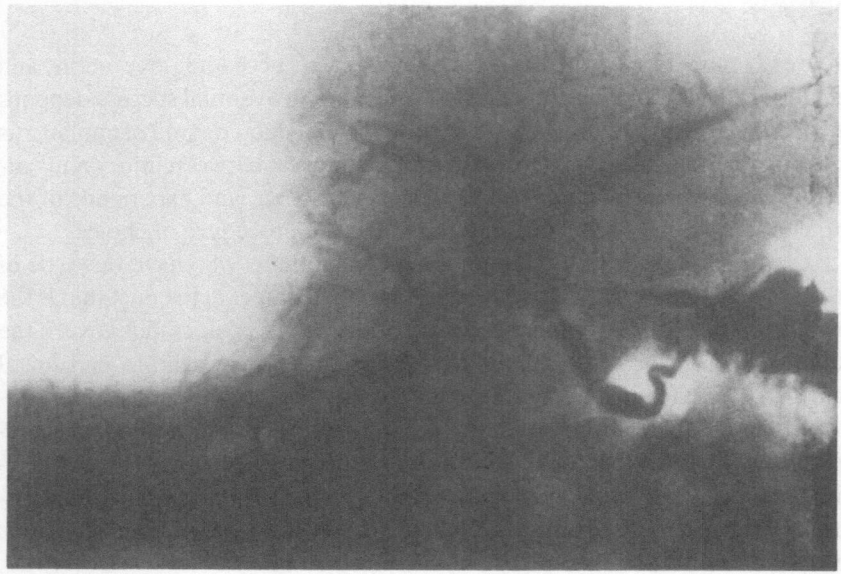

Fig. 11. Operative cholangiogram showing short strictured area in the common hepatic duct with dilatation of the proximal hepatic ducts and normal distal common duct treated by excision of the stricture and end-to-end anastomosis.

Roux-en-Y hepaticojejunostomy. The Roux-en-Y anastomosis is preferred by most surgeons experienced in the repair of large numbers of common bile duct strictures. The defunctionalized jejunal limb should be approximately 50 cm in length. I prefer an end-to-side hepaticojejunostomy than to use the end of the divided jejunum. If the caliber of the proximal duct is sufficiently large, no stent will be necessary. If the caliber of the proximal duct is small and if considerable evidence of cholangitis is present, I use a stent. The choice of a stent may vary from a segment of straight latex tubing traversing the anastomosis and brought to the outside through a stab wound in the jejunum or in the proximal duct. Other stents include a T tube, a buried Y tube, a modified Y tube, or transhepatic tubes. They may be of latex or silicone; the choice is an individual one. The anastomosis must involve mucosa-to-mucosa approximation.

For many years, a Y tube with special configuration was employed at the Lahey Clinic and was accepted in other clinics around the world. The disadvantage of the buried Y tube was the necessity for reoperation for its removal when recurrent cholangitis developed as a result of occlusion of the Y tube. Despite this disadvantage, the Y tube gave excellent results in 97% of patients who had a two-stage procedure when the Y tube was used at the initial repair and was subsequently removed when recurrent cholangitis occurred. Because the results were good after operation, the Y tube was modified so that it could

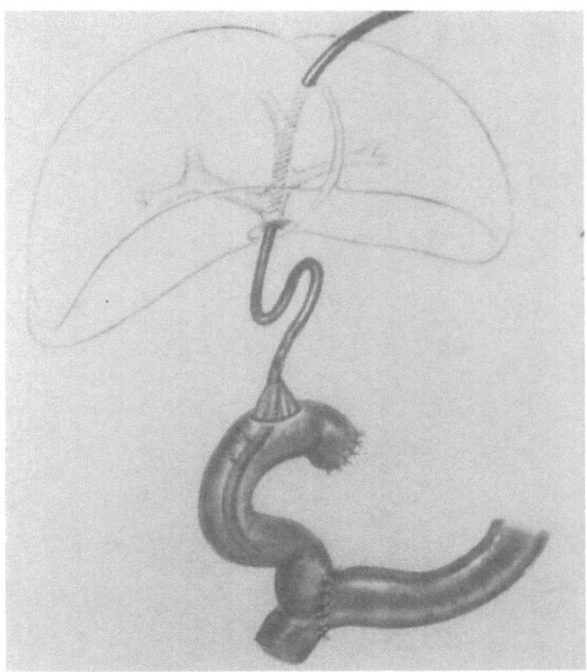

Fig. 12. Mucosal graft technique of Rodney Smith. Seromuscular ellipse has been removed from the Roux-en-Y limb of the jejunum. A transhepatic tube has been drawn through the left ductal system and inserted into the jejunum through the mucosal pouch. The tube has been anchored in the jejunum with two interrupted sutures of chromic catgut.

be removed in the office. I have utilized this tube for many years and find it extremely satisfactory.

Transhepatic stenting
Interest in the use of transhepatic stenting has been stimulated primarily by the work of Praderi and Lord Smith. Praderi has published an excellent historical review of the use of transhepatic tubes. Smith has modified the use of the transhepatic tubes by a method he described as the mucosal graft repair and one he ultimately adopted for routine use in the repair of high common duct strictures. This technique is demonstrated in Figs. 12 through 14. I have used the mucosal graft technique in many instances and have found it to be an excellent method of repairing high common bile duct injuries. This technique has been criticized particularly by surgeons who have never learned to perform the operation properly.

18

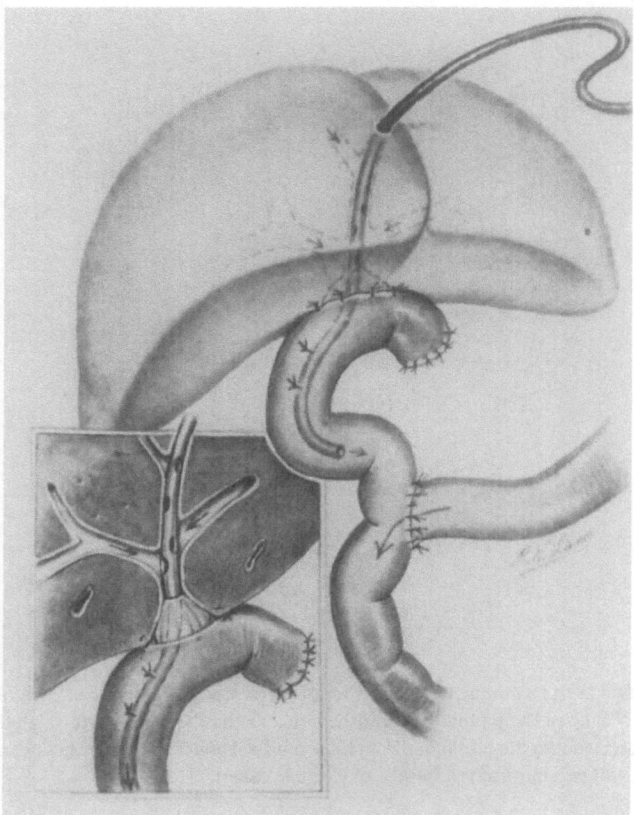

Fig. 13. The mucosal pouch has been drawn into the proximal common hepatic duct. The sero-muscular layer of the jejunum has been anchored to the periductal tissue.

Complications

Biliary fistula
A small biliary fistula is not uncommon after repair of a common duct injury. It usually closes spontaneously within a few days. Since a fistula is possible, I always use suction drainage in the subhepatic space.

Hemorrhage
Postoperative hemorrhage is another annoying and occasionally life-threatening complication. If the postoperative hemorrhage is arterial, operation should be performed immediately. If the bleeding is venous in character, it frequently will stop if the patient is given appropriate transfusions.

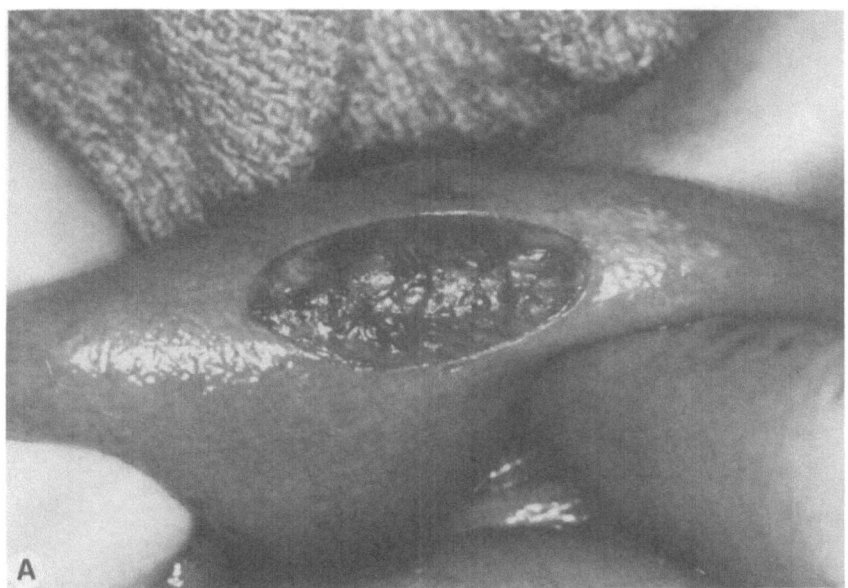

Fig. 14. A. Preparation of the mucosal pouch.

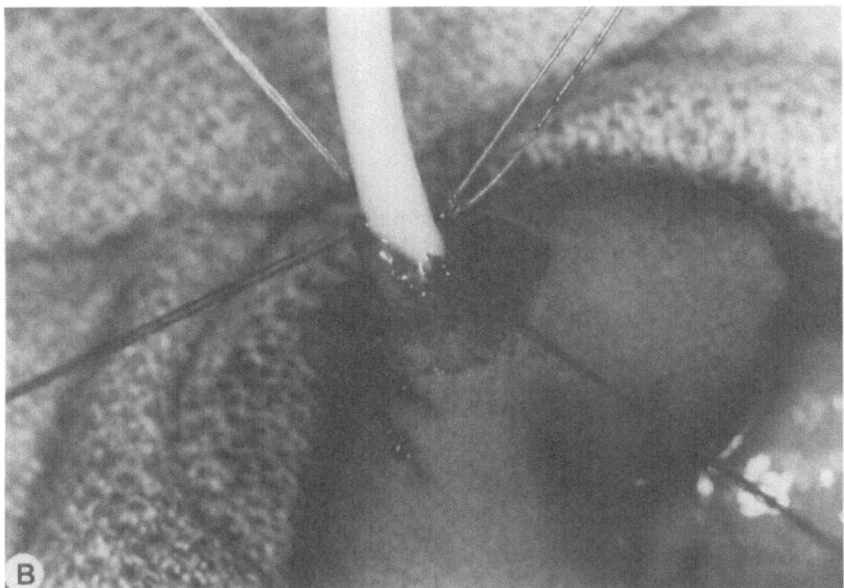

Fig. 14. B. Insertion in and anchoring of transhepatic tube to the mucosal pouch.

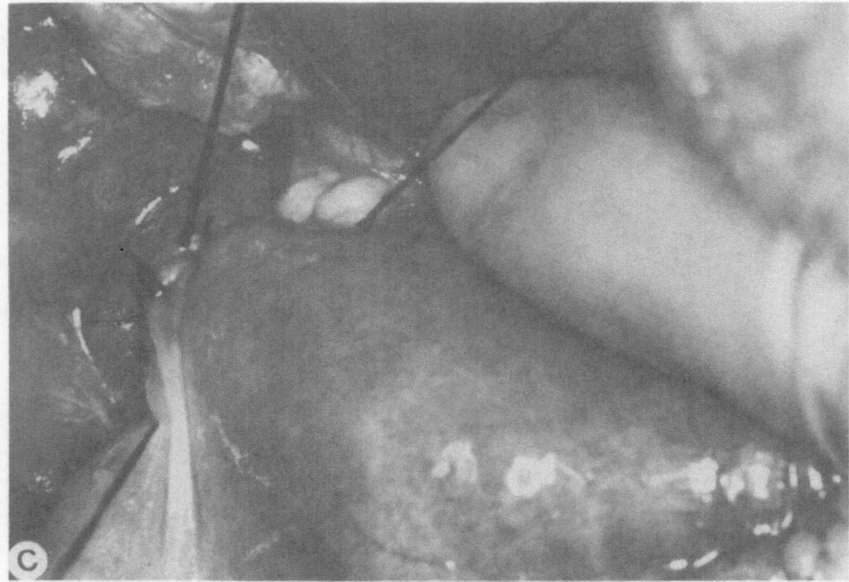

Fig. 14. C. Complete procedure. The seromuscular layer of jejunum has been approximated to the periductal tissues.

Wound infection
Wound infections can be minimized by careful technique and proper drainage of the deep wound.

Coagulation defects
Coagulopathy should always be anticipated, and prophylactic treatment should be utilized. When serious infection develops, the patient is a candidate for rapid platelet destruction. Consequently, the platelet count must be checked carefully in any patient who has postoperative complications.

Malnutrition

In recent years, most of my patients have had some type of intravenous hyperalimentation. In addition, feeding jejunostomies have been used with increasing frequency in patients who are debilitated and whose preoperative evaluation indicated serious nutritional deficiencies.

Bronchobiliary and pleurobiliary fistulas
Bronchobiliary fistula, fortunately rare, is one of the most dramatic and potentially devastating complications of injury to the bile duct. I have recently re-

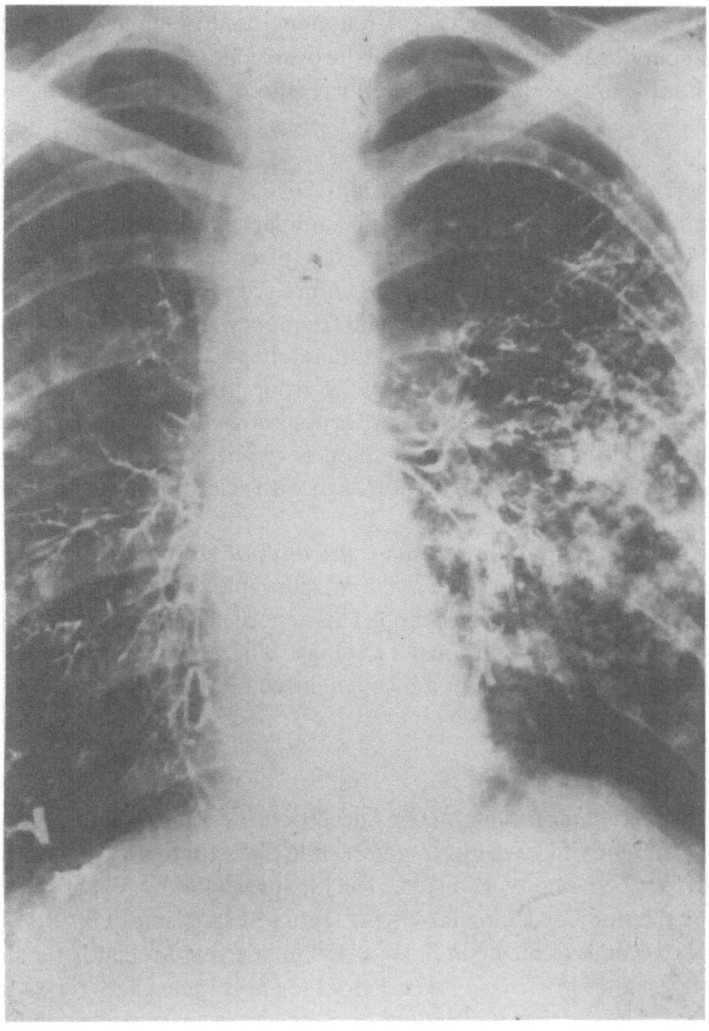

Fig. 15. Bronchogram showing diffuse bronchial involvement from rupture of biliary pleu-robronchial fistula.

ported 15 instances of this complication treated over a 30-year period at the New England Baptist Hospital (Fig. 15). Biliary obstruction was present in all patients with bronchobiliary fistulas.

The symptoms can be divided into two phases, acute and chronic. In the acute phase, the patient's lungs are suddenly flooded with infected bile. The patient requires immediate operation. In the chronic phase, the patient has periodic opening of the fistula, and the symptoms are much less dramatic but nevertheless annoying. The surgical treatment is one of immediate drainage to the subhepatic space and correction of the obstruction in the biliary tract if possible. Multiple operations are frequently required. There have been no deaths in this series.

Biliary cirrhosis and portal hypertension
Unfortunately, biliary cirrhosis and portal hypertension develop in some patients with benign biliary strictures. Not infrequently, these serious complications are the result of neglect and failure to reoperate on the patient who has recurrent cholangitis with sufficient frequency and severity that invite the development of biliary cirrhosis and ultimately portal hypertension. In these patients who represent 10% to 15% of the group, the precise incidence of portal hypertension secondary to stricture is not known, but occasionally patients require a shunting procedure. If a shunt is required, a splenorenal shunt is best. Attempts to control the hemorrhage with sclerotherapy are justifiable.

Balloon dilatation of recurrent benign strictures of bile ducts
Interventional radiologists have made considerable progress in the temporary management of bile duct obstruction. This experience has led to further extension of the use of interventional radiology. The precise place of such procedures can only be determined by cumulative future experience.

Comments

The results of repair of common bile duct strictures depend on the patient population. Patients who have high common bile duct strictures will have the least prospect for good long-term results. The longer the follow-up period, the lower will be the number falling into the category of satisfactory results. The importance of time is reflected in the fact that in one year I recently repaired two common bile duct strictures I had repaired 13 and 19 years ago, respectively. It is premature to say that if a patient does not have a recurrence within three years that patient will never have another recurrence. On the other hand, it is true that if patients live three years without symptoms of cholangitis, 85% will have a good long-term result.

Sclerosing cholangitis

Much of the mystery and confusion surrounding sclerosing cholangitis can be clarified if it is appreciated that the bile ducts can react only in limited ways to pathologic stimuli. The ducts may become dilated or stenotic, and the dilatation and stenosis may be localized or diffuse. Sclerosing cholangitis is characterized by severe narrowing of the lumen caused by intense subepithelial fibrosis. As a result of progressive sclerosis of the bile ducts, patients with sclerosing cholangitis exhibit progressive biliary obstruction and its sinister sequelae. Confusing diagnostic criteria have appeared in the literature and include progressive obstructive jaundice, absence of common duct calculi, no previous biliary surgery, cholangiographic evidence of diffuse multifocal strictures with irregularity and tortuosity of the ductal system, and the absence of coexistent bile duct cancer. These criteria are much too restrictive. Most patients I see have had previous operations, and many of them have gallstones. Also adding to the confusion are the synonyms used in describing this condition: primary sclerosing cholangitis, stenosing cholangitis, primary cholangitis, sclerosing obliterative cholangitis, chronic fibrosing choledochitis, sclerosing pericholedochitis, and chronic obliterative cholangitis.

Etiology

The cause of sclerosing cholangitis is unknown. Bacterial infection would appear to be important. In my series of patients previously reported, 34% had ulcerative colitis. As more clinical material is accumulated, a few patients with Crohn's disease have also been observed to have sclerosing cholangitis. In addition to its association with ulcerative colitis and Crohn's disease, sclerosing cholangitis has been observed in retroperitoneal fibrosis, Riedel's struma, and lymphoma. For the purpose of analysis in a previous paper, I have grouped the patients into the following three categories: those with ulcerative colitis, those with no known association, or those with associated gallstones.

The gallstones are probably the result of sclerosing cholangitis and not the cause. The relationship between ulcerative colitis or Crohn's disease and sclerosing cholangitis is purely speculative. Although the liver is bombarded with showers of bacteria by way of the portal system, a large number of patients with ulcerative colitis never have sclerosing cholangitis.

Pathology

The entire biliary tree, including the gallbladder, may be involved with sclerosis. The common bile duct is frequently converted into a thickened cord with a small lumen. No diagnostic pathologic changes are seen, but a liver biopsy will often show a paucity of ductal elements in addition to irregularity of the ducts.

Clinical features

The clinical manifestations of 84 patients with sclerosing cholangitis are shown in Table 3. Jaundice, the most common feature, was present in 93% of patients. Pain occurred in 69% and weight loss in 63%. Anorexia and malaise are frequent features and occurred in 59% of patients.

The prominent physical findings included jaundice, liver enlargement, and localized tenderness in the area of the liver. The jaundice may be intermittent, but ultimately it becomes chronic. Chills and fever may occur in episodic fashion.

Of patients who had associated ulcerative colitis, the interval between onset of the ulcerative colitis and the onset of sclerosing cholangitis ranged from less than one to more than 20 years. In two patients, it appeared the sclerosing cholangitis antedated the ulcerative colitis.

Diagnosis

The diagnosis is usually made during a careful evaluation of the patient with vague gastrointestinal symptoms and especially the investigation of a patient who has jaundice. With newer imaging techniques, the diagnosis is more readily made. Ultrasound may be of limited value. Endoscopic retrograde cholangiopancreatography will give the highest percentage of diagnostic accuracy because percutaneous cholangiography may be unsatisfactory owing to the small caliber of the intrahepatic ducts. The classic examples of sclerosing cholangitis are shown in Figs 16 and 17.

Table 3. Clinical manifestations of 84 patients with sclerosing cholangitis treated at Lahey Clinic.

Clinical feature	Number of patients	Percent of series
Historical features		
Jaundice	78	93
Pain	58	69
Weight loss	53	63
Anorexia and malaise	50	59
Chills and fever	42	50
Pruritus	41	48
Nausea and vomiting	40	45
Colitis	27	32
Physical findings		
Jaundice	48	57
Liver enlargement	37	44
Local tenderness	29	34
Ileostomy	5	6

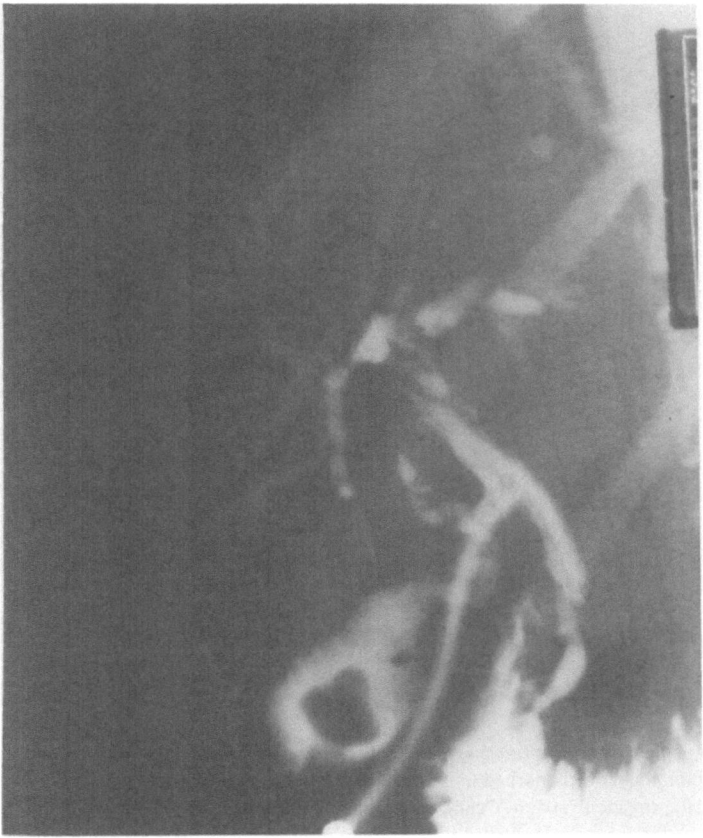

Fig. 16. T-tube cholangiogram showing characteristic irregular narrowing of the extrahepatic and intrahepatic ductal system and the presence of calculi in the gallbladder.

Treatment

Given that no definitive cause of sclerosing cholangitis is known in most instances, treatment is empirical and is based mainly on demonstration of structural alterations in the extrahepatic and intrahepatic ductal systems. The primary aim is to relieve biliary obstruction.

During the surgical procedure, the common bile duct is identified, and operative cholangiography is performed to define the anatomy of the biliary tree. The common duct is then opened. This may be a difficult procedure because the lumen may be small compared with the external diameter of the bile duct. Occasionally it will be necessary to open the duodenum and identify the common bile duct by probing the duct through the papilla of Vater. If the gallbladder is present, it is removed. Calculi should be removed from the extra-

26

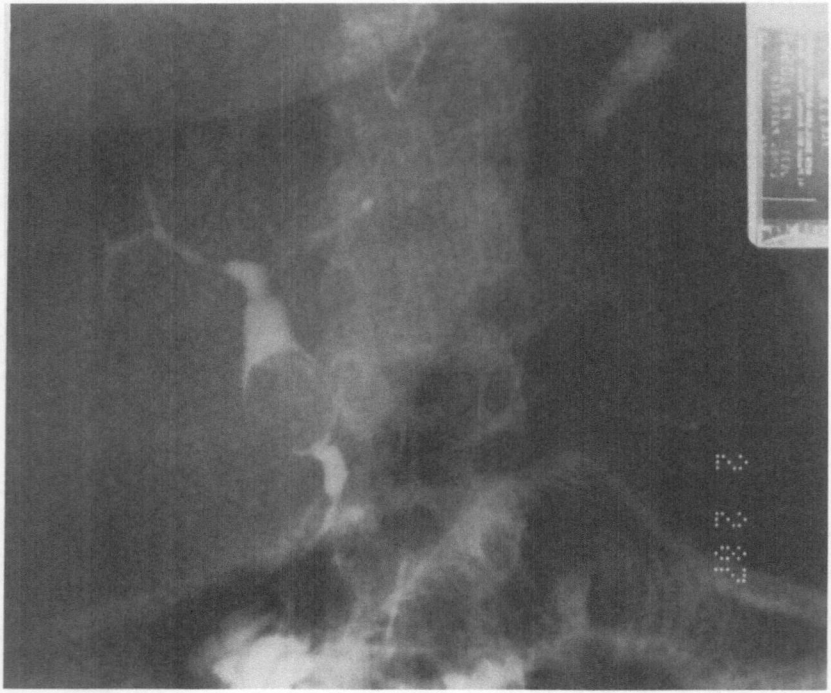

Fig. 17. Cholangiogram performed by retrograde endoscopy showing large calculus almost occluding the common duct with marked narrowing of intrahepatic ducts treated by removal of the calculus and side-to-side Roux-en-Y choledochojejunostomy.

hepatic and intrahepatic ductal system. The proximal duct should be dilated carefully starting with special lacrimal duct probes or graduated Coude catheters. If the segment of the extrahepatic ductal system is of sufficient caliber, a bypass should be performed, preferably with a Roux-en-Y choledochojejunostomy. Since the tendency is for ductal strictures to be progressive, easy access to the Roux-en-Y is ensured by anchoring the inverted end of the Roux-en-Y loop in a subcutaneous position.

Despite the small caliber of the ducts, it is frequently beneficial to have a stent, such as a T tube, modified Y tube, or transhepatic U tube, of appropriate size. The interventional radiologist can sometimes be helpful over a period of months in managing these tubes and minimizing the progression of the intrahepatic stricture.

Colectomy in the presence of ulcerative colitis has no apparent impact on the natural history of sclerosing cholangitis. Corticosteroids have been used widely in the medical management of patients with this disease, but in my experience they have not been beneficial.

Sclerosing cholangitis is a serious condition. Some patients have rapidly progessing disease with early onset biliary cirrhosis leading to portal hypertension and liver failure. It is not uncommon for the terminal event to be massive hemorrhage associated with hepatic encephalopathy and ultimate death. On the other hand, many patients live for many years even after chronic hyperbilirubinemia develops. One of my patients went 19 years after my first operation, but ultimately died of cirrhosis, portal hypertension, and hemorrhage.

In an analysis of the 84 patients previously reported, only 13% had no further problem at the time of publication of these data. In this group of patients, postoperative complications included bacterial cholangitis in 12%, biliary fistula in 7%, postoperative gastrointestinal bleeding in 7%, subphrenic abscess in 6%, hepatic coma in 3%, and septic shock in 3%.

Primary carcinoma of bile ducts

It is estimated that carcinoma of the bile ducts accounts for 3% of all cancer deaths in the United States. It is slightly more common in men than in women. The highest frequency is in the sixth and seventh decades of life.

Etiology

The cause of bile duct carcinoma is unknown. Although the incidence of associated gallstones has been reported from 20% to 50%, no direct evidence exists to establish that gallstones cause ductal carcinoma. In a few patients, carcinoma results from malignant transformation of papillomas of the bile duct. An association between ulcerative colitis and bile duct carcinoma has been reported.

In patients who have had carcinoma of the bile duct associated with chronic inflammatory bowel disease, the carcinoma occurred at a much earlier age than the group as a whole. The incidence of malignant transformation in choledochal cysts, Caroli's disease, and other cystic conditions of the bile duct is appreciable.

Pathology

Bile duct carcinoma has a tendency to infiltrate extensively. These tumors may be multicentric. It is occasionally difficult to distinguish between a malignant and a benign stricture of the bile ducts.

Secondary effects of the tumor are important. Obstruction of the bile duct gives rise to jaundice, and obstruction of the cystic duct may result in a mucocele of the gallbladder or in acute cholecystitis. A carcinoma at the terminus of the common duct may obstruct the pancreatic duct and give rise to pancreatitis. By the time operation is performed, one third of all patients have lymph node metastases, one third have involvement of the liver and hilar structures, and one half of the patients demonstrate nerve sheath invasion. The histology is almost invariably adenocarcinoma of varying degrees of differentiation.

Clinical features

Clinical features of 173 patients with carcinoma of the extrahepatic ducts seen at the Lahey Clinic are shown in Table 4. The most common presentation is progressive obstructive jaundice. Usually the patient does not have associated chills or fever, but if the cystic duct becomes obstructed, the patient may have typical acute cholecystitis.

Diagnosis

Jaundice, pruritus, pale stools, and dark urine are often coupled with an obstructive pattern of liver function tests. The diagnosis depends primarily on radiologic techniques. Ultrasonography can yield useful information regarding the gallbladder, the liver, and the bile ducts. The demonstration of ductal dilatation is particularly useful in separating surgical from nonsurgical causes of jaundice. Better anatomic definition is obtained by endoscopic retrograde cholangiography or percutaneous transhepatic cholangiography.

Surgical exploration remains the principal method of diagnosis, although it may still be impossible at operation to distinguish a benign from a malignant stricture and to differentiate between the various forms of periampullary cancer.

Table 4. Clinical features of 173 patients with extrahepatic bile duct carcinoma.

Symptoms and signs	Percent
Symptoms	
Upper abdominal pain	57
Weight loss	46
Pruritus	31
Chills and fever	12
Signs	
Jaundice	82
Palpable liver	37
Abdominal mass	10
Palpable spleen	5

Treatment

Operation offers the only hope of cure and the best prospect of palliation. Four features warrant emphasis:
1. Mucosal spread may be extensive without any external sign. Resection should, therefore, be generous.
2. Although the affected duct lumen may permit moderate-size dilators to pass freely, obstructive jaundice may persist after operation. This probably means that the obstruction was not completely overcome.
3. The presence of a collapsed gallbladder usually indicates the tumor is above the choledochocystic junction, but a tumor below this junction may also produce collapse of the gallbladder.
4. Histology of these tumors is often difficult to interpret. Intense stromal re-action can obscure malignant cells, resulting in a diagnosis of benign biliary stricture. Therefore, a tissue biopsy should be adequate in amount and taken from the most representative sites and should include the entire duct wall when possible. It may be necessary to take several biopsies to establish the correct diagnosis. Cytologic examination of mucosal scrapings occasionally may reveal the presence of a malignant tumor.

The tumor should be resected when technically possible. Recently, extensive resection has been advocated for malignant tumors occurring at the bifurcation of the major biliary ducts. Formal lobectomy or extended lobectomy has been performed in many instances, but a sufficient number of these extended operations have not been followed long enough to warrant a definite conclusion as to the merit of these procedures.

In general, tumors of the distal common bile duct are most amenable to resection by pancreatoduodenectomy. By far the best results in treating carcinoma of the bile duct have been obtained after this operation. About 30% of my patients having pancreatoduodenectomy for carcinoma arising in the distal common bile duct have survived five years.

When a low-lying tumor cannot be resected, palliative biliary enteric bypass should be performed. For tumors in the middle segment, resection may be curative. Cholecystectomy should be performed to prevent any complication from cystic duct obstruction. In general, the proximal divided duct should be anastomosed to the jejunum.

If tumors in the upper segment cannot be resected, palliation may be difficult, but efforts to overcome the obstruction should be pursued. If the dissection can be carried out above the point of obstruction, an anastomosis between the proximal right or left hepatic duct and the jejunum should be performed.

Under more difficult circumstances, palliation may be limited to transtumor dilatation of the duct with the insertion of an appropriate stent (Fig. 18). Transhepatic tubes offer the best palliation. They can be replaced easily and

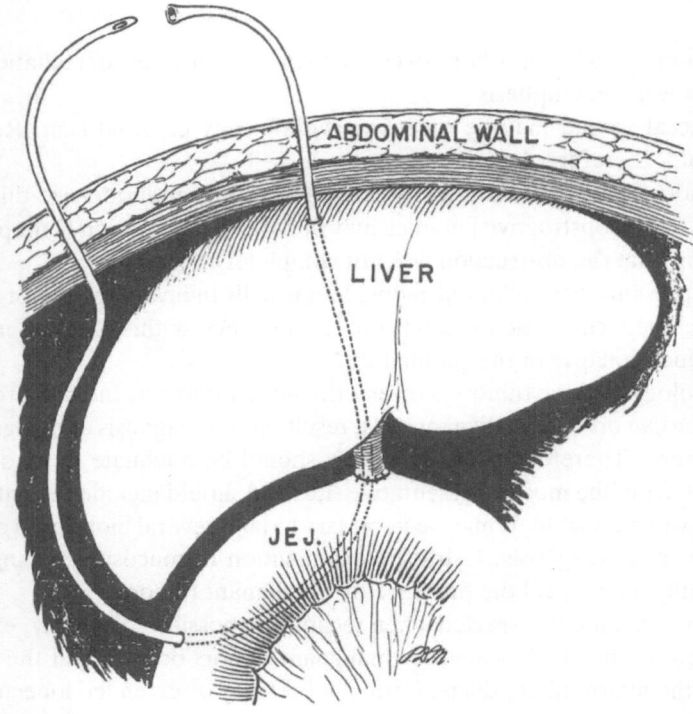

Fig. 18. Method of insertion of transhepatic U tube after hepaticojejunostomy. Frequently it will be necessary to use bilateral transhepatic tubes to overcome the obstruction due to the tumor.

offer access to the interventional radiologist who may wish to change or otherwise manipulate these nonresectable tumors. Percutaneous or endoscopic drainage is increasing in popularity. The interventional radiologist and the endoscopist are showing increasing ingenuity in the application of these techniques. Occasionally these maneuvers are employed as an initial step when a surgical procedure might offer better palliation.

Prognosis

The prognosis is poor, and the overall five-year survival rate is only 5%. In contrast, as stated earlier, approximately 25% of patients with a malignant tumor of the distal common bile duct that is resectable live five years. The length of survival is determined by the degree of tumor differentiation. Death commonly occurs as a result of unrelieved ductal obstruction complicated by septicemia.

Periampullary carcinoma

Malignant tumors arising in the ampulla of Vater, the distal common bile duct, the duodenal mucosa around the papilla of Vater, and ductal carcinoma of the head of the pancreas should be considered together because these patients have similar clinical histories and physical and laboratory findings.

For prognostic purposes, a distinction should be made between tumors arising in the ampulla of Vater, the distal common bile duct, and the duodenal mucosa surrounding the papilla of Vater on the one hand and ductal carcinoma arising in the head of the pancreas on the other. A further distinction should be made between ductal carcinoma of the head of the pancreas and other types of malignant tumors arising in the head of the gland. Tumors arising in the ampulla of Vater, the distal common bile duct, and the duodenum are much more favorable than ductal carcinoma arising in the head of the pancreas. Nonductal malignant tumors, such as malignant islet cell tumor, cystadenocarcinomas, lymphomas, and fibrosarcomas, are more favorable than ductal carcinomas.

In 150 of 348 patients previously reported on by me, the tumor arose in the head of the pancreas, 112 arose in the ampulla of Vater, 47 arose in the common bile duct, and 39 arose in the duodenum (Table 5).

The histologic types of these tumors are listed in Table 6. The operative mortality rate in the group of patients operated on between 1962 and 1971 is shown in Table 7. The overall mortality rate was 10.7%. The overall mortality rate for 348 resections was 14.9%. In a personal series of pancreatoduodenectomies performed for ductal carcinoma of the head of the pancreas between 1971 and 1980, the mortality rate was 3.4%.

Of 150 patients with cancer of the head of the pancreas, 12 had tumors other than adenocarcinoma, and six of them had islet cell cancers. Of the ten patients eligible for follow-up, the five-year survival rate was 40% (Table 8).

Relative survival rates according to site of tumor are listed in Table 9. The relative survival rates according to site of tumor without lymph node metastasis are listed in Table 10. The relative survival rates according to site of tu-

Table 5. Patients treated by pancreatoduodenectomy or total pancreatectomy.

Site	Malignant tumors	Benign	Total
Pancreas	150	4	154
Ampulla	112	1	113
Common bile duct	47	2	49
Duodenum	39	0	39
Total	348	7	355

mor with lymph node metastasis are listed in Table 11. Analysis of these data confirm the previous statement of the relatively favorable results with resection of carcinoma of the ampulla of Vater, distal common bile duct, and duodenum and the poor survival rate associated with ductal carcinoma of the head of the pancreas. It will also confirm the more favorable survival for patients with tumors arising in the head of the pancreas that are nonductal in origin.

Efforts to improve the long-term results of the surgical treatment of per-

Table 6. Histologic types of tumor.

Type of tumor	Pancreas	Ampulla	Common bile duct	Duodenum	Total
Adenocarcinoma	138	109	47	37	331
Islet cell tumors	6	0	0	0	6
Carcinoid	1	2	0	1	4
Cystadenocarcinoma	2	0	0	0	2
Adenoacanthoma	1	1	0	0	2
Neurofibrosarcoma	1	0	0	0	1
Melanoma	1	0	0	0	1
Leiomyosarcoma	0	0	0	1	1
Total	150	112	47	39	348

Table 7. Operative mortality (1962–1971).

Site	Number of cases	Operative deaths	Percent
Pancreas	58	6	10.3
Ampulla	39	3	7.6
Common bile duct	23	4	17.4
Duodenum	19	2	10.5
Total	139	15	10.7

Table 8. Comparison of survivals between adenocarcinoma and other malignant tumors of head of pancreas.

Type	Number of cases	1 year	3 years	5 years	10 years	15 years
Adenocarcinoma	110	44.2%	10.2%	9.0%	3.8%	1.8%
Other cancers	10	70.0%	60.0%	40.0%	40.0%	10.0%

iampullary tumors has led to more radical operations, including total pancreatectomy and extended regional pancreatectomy. Brooks has advocated total pancreatectomy for ductal carcinoma. His data show a slight improvement in the five-year survival rate for patients with ductal carcinoma compared with patients who had a Whipple procedure. The series from the Mayo Clinic, which was at one time interpreted as showing superiority of total pancreatectomy, later indicated survival rates were not increased after total pancreatectomy compared with results after a Whipple procedure.

Table 9. Relative survival rates site of tumor.

Site	Five-year survivals, %
Pancreas	12.5
Ampulla	32.0
Common bile duct	25.0
Duodenum	41.3

Table 10. Relative survival rates site of tumor – no lymph node metastases.

Site	Five-year survivals, %
Pancreas	16.8
Ampulla	40.0
Common bile duct	27.5
Duodenum	50.0

Table 11. Relative survival rates site of tumor – lymph node metastases.

Site	Five-year survivals, %
Pancreas	7.4
Ampulla	9.5
Common bile duct	0
Duodenum	22.2

Surgical management of chronic relapsing pancreatitis

Chronic relapsing pancreatitis is characterized by recurrent attacks of upper abdominal pain associated with varying degrees of exocrine and endocrine pancreatic dysfunction. The disease produces a wide variety of progressive and irreversible structural changes in the pancreas. At present, the most controversial aspect of the disease is a choice of an appropriate operative procedure. Because there is no single cause and no consistent lesion, there can be no ideal surgical procedure. Even when the appropriate operation is chosen for each patient, the nature of the disease hinders the prospect of an excellent result.

Histology

Certain clinical antecedents, such as cholelithiasis, alcoholism, trauma of the pancreas, and obscure congenital factors are associated with both acute and chronic pancreatitis, but the precise causal relationships are difficult to prove. Cholelithiasis was associated with 28% of patients operated on for chronic relapsing pancreatitis; 41% were chronic alcoholics, and severe trauma was responsible in 3%. In 37% of patients, no apparent cause was known. Gallstones and chronic alcoholism were present in 10%. Pancreatitic cysts were present in 27% and pancreatolithiasis in 22%; 18% had diabetes mellitus, 16% had peptic ulcers, and 14% were jaundiced. Intractable pain was the principal reason for operation in almost all of the patients.

Surgical treatment

With increasing experience, the wide variety of pathologic changes and metabolic consequences of chronic pancreatitis became evident, and I began to realize the necessity for operating directly on the pancreas and selecting the appropriate operation for each patient. Consequently, I now relate the surgical management of chronic relapsing pancreatitis to the pathologic manifestations of the disease and make every effort to tailor each operation to the pathologic findings.

Follow-up studies of all patients have been made from one to 23 years, and in 421 patients (79%) the follow-up period was three years or more. A satisfactory result was recorded when the patient was asymptomatic or had mild symptoms compatible with full activity. Patients who had disabling symptoms that interfered with their activities were classed as having poor results. Peptic ulcer in 84 patients was added for 16% of the group (Table 12).

Indirect procedures
Of the indirect procedures, 70 patients had cholecystectomy, exploration of

the common bile duct, or some form of biliary diversion, such as choledocho-duodenostomy. Satisfactory long-term results were obtained in 61%. Biliary tract procedures were performed in 70 patients with satisfactory results in 61%. Sphincterotomy or sphincteroplasty was performed in 39 patients with satisfactory results in 49%. Autonomic nervous system procedures gave the poorest results with only 15% having a satisfactory outcome. Gastrointestinal diversion alone was performed in six patients with a satisfactory result in 67%. In these patients, however, the primary indication for gastrointestinal diversion was gastric outlet obstruction or partial duodenal obstruction. A variety of procedures for pancreatic cyst and abscesses were performed in 70 patients, and good results were obtained in 71%. Some type of anastomosis for external fistulas was performed in five patients with excellent results in 80%. Transpancreatic decompression was carried out in 25 patients with good results in 60%. Distal pancreatectomy was performed in 73 patients with good results in 78%. Pancreatoduodenectomy was the operation performed in 82 patients with satisfactory results in 68%. Total pancreatectomy was performed in eight patients with preliminary good results in 88%.

The satisfactory or good results achieved with total pancreatectomy do not hold up well with the passage of time. Most of these patients required readmission to the hospital for a variety of symptoms, usually with severe abdominal pain. Biliary tract surgery alone is valueless in the absence of biliary tract disease and is of little benefit in patients with advanced chronic pancreatitis.

Sphincterotomy/sphincteroplasty. Sphincterotomy alone or combined with cholecystectomy or choledochostomy was performed in 39 patients with a satisfactory result in only 49%. Many years ago I abandoned procedures on the autonomic nervous system for the relief of pain of pancreatitis.

Table 12. Clinical features in 530 patients with chronic relapsing pancreatitis.

Clinical feature	Number of patients	Percent
Pain	527	99
Weight loss	417	79
Previous operation	370	70
Alcoholism	216	41
Narcotic addiction	185	35
Cholelithiasis	150	28
Pancreatic cysts	143	27
Pancreatolithiasis	114	22
Diabetes	96	18
Peptic ulcer	84	16
Jaundice	73	14

Direct pancreatic procedures

Current operations for chronic relapsing pancreatitis may be divided into those that aim to drain cystic collections in or around the pancreas that have resulted from recurrent attacks of pancreatitis and those that attempt to relieve duct obstruction by some form of ductal decompression or pancreatic resection. Effective operations include internal or external drainage of pancreatic cysts, drainage of chronic pancreatic collections, transduodenal exploration and manipulation of the pancreatic ducts, transpancreatic exploration, and decompression of the duct of Wirsung by some modification of the Puestow procedure. Further direct operations include distal pancreatectomy, pancreatoduodenal resection, and total pancreatectomy.

Procedures on pancreatic cysts and abscesses

Seventy patients had some type of external or internal drainage of pancreatic cysts or chronic pancreatic or peripancreatic abscesses that were found in association with chronic pancreatitis. The results of treatment in this group are analyzed in Table 13.

In an early experience, drainage of abscesses was performed in 14 patients with satisfactory results in 71%. External drainage of cysts was performed in 23 patients with satisfactory results in 61%. Internal drainage of cysts was carried out in 29 patients with 79% satisfactory results, and excision of cysts was performed in three or four patients with satisfactory results in 75%.

External drainage of pancreatic cysts is recommended when the cystic collection is recent, and no firm wall is suitable for internal anastomosis to the gastrointestinal tract (Fig. 19). It is also employed if the cyst is in an unusual anatomic position. Satisfactory results were achieved in 61% of the patients.

Internal drainage of pancreatic cysts was carried out by transgastric cystogastrostomy in 23 patients (Fig. 20) and by cystojejunostomy in six; the results were superior with cystogastrostomy.

Table 13. Results of 70 procedures on cysts and chronic abscesses.

Procedure	Number of patients	Satisfactory result	
		Number	Percent
Drainage abscess	14	10	71
External drainage cyst	23	14	61
Internal drainage cyst	29	23	79
Excision cyst	4	3	75
Total	70	50	71.4

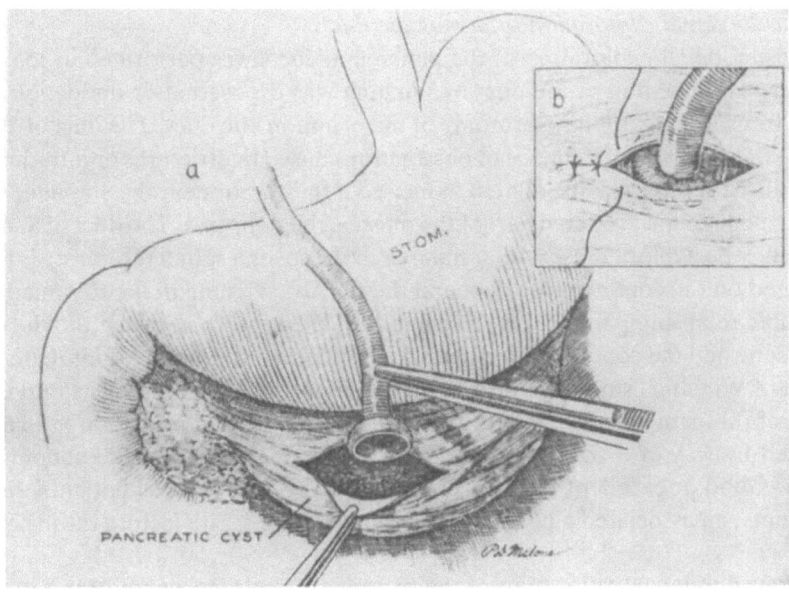

Fig. 19. External drainage of pancreatic cyst. Opening made in the cyst, the contents evacuated, and a catheter inserted. Inset, Opening in cyst loosely closed around catheter.

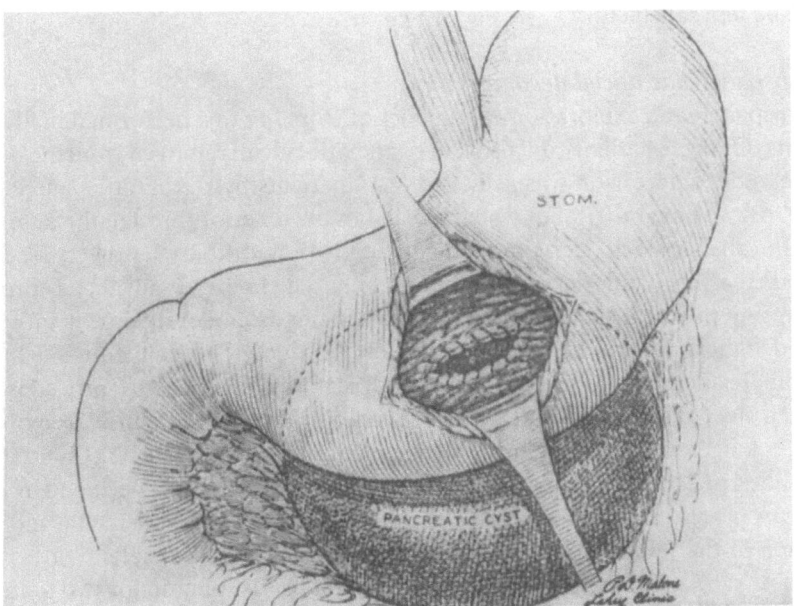

Fig. 20. Cystogastrostomy. Anterior gastrotomy permits opening into cyst through the posterior wall of the stomach. A continuous interlocking suture of 3–0 Dexon secures the anastomosis.

Transduodenal exploration of pancreatic ducts

Transduodenal exploration of the pancreatic ducts was performed in 155 patients. The opening of the duct of Wirsung was exposed after duodenotomy and transduodenal sphincterotomy of the common bile duct. The duct of Wirsung was probed for evidence of obstruction caused by strictures or intraductal calculi. Strictures may be dilated or incised if they occur near the ampulla, and any calculi in the proximal part of the duct can be removed. The duct of Santorini may be explored in a similar manner. Whenever a sphincteroplasty is performed on the common bile duct and the duct of Wirsung in the treatment of chronic relapsing pancreatitis, a segment of the septum between the duct of Wirsung and the common bile duct is excised. Not infrequently, I intubate the duct of Wirsung using a ureteral catheter of appropriate caliber. The opposite end of this catheter may be left within the lumen of the duodenum or exteriorized by way of a small duodenotomy and a stab wound in the abdominal wall. Good or excellent results were obtained in 72% of these patients. In 21 patients, an associated gallstone was treated also with satisfactory results in 18 (86%).

Transduodenal exploration of the pancreatic ducts is reserved for patients who have mild or moderately advanced pancreatitis and for those in whom pancreatic ductal obstruction is thought to be present in the proximal part of the duct. In the presence of advanced disease, the results of sphincteroplasty will be less satisfactory.

Transpancreatic ductal decompression

Transpancreatic exploration of the duct of Wirsung was performed in 25 patients. Of these patients, 13 also had pancreatic calculi removed from the duct. Ductal decompression was achieved in 14 patients by retrograde pancreatogastrostomy over a T tube, which was led to the exterior through the anterior wall of the stomach. Longitudinal pancreaticojejunostomy has been used by me increasingly and is currently the treatment of choice for advanced chronic relapsing pancreatitis when the duct of Wirsung is moderately or greatly dilated indicating proximal obstruction of the duct. The conventional longitudinal pancreaticojejunostomy is a modification of the Puestow procedure in which most of the length of the duct of Wirsung is opened, calculi are removed, and a long pancreaticojejunostomy is performed. In most instances, an anastomosis of 2 to 3 inches is sufficient unless much of the duct is occluded by calculi. A precise anastomosis between the lining of the duct of Wirsung and the lumen of the jejunum must be performed for satisfactory results. Unless the duct of Wirsung is greatly dilated, this anastomosis is splinted for two to three months with a T tube, which has been exteriorized (Fig. 21).

Long-term results have been satisfactory in 60% of patients. This percentage of satisfactory results has been improved by more careful selection of patients for this procedure.

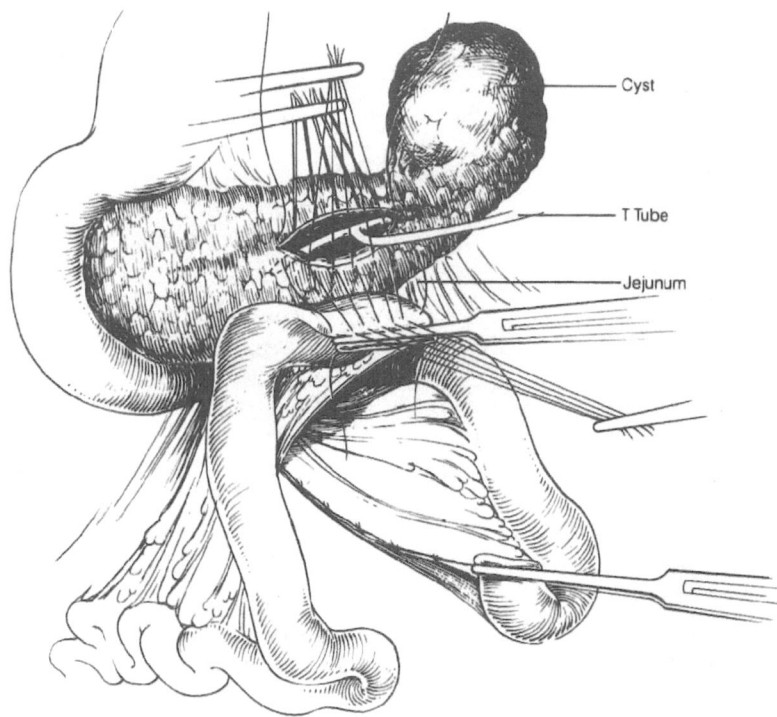

Fig. 21. Longitudinal pancreatojejunostomy, Roux-en-Y, splinted by a T tube. The cyst was drained by insertion of a catheter.

Distal pancreatectomy

Distal pancreatectomy, splenectomy, and resection of the body and tail of the pancreas were performed in 73 patients. The primary indication for distal pancreatectomy is chronic pancreatitis confined to the distal segment of the gland, but such ideal circumstances are encountered only occasionally. Distal pancreatitis was the indication for distal pancreatectomy in 39 of 73 patients while post-traumatic distal pancreatitis was present in 15 patients (Table 14). Severe

Table 14. Indications for distal pancreatectomy in 73 patients with chronic relapsing pancreatitis.

Indication	Number of patients
Distal pancreatitis	39
Post-traumatic distal pancreatitis	15
Severe pancreatitis (entire gland)	14
External pancreatic fistula	5
Total	73

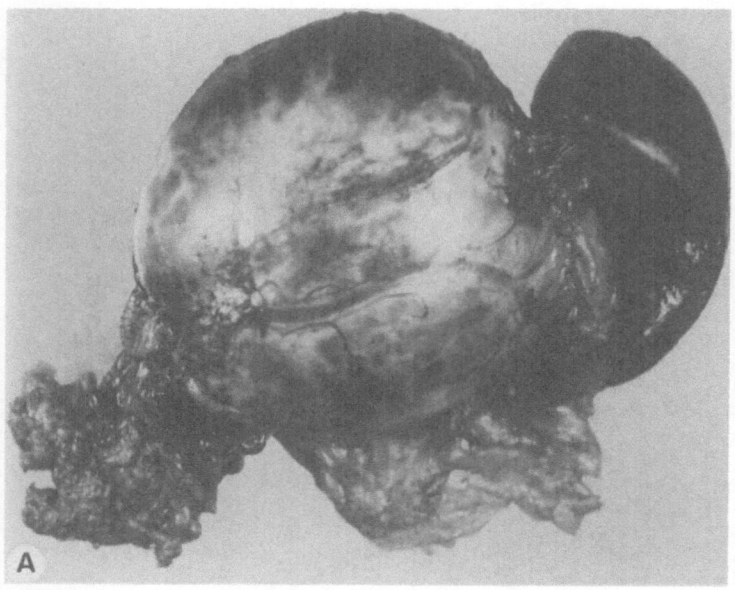

Fig. 22. A. Large retention cyst occupying the distal half of the pancreas treated by splenectomy and distal pancreatectomy.

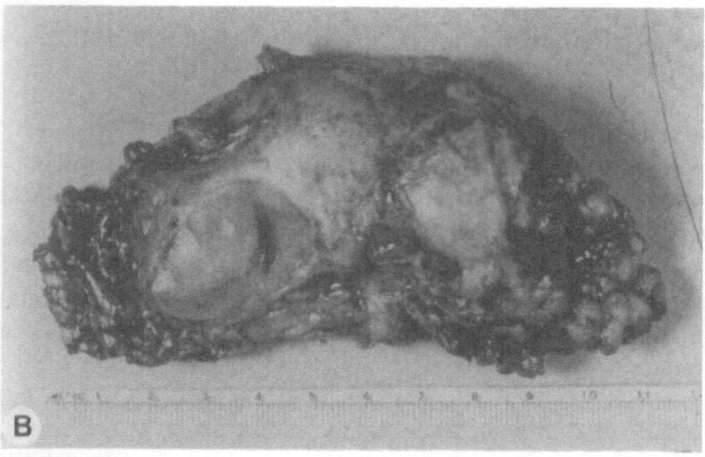

Fig. 22. B. Multilocular cysts of pancreas treated by distal pancreatectomy.

pancreatitis of the entire gland was present in 14. An external pancreatic fistula was present in five patients.

Distal pancreatectomy is the treatment of choice when the disease is confined to the distal segment of the pancreas (Fig. 22). Under those circum-

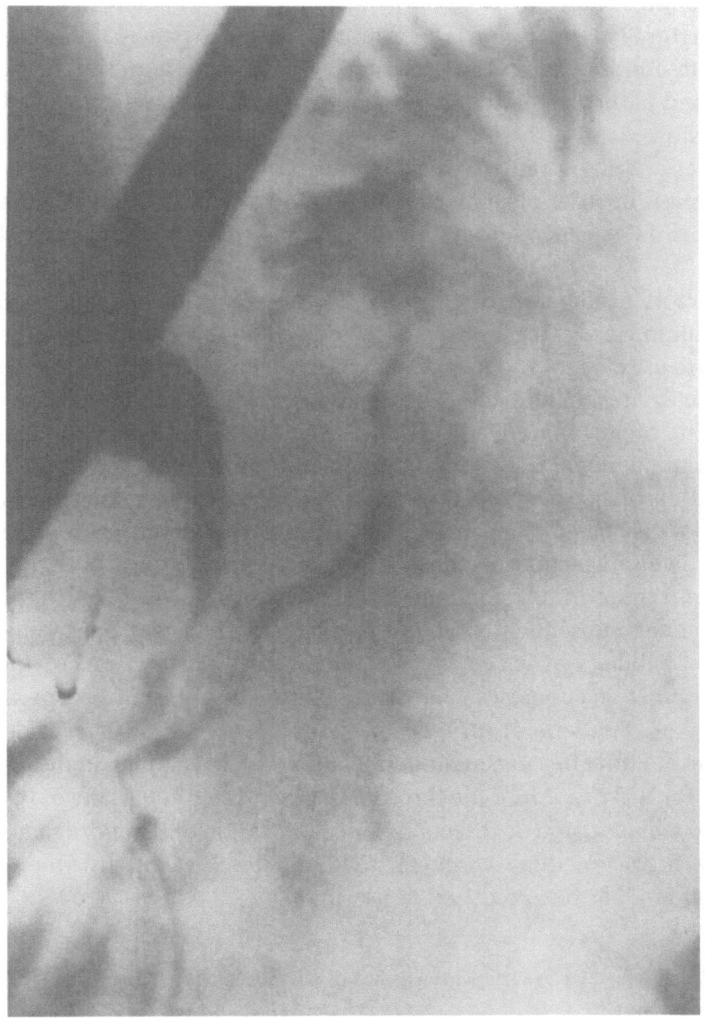

Fig. 23. Endoscopic retrograde cholangiopancreatogram showing tapering of distal common bile duct and patency of distal pancreatojejunostomy after distal pancreatectomy.

stances, excellent results can be anticipated in most of these patients. On the other hand, distal pancreatectomy performed for diffuse chronic pancreatitis gives poor results and should not be employed unless retrograde pancreaticojejunostomy is performed simultaneously (Fig. 23).

Pancreatoduodenectomy
Pancreatoduodenal resection was carried out in 82 patients. The important

clinical features shown in Table 15 indicate the severity of the pancreatitis in these patients. This operation is appropriate for severe pancreatitis of long duration with multiple points of intrapancreatic obstruction present in the head of the gland particularly when more limited operations have previously been unsuccessful.

Pain was present in 100% of the patients, previous operations in 81%, pancreatolithiasis in 66%, alcoholism in 61%, diabetes mellitus in 50%, narcotic addiction in 43%, pancreatic cysts in 39%, jaundice in 29%, and weight loss in 9%.

Satisfactory results were obtained in 68% of these patients, which is a gratifying result in view of the severity of the disease in this group. These patients continue to use alcohol and to take narcotics, which makes a higher percentage of satisfactory results difficult. Of 82 patients, two died in the postoperative period: one of postoperative pancreatitis and one of pulmonary embolus.

Pancreatoduodenal resection continues to be my treatment of choice for far-advanced chronic pancreatitis associated with total disorganization of the anatomy of the head of the pancreas and in patients in whom lesser procedures failed to give satisfactory results. This experience has grown over the years, and the current mortality continues at an acceptable level.

Two patients subsequently required revision of a stenosed pancreaticojejunostomy. A biliary stricture in one patient required revision of the choledochojejunal anastomosis. Diabetes mellitus, not present preoperatively, developed in 12 patients at varying times after the operation. The incidence of jejunal ulceration after pancreatoduodenal resection was high in the early experience for this procedure for chronic pancreatitis (17%). Many of these patients had a limited gastric resection. Since utilization of the more radical gastrectomy or gastrectomy combined with bilateral vagotomy, the jejunal ulceration rate has been reduced to less than 7%.

Table 15. Clinical features in 82 patients who had pancreatoduodenectomy for chronic relapsing pancreatitis.

Clinical feature	Number	Percent
Pain	82	100
Weight loss	65	79
Previous operation	66	81
Pancreatolithiasis	54	66
Alcoholism	50	61
Narcotic addiction	35	43
Cysts	32	39
Diabetes	41	50
Jaundice	24	29

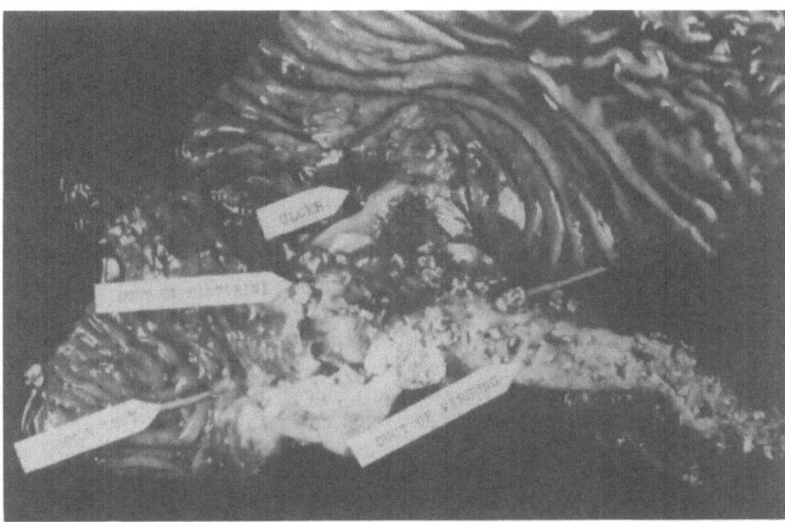

Fig. 24. Total pancreatectomy for diffuse pancreatolithiasis with almost total destruction of the pancreas.

Total pancreatectomy

Total pancreatectomy for chronic pancreatitis has been performed in 40 patients. We reserve this operation for patients with the most extensive type of chronic pancreatitis associated with innumerable points of pancreatic obstruction and usually with extensive pancreatolithiasis (Fig. 24). It has also been performed when disabling symptoms are present after partial resection of the pancreas. The long-term results have been discouraging.

Conclusions

Despite the passage of time, the advancement of frontiers of scientific knowledge, the development of new surgical techniques, and the refinement of old ones, the validity of the quotation by the late Dr. Frank H. Lahey from the preface to the first edition of *Surgical Practice of the Lahey Clinic** is apparent: 'It has been our experience that as we have standardized operations, we have widened operability, decreased mortality, and improved end-results.'

In assessing abandoned principles and techniques of yesteryear, one should not lose sight of the important fact that an outmoded procedure may have bridged a historical gap in the evolution of the art and science of surgery and may have reduced morbidity or saved a human life.

* Surgical Practice of the Lahey Clinic. Philadelphia, W B Saunders Co, 1941

44

Suggested reading

Brooks JR: Cancer of pancreas. In: Brooks JR (ed) Surgery of the Pancreas. Philadelphia, W B Saunders Co, 1983, pp 263–298

Caroli J, Soupalt R, Kossakowski J, Plocker L, Pardowska: La dilatation polykystique congénitale des voies biliaires intra-hépatiques: essai de classification. [Congenital polycystic dilation of the intrahepatic bile ducts: attempts at classification.] Sem hôp Paris 34: 488–495, 1958

Praderi RC, Estefan AF, Tiscornia E: Transhepatic intubation in benign and malignant lesions of the biliary ducts. Current Problems in Surgery 22, (12) December 1985

Smith R: Mucosal graft operations for hilar strictures of the hepatic ducts. In: Maingot R (ed) Abdominal Operations, ed 6. New York, Appleton-Century-Crofts, 1974

Warren KW: Cysts of the pancreas. In: Bockus HL (ed) Gastroenterology, ed 3. Vol 3, Philadelphia, W B Saunders Co, 1976, pp 1166–1169

Warren KW, Tan ECG, Williams CI: The gallbladder and bile ducts. In: Schiff L, Schiff B (eds) Diseases of the Liver, ed 6. Philadelphia, J B Lippincott Co, in press

Warren KW, Choe DS, Plaza J, Relihan M: Results of radical resection for periampullary cancer. Ann Surg 181: 534–540, 1975

Warren KW, Viedenheimer MC, Athanassiades S, Frederick PL: Pancreatic cysts occurring secondary to ductal carcinoma of the pancreas. Lahey Clin Found Bull 15: 13–15, 1966

2. Radiology in hepato-pancreatico-biliary disease

A. LUNDERQUIST

Diagnosis of focal lesions in the liver parenchyma

Benign liver cysts have since the availability of ultrasonography (US) and computerized tomography (CT) been rather common findings when patients are
examined for suspected lesions within the liver. Examined with US these cysts
are non-echogenic, they have a smooth outlining without a capsule and with a
marked echo extending from the opposite side. These cysts can be single, they
can be multiple, and fill almost the whole liver. Cysts may be present at the
same time in the pancreas and kidneys.

Examined with CT (Fig. 1) the cysts appear as well outlined lesions with low
attenuation (0–10 HU). Small cysts, up to the diameter of 1 cm might be more
difficult to separate from other lesions as partial volume effect makes the measurement of the attenuation uncertain.

Echinococcus cysts have a characteristic picture both on US and CT (Fig. 2).
With both examination techniques a capsule can easily be seen and this may
some times be calcified. On ultrasound the cyst shows a more echogenic content than the simple cyst. Diagnostic percutaneous puncture of these cysts is
not to be recommended because of the risk of anaphylactic reaction. An early
diagnosis of *liver abscess* is essential to reduce the otherwise high mortality.
Examined with ultrasound the abscess can appear as either low echogenic or
high echogenic lesion with diffuse margin to normal liver parenchyma. At CT
the abscess appears as a low attenuated lesion with diffuse margin to normal
liver. If the examination is repeated after intravenous administration of contrast material an increased attenuation is found in the periphery of the abscess
depending on the increased vascularity in this region. Neither ultrasound nor
CT can, however, give a specific diagnosis, why percutaneous aspiration biopsy has to be performed for cytology and culture.

Primary and secondary tumors of the liver. Technetium sulphur colloid scintigraphy can localize lesions down to the size of 2 cm unless the lesion is not

46

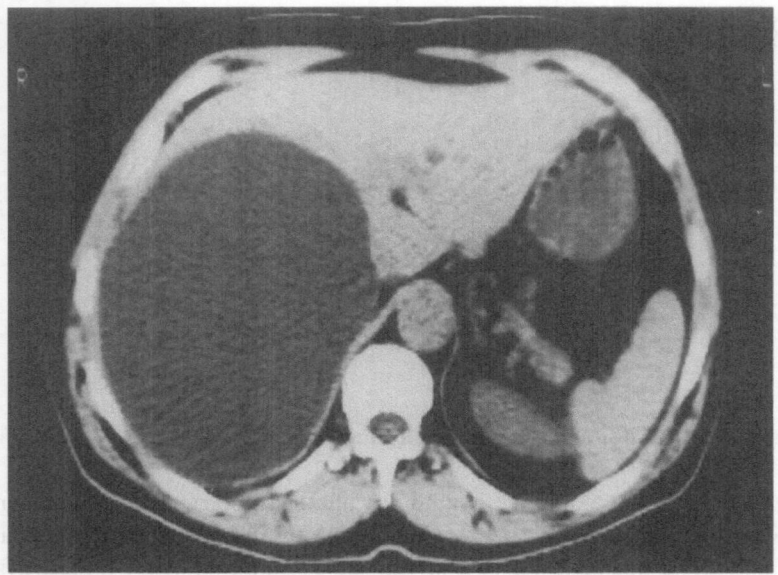

Fig. 1. CT of the liver demonstrating a large benign cyst.

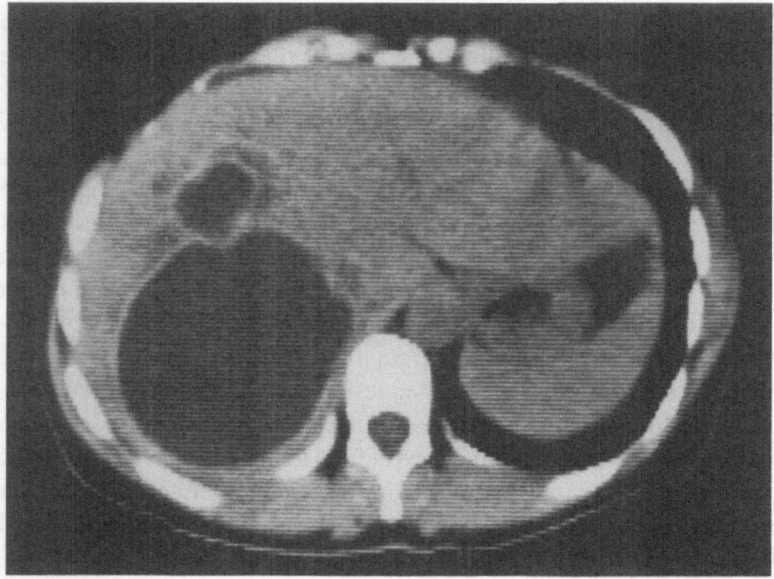

Fig. 2. CT of the liver in a patient with two echinococcal cysts in the right lobe of the liver. Observe the capsule of the cysts.

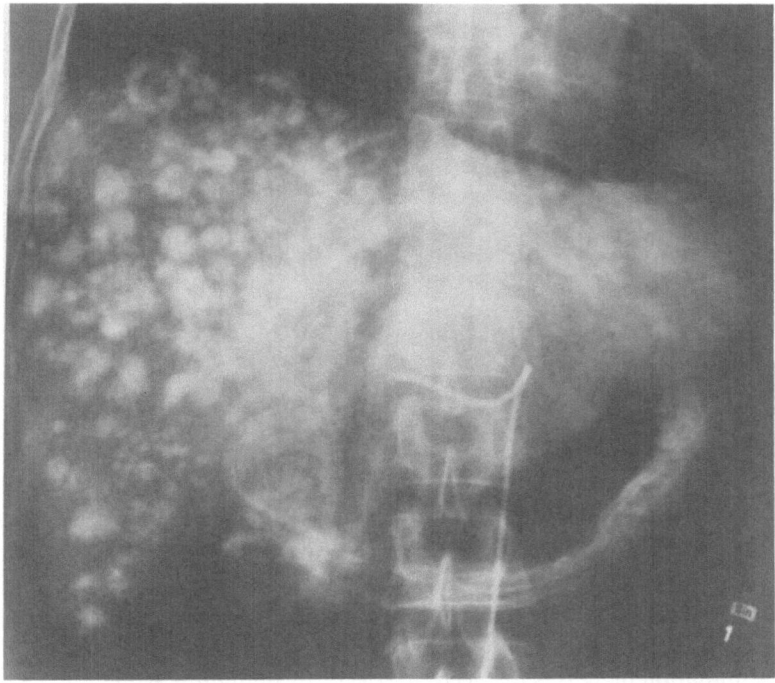

Fig. 3. Selective hepatic angiography in a patient with metastasis to the liver of a carcinoid tumor. Very small tumors can be demonstrated because of the high vascularity.

localized within the thickest part of the liver. Scintigraphy is unspecific and has a reduced value when diffuse parenchymal disease is present within the liver [1].

Angiography can demonstrate small tumors, 3–4mm in diameter, in the case the tumors are highly vascularized (Fig. 3). This is the case with metastases from endocrine tumors and some renal tumors. However, most secondary tumors in the liver, as metastases from colonic carcinoma, are low vascularized and thus difficult to diagnose with angiography. This, however, is now compensated by the high diagnostic accuracy of US and CT. Ultrasonography can localize tumors down to 1cm in diameter. Most tumors have an echogenecity lower than the normal liver parenchyma (Fig. 4). Fortunately, cavernous hemangioma appear as rather characteristic high echogenic lesions frequently adjacent to a vein. Sometimes, however, a cavernous hemangioma may appear as a low echogenic lesion and can then not be separated from a malignant tumor. In these cases, dynamic CT after intravenous injection of contrast medium may become diagnostic. Early after injection of contrast medium the lesion then appears with a highly attenuated periphery and slowly during a period of up to 1 hour, the lesion is filled with contrast to become isodense with the normal liver parenchyma [2].

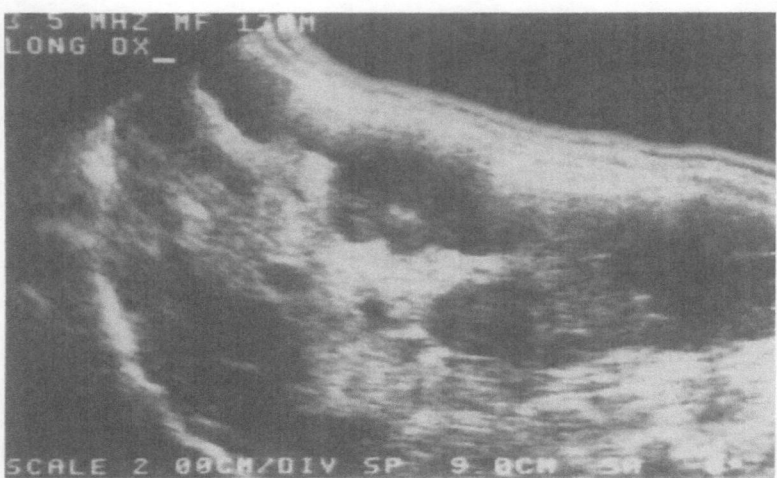

Fig. 4. Ultrasonography of the liver in a patient with metastasis from colonic carcinoma. The metastases have low echogenecity to be compared with the normal liver parenchyma.

Small lesions down to a diameter of 1 cm can also be localized with CT. Intravenous or intraarterial injection of contrast medium combined with the CT-examination increases the accuracy of the examination even more. As the only curative treatment of malignant primary and secondary tumors of the liver is liver resection, it is very important to make sure that the tumor is confined to one liver lobe. Prior to surgery angiography is often performed to demonstrate the vascular anatomy. Combined with this angiography, angio-CT of the liver can be performed and this gives the best demonstration of the extension and location of the tumors (Fig. 5). It is important to be aware of that none of the diagnostic methods is specific enough to suggest the microscopic diagnosis. To prevent serious mistakes, percutaneous biopsy for cytology is therefore important.

Budd-Chiari's syndrome is produced by an obliteration of the hepatic veins either by tumor or thrombosis. Technetium sulphur colloid scintigraphy in these cases shows a normal uptake of the isotope in the central part of the liver around the inferior vena cava, but a low uptake in other parts of the liver. This is to be compared with contrast enhanced CT examination which shows a normal attenuation in the central parts of the liver but a reduced attenuation in more peripheral parts. Ultrasonography can demonstrate the obliterated hepatic veins [3] and they can also be demonstrated by direct injection of contrast medium into the hepatic veins after catheterization through the inferior vena cava (Fig. 6).

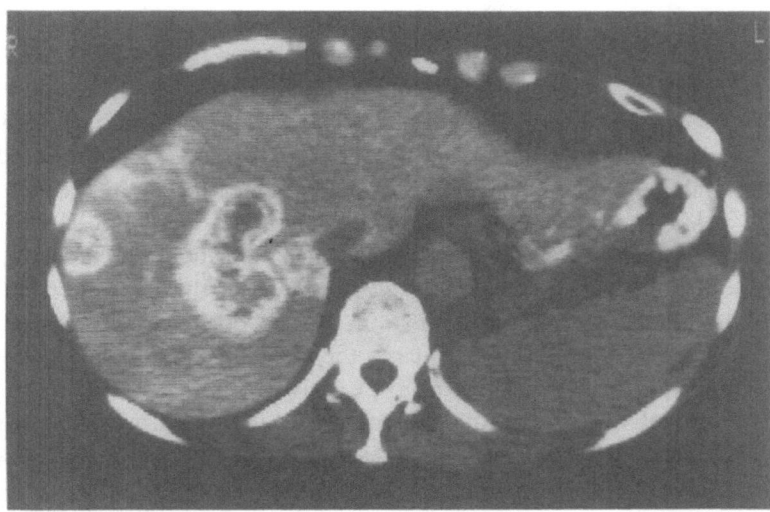

Fig. 5. Angio-CT of the liver in patient with metastases from colonic carcinoma. Angio-CT gives the best demonstration of the tumors because of the increased attenuation in the vascular periphery of the tumors.

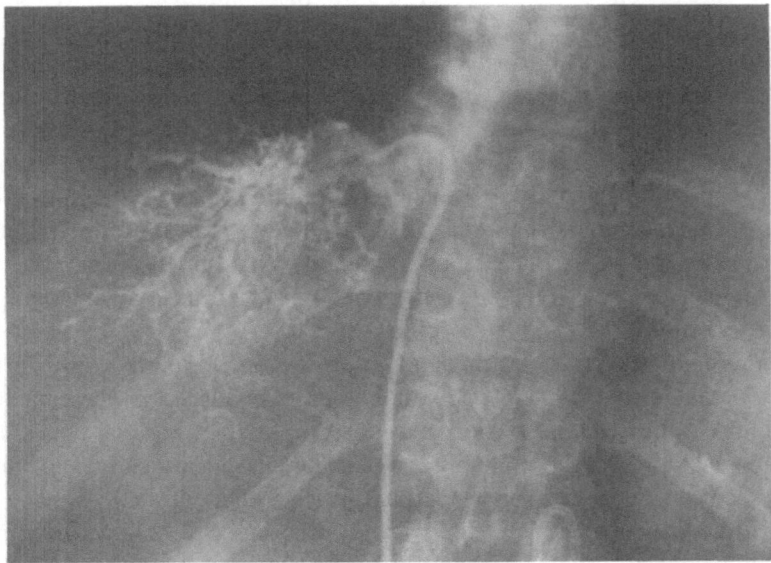

Fig. 6. Selective hepatic venography in Budd-Chiari syndrome demonstrating the venous collateral network after thrombotization of the normal hepatic veins.

Liver trauma

Rupture of the liver caused by blunt trauma to the upper part of the abdomen has been a clear indication for laparotomy after peritoneal lavage has shown blood in the peritoneal cavity. Immediate laparotomy is no longer indicated if clinical examination does not suggest continuous hemorrhage, and the patient can be kept stable on substitute of blood and fluid. CT examination of the upper part of the abdomen gives an important information about the extent of the damage to the liver, spleen and kidneys. In addition, intravenous injection of contrast, at the time of the CT examination, can show the location of an eventual hemorrhage. However, in many cases the bleeding has stopped when the examination is performed, and also a quite extensive rupture of the liver can be treated conservatively. In the follow-up of these patients CT as well as ultrasonography or scintigraphy can be quite useful. At the time of the acute trauma ultrasonography, however, has shown to be less valuable.

Bile ducts

Severly years ago *intravenous cholangiography* was used quite frequently to demonstrate the bile ducts. However, the contrast medium used as well as the technique of administration caused several side-effects which made the method less attractive. New contrast materials and other techniques of administration of the contrast medium have reduced the side-effects markedly, why intravenous cholangiography again has been considered as a method of value. At some institutions intravenous cholangiography has been used as a preoperative examination prior to elective cholecystectomy. In this way information has been gained about the anatomy of the bile ducts as well as eventual stones. It has been possible to reduce the operation time and, hopefully, also the risk for iatrogenic damage to the bile ducts when intraoperative cholangiography can be excluded.

Scintigraphy after intravenous injection of isotopes excreted through the liver together with the bile (HIDA-or DISI-DA-scintigraphy) have made it possible to interpret the function and gross anatomy of the bile ducts. The function of bilio-digestive anatomoses, posttraumatic or surgical leak of bile as well as bile reflux to the stomach can thus be investigated.

Ultrasonography of the gallbladder is now an accepted technique to examine the gallbladder in case of suspected stones or cholecystitis. The technique is more accurate than peroral cholecystography or intraveneous examination of the gallbladder. In case of carcinoma of the gallbladder, ultrasonography has the advantage compared with peroral cholecystography to be able to demonstrate infiltration in the tissue outside the gallbladder and into the liver.

51

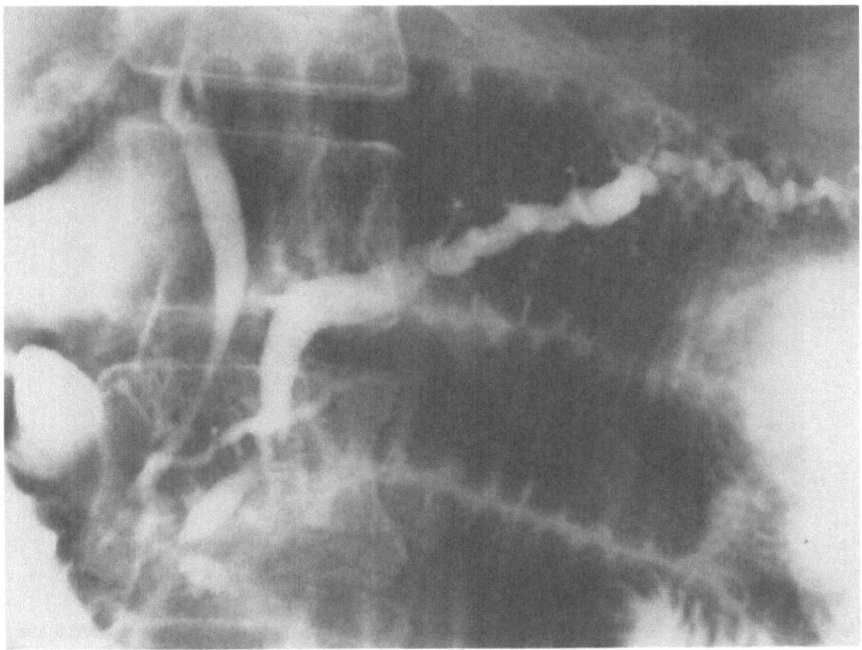

Fig. 7. ERCP in a patient with pancreatitis. Wide irregular pancreatic duct with irregular side branches. Tapered distal part of the common bile duct produced by a benign pseudocyst.

Radiologic examination of the pancreas

With the availability of new diagnostic modalities, angiography has lost almost all of its importance as a diagnostic procedure in the workup of pancreatic lesions. Ultrasonography, computerized tomography and endoscopic retrograde cholangio-pancreatography (ERCP) are now the methods of choice often combined with percutaneous biopsy for cytology. Magnetic resonance has not yet an established place in pancreatic imaging. In acute pancreatitis US and CT will show the enlarged and edematous pancreas and sometimes the presence of pseudocysts. In chronic pancreatitis ERCP will show the extent of the damage to the pancreatic ducts (Fig. 7). Pancreatic adenocarcinoma can be demonstrated with US as well as CT. Percutaneous biopsy guided by CT (Fig. 8) or US can provide the specific diagnosis. In the case of obstruction of the bile ducts, the dilated ducts can be visualized both with US and CT. In patients with endocrine tumors of the pancreas angiography, however, still plays an important role in the localization of the tumor. Angiography can localize these tumors in about 60% of the cases, and if angiography is negative, transheaptic catheterization of the pancreatic veins and venous sampling for hormone assay

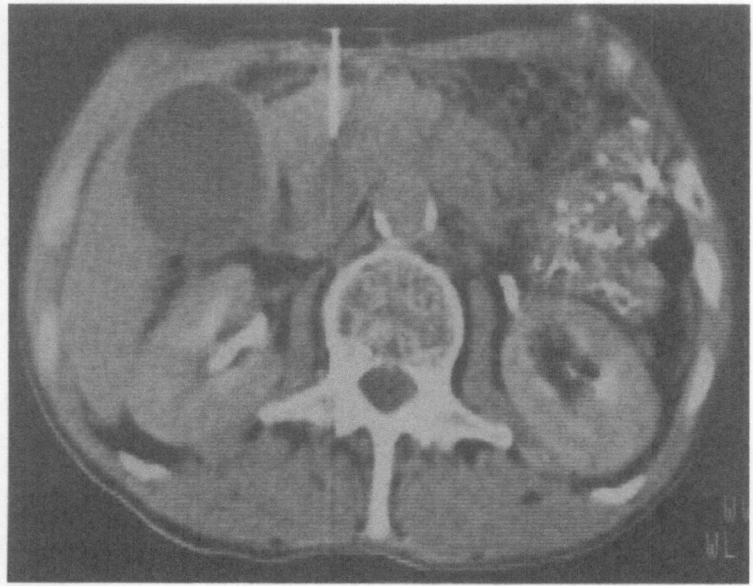

Fig. 8. CT of the liver in patient with carcinoma of the head of the pancreas. CT guided percutaneous biopsy with the needle demonstrated within the tumor. Distended gallbladder.

can be performed. This additional technique can correctly localize the endocrine tumors in more than 80% of the cases [4].

Radiologic interventional techniques in hepatico-pancreatico-biliary disease

During the last 15 years a large number of therapeutic radiological techniques have developed, some of them have survived – some have disappeared. It is very important for us to be critical in the evaluation of the methods we are using, compare success rate and complications with other methods including surgery, and not persist to do a procedure when better and safer alternatives are available. In this connection we also have to keep in mind the quality of life we may give the patient, or, if an increased survival time may only be exchanged to more days in the hospital.

Bile ducts

Percutaneous transhepatic drainage of the bile ducts (PTCD) is now an accepted treatment to decompress the bile ducts prior to surgery. After many years of excitement over this non-surgical treatment, the materials have been analyzed with regard to complications and benefits.

Complications are not infrequent, but most of them fortunately not serious.

Complications from PTCD

Bleeding into bile ducts
Subcapsular or intraparenchymal hematomas
Bleeding into peritoneum or pleura
Infections – septicemia
Bile leakage
Displacement of a drainage catheter
Occlusion of drainage catheter

The most serious complications encountered are hemorrhage and septicemia. Life-threatening hemorrhage can occur if an hepatic artery is damaged when puncture of the bile duct is attempted. The hemorrhage can be stopped by a transcatheter embolization which has to be performed quite selectively if parenchymal damage should be avoided [5].

If bile is infected septicemia can often not be prevented even if the patient is covered with antibiotics. On the other hand, percutaneous drainage offers an effective method of decompression in patients with septic cholangitis [6].

Palliative surgery with biliary bypass has a high mortality rate (15–22%). Therefore the surgical procedure has often been exchanged to permanent percutaneous drainage of the bile ducts, or insertion of an endoprosthesis. Endoprostheses have been used particularly in patients with nonresectable tumors causing jaundice (Fig. 9). When more experience was gained it became clear that the endoprosthesis frequently obliterated usually after 4–6 months in position. Consequently it should not be used if patients are expected to live longer than this period of time [7, 8].

It has been taken for granted that the jaundiced patient should gain from biliary drainage prior to surgery. Now, however, this has been questioned. There are several factors more than high bilirubin that influence the outcome of an operation. Few randomized studies compare immediate surgery and surgery after biliary drainage. These studies, however, do not suggest that biliary drainage reduced the surgical complications and mortality. In addition, it has been shown that preoperative biliary drainage may increase the hospitalization time and therefore also the cost [9]. In the future, there will be a marked reduction in number of PTCD-procedures as they will be replaced by endoscopic techniques. The endoscopists can not only place naso-biliary catheters for drainage but also stents up to the size of F12–14. They can also remove stones and dilate strictures. An experienced endoscopist fails only in about

54

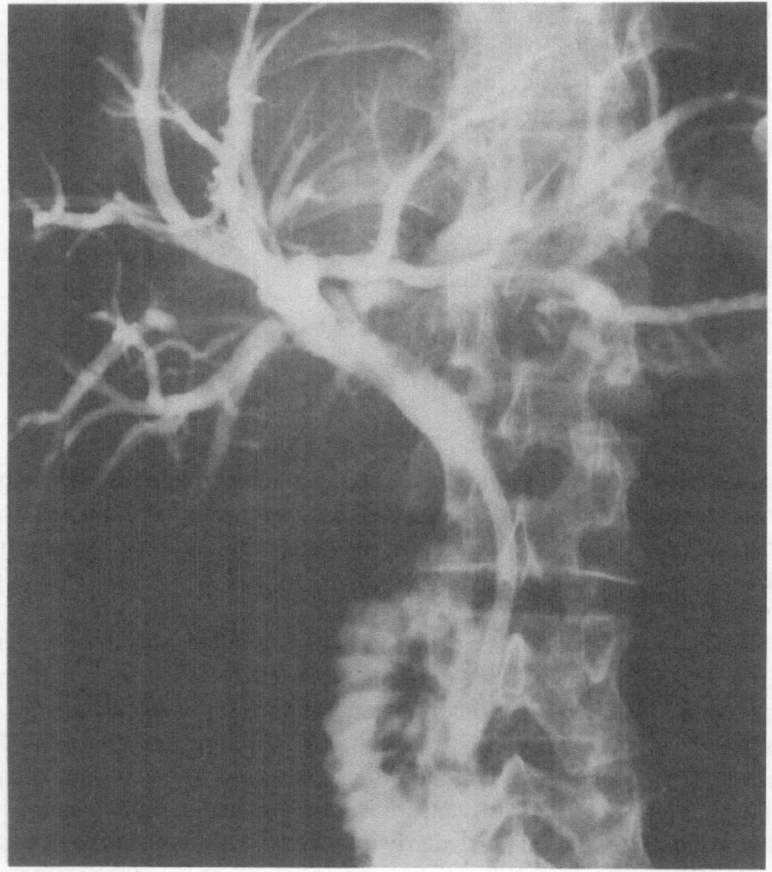

Fig. 9. Patient with a pancreatic carcinoma. Biliary endoprosthesis placed percutaneously into the bile duct and with its tip into the duodenum.

20% of cases, and here the transhepatic technique will still have its place.

Liver trauma. Trauma to the liver, blunt or penetrating can produce a life-threatening hemorrhage. It has been a rule to perform laparotomy if perito-neal lavage demonstrated bleeding into the peritoneal cavity. At the time of surgery bleeding has often stopped, but it is again activated when the surgeon removes the clots in order to evaluate the extent of the lesion. To stop the bleeding from a ruputured liver he either has to ligate the hepatic artery or per-form a lobe resection.

New imaging and interventional radiologic techniques have changed this ap-proach. If the patient can be kept stable, CT in an excellent way demonstrates the extent of the lesion. If CT with contrast enhancement shows continuous bleeding, angiography can be performed and the bleeding vessel can be localized. Already 14 years ago Dotter, Rösch and Brown [10] demonstrated that bleeding arteries could be safely embolized and occluded provided they are not end-arteries. Liver arteries are not end-arteries, and in addition, the portal blood supply prevents ischemia to develop if branches of the hepatic artery are obliterated. Transcatheter embolization to control hepatic hemorrhage has now become an accepted treatment [11]. Frequently surgery can be prevented and only left for cases in critical conditions, where the delay to perform angiography can not be tolerated.

In penetrating trauma infection often develops in the hematoma in or around the liver. However, when the bleeding has stopped this infected hematoma can be drained either percutaneously or surgically.

Drainage of abscesses. A liver or pancreatic abscess localized by US or CT can be percutaneously punctured and its content aspirated. When a simple needle aspiration is unsuccessful an ordinary angiographic catheter with multiple side-holes can be introduced for continuous drainage, and even large sump drains may also be introduced percutaneously to drain more thick fluid with much debris. Improved imaging and percutaneous drainage has markedly reduced the mortality from liver abscesses. Before the era of radionuclide scanning, operative mortality was more than 40% and was reduced to 20% when ultrasonography and CT became available. Percutaneous drainage has given another marked improvement and reduced the mortality rate to below 4% [12].

Treatment of liver tumors. Primary and secondary tumors of the liver have been treated with intravenous cytostatic drugs for many years. Response rate has been low. Intraarterial cytostatic infusion was presumed to reduce side-effects and improve the response rate, but this was found to be only marginal. A combination of temporary liver ischemia and drug infusion into the hepatic artery has also been tried with some success. In the intraarterial drug infusion the radiologist can assist the surgeon in placing a catheter into the hepatic artery percutaneously and in this way prevent repeated surgery.

Liver metastasis from hormone producing endocrine tumors have been treated surgically with liver dearterialization. These hypervascular metastases respond with partial necrosis and reduced hormone release. In this way the patient's quality of life can be improved even if the length of survival is not markedly increased.

It has been demonstrated that transcatheter hepatic artery embolization for temporary obliteration of the hepatic artery can be an alternative to surgical dearterialization. When the embolization is performed with gelfoam powder the obliteration of the hepatic arteries will only persist for 1–2 days, thus

56

producing a short-term ischemia. Tumor response to this transcatheter embolization has been about the same as from surgical dearterialization.

References

1. Reba RC, Chen DCP, Fajman WA: Hepatic scintigraphy. In: Bernardino ME and Sones PJ (eds) Hepatic Radiography. MacMillan Publishing Company, New York, 1984
2. Freeny PC, Marks WM: Patterns of contrast enhancement of benign and malignant hepatic neoplasms during bolus dynamic and delayed CT. Radiology 160: 613, 1986
3. Menu Y, Allison D, Lorphelin J-M, Valla D, Belghiti J, Nahum H: Budd-Chiari syndrome: US evaluation. Radiology 157: 761, 1985
4. Lunderquist A, Eriksson M, Ingemansson I, Larsson L-I, Reichardt W: Selective pancreatic vein catheterization for hormone assay in endocrine tumors of the pancreas. Cardiovascular Radiology 1: 117, 1978
5. Doppman JL, Girton M, Vermess M: Risk of hepatic artery embolization in the presence of obstructive jaundice. Radiology 143: 37, 1982
6. Gould RJ, Vogelzang RL, Neiman HL, Pearl GJ, Poticka SM: Percutaneous biliary drainage as an initial therapy in sepsis of the biliary tract. Surg Gynec Obstet 160: 523, 1985
7. Lammer J: Perkutane transhepatische Gallengangsendoprosthese. Fortschr Röntgenstr 142: 243, 1985
8. Mueller PR, Ferrucci JT, Teplick SK, van Sonnenberg E, Haskin PH, Butch RJ, Papanicolaou N: Biliary stent endoprosthesis: Analysis of complications in 113 patients. Radiology 156: 637, 1985
9. Pitt HA, Gomes AS, Lois JF, Mann LL, Deutsch LS, Longmire WP: Does preoperative percutaneous biliary drainage reduce operative risk or increase hospital cost? Ann Surg 201: 545, 1985
10. Rösch J, Dotter CT, Brown MJ: Selective arterial embolization. A new method for control of acute gastrointestinal bleeding. Radiology 102: 303, 1972
11. Rubin BE, Katzen BT: Selective hepatic artery embolization to control massive hepatic hemorrhage after trauma. Amer J Roentgenol 129: 253, 1977
12. Gerzof SG, Johnson WC, Robbins AH, Nabseth DC: Intrahepatic pyogenic abscesses: Treatment by percutaneous drainage. Amer J Surg 149: 487, 1985

3. Endoscopic approach to management of hepatico-pancreatico-biliary disorders

J.H. SIEGEL

The endoscopic evaluation and treatment of patients presenting with diseases of the liver and pancreas has gained considerable attention since the introduction of Endoscopic Retrograde Cholangiopancreatography [ERCP], sphincterotomy and placement of endoprostheses for the diagnosis and treatment of diseases of these organ systems [1–16]. Early utilization of ERCP for the management of patients with these disorders is increasing in most medical centers throughout the world.

The complete spectrum of interventional endoscopic techniques currently employed in the evaluation of patients with pancreaticobiliary tract disorders are listed in Table 1. As seen from this expansive list, the numbers of procedures and modalities has increased in recent years because of the successful performance of these procedures, their effective utilization and cost effectiveness.

ERCP

The indications for ERCP are well-established and known to most gastroenterologists and surgeons (Table 2). ERCP is most useful in the evaluation of patients with cholestasis. Its value in distinguishing intrahepatic from extrahepatic disorders is well known [4, 5, 10, 17]. Table 3, an algorithm, offers the

Table 1.

Endoscopic retrograde cholangiopancreatography [ERCP]	
Duodenoscopic sphincterotomy [DS]	
Percutaneous endoscopic extraction of retained stones [PEERS]	
Balloon dilatation	
Prostheses	Nasobiliary
	Endoprostheses

58

most practical and expeditious pathway for evaluating patients with cholestasis
[18]. Following historical review, physical examination and biochemical testing, the work-up of cholestasis should proceed initially with non-invasive
imaging techniques, i.e., ultrasonography, scintigraphy and CT scans. These
tests are then followed by the more invasive techniques of percutaneous cholangiography and/or ERCP. This expeditious evaluation employing non-in-

Table 2.

Indications for ERCP

I.   Jaundice
     A.   Intrahepatic
          1. Hepatocellular (virus, drug, alcohol)
          2. Cirrhosis
          3. Tumor
          4. Abscess
     B.   Extrahepatic
          1. Choledocholithiasis
          2. Tumor
          3. Other (nodes, pseudocyst)

II. Pancreatic disease
     A.   Recurrent
     B.   Chronic relapsing
     C.   Pseudocyst
     D.   Abscess
     E.   Tumor

III. Gallbladder disease

IV. Pre- and postoperative evaluation of biliary tract and pancreatic duct

V.   Abdominal pain of unknown cause

VI. Other applications of ERCP
     A.   Collection of pancreatic secretions for cytology, CEA, Chemistries
     B.   Biopsy
     C.   Research

VII. Therapeutic applications of ERCP
     A.   Sphincterotomy
     B.   Stone removal
     C.   Balloon dilatation
     D.   Endoprostheses
     E.   Placement of radioactive material
     F.   Perfusion of medicaments

Contraindications for ERCP

I.   Acute pancreatitis

---

vasive techniques should be completed prior to hospital admission. Then, on the first hospital day, I suggest that ERCP be performed. During the performance of ERCP, appropriate therapeutic procedures can be performed if indicated, i.e., sphincterotomy for stone extraction and placement of prostheses for obstruction. If the ERCP fails in providing a diagnostic cholangiogram or in providing decompression, a percutaneous transhepatic cholangiogram should then be attempted. This approach facilitates both diagnosis and definitive therapy on Day 1.

In experienced hands, ERCP provides diagnostic information in approximately 88% of procedures attempted. ERCP offers selective opacification of the duct of intention, establishing the diagnosis with a high degree of success (Table 4) [12]. Obviously, the experienced endoscopist is the most important component in accomplishing these high rates of accuracy. In addition to the standard techniques, the endoscopist can employ more aggressive endoscopic techniques, i.e., guide wires, precut techniques and fistulotomy, increasing

Table 3. Workup of cholestasis.

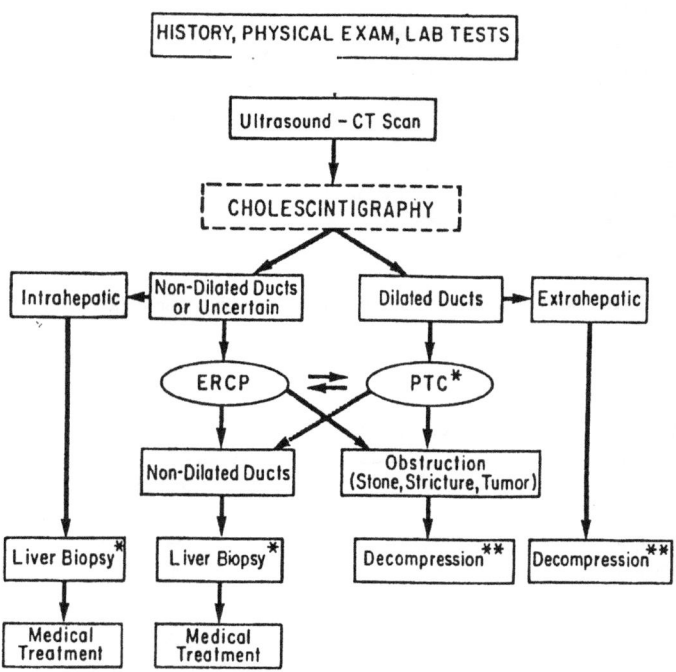

* Normal coagulation
** Percutaneous drainage, Duodenoscopic sphincterotomy, Transpapillary Drainage, Surgery.

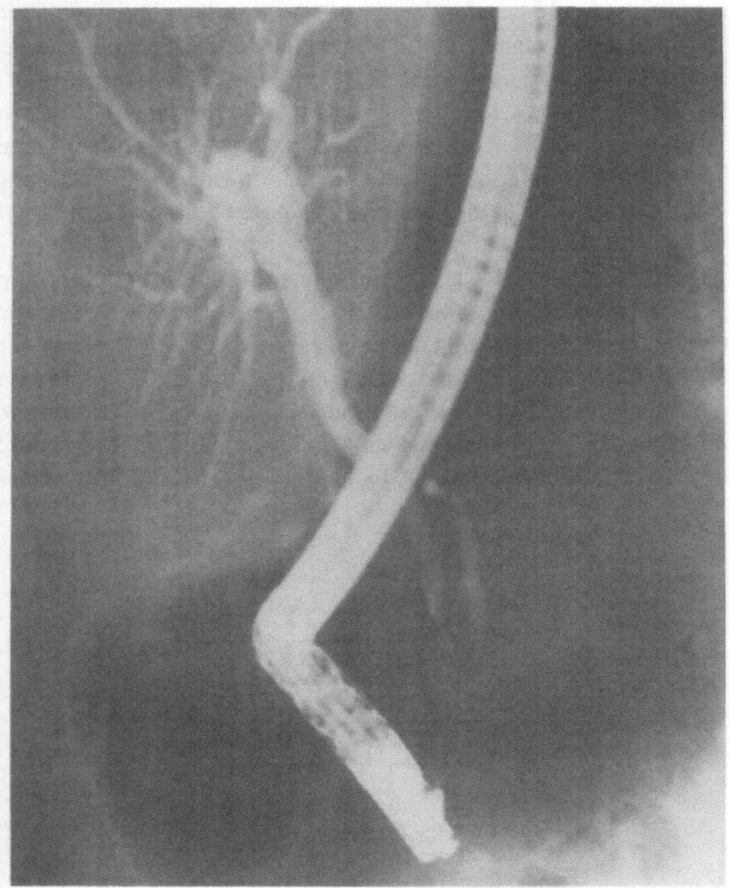

Fig. 1. Normal ERCP with opacification of both biliary tree and pancreatic duct.

Table 4. ERCP specificity in 4936 examinations.

	Attempted	Cannulated	% Success
Pancreatic disease	1530	1484	97
Biliary disease	3406	3236	95
Single duct cannulated		628	
Both ducts cannulated		4245	86
Total		4873	98.7
Duct of intention		4288	87.9

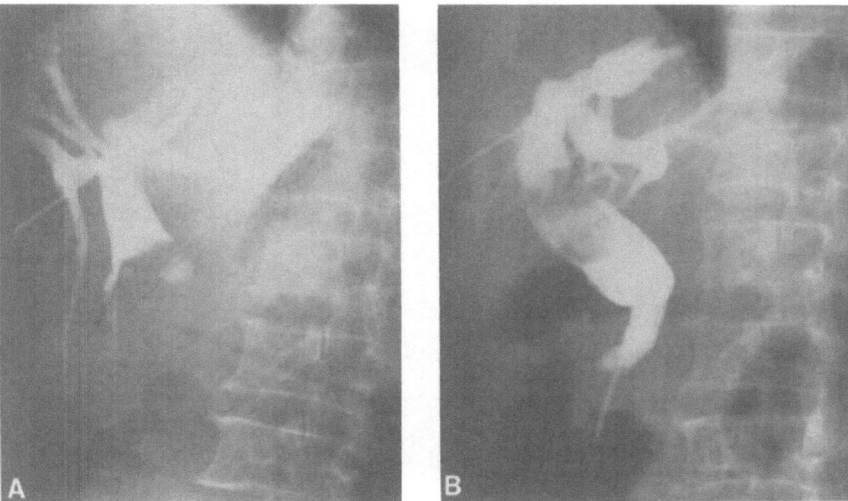

Fig. 2. A. Percutaneous cholangiogram showing dilated common hepatic duct with obstruction noted at mid common bile duct. B. ERCP clearly demonstrating distal common bile duct with large lucency noted in mid common duct which is calculus. Endoprosthesis placed for drainage and decompression prior to removal. Prosthesis seen exiting from distal common bile duct.

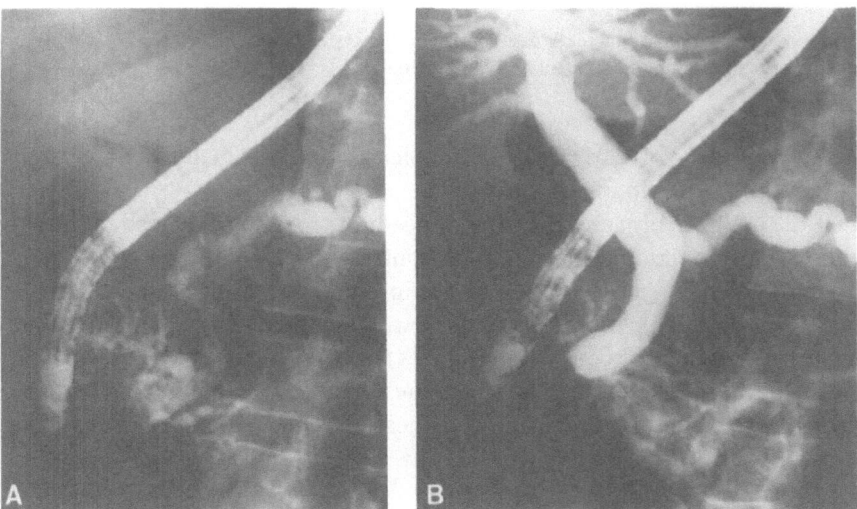

Fig. 3. A. Dilated pancreatic duct seen on ERCP. Note branching of accessory duct and uncinate process consistent with obstructive disease. B. Dilated bile duct and biliary tree in same patient. Note indentation of ampullary segment of distal duct consistent with lesion of ampulla.

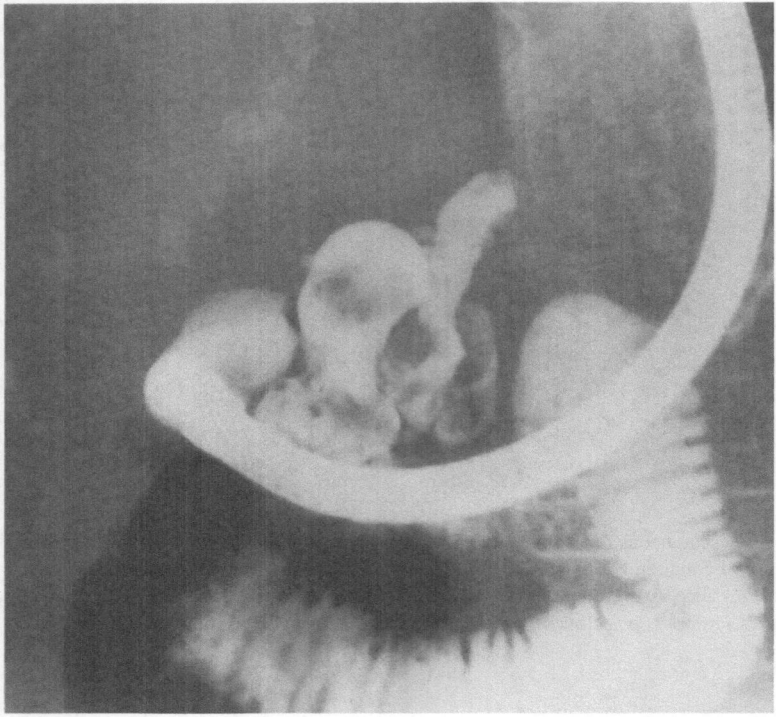

Fig. 4. Cystic dilatation of pancreatic duct consistent with cystadenoma. Note lucencies within cystic structure representing solid neoplastic components.

the success rate to nearly 98%. Examples of diagnostic cholangiopancrea-
tograms are shown in Figs. 1 through 4.

ERCP has been proven to be a safe procedure providing diagnostic accuracy
with low morbidity and mortality. In contrast to percutaneous cholangiography, ERCP is the procedure of choice in: 1) uncooperative patients, 2) patients with a coagulopathy, 3) individuals with ascites, and 4) patients in whom
sensitivity to iodinated contrast substances has been documented. In addition,
ERCP is the only nonsurgical technique which provides pancreatography
through selective cannulation and opacification of the pancreatic duct system
[3, 5, 15].

Duodenoscopic sphincterotomy [DS]

Duodenoscopic sphincterotomy [DS] became a natural extension of ERCP.
Indications for employing the technique are listed in Table 5. Gallstone (bili-

ary) pancreatitis has become firm indication for ERCP, whereas idiopathic pancreatitis is considered a contraindication for the procedure. The incorporation of ERCP into the work-up of patients with biliary pancreatitis expedites the evaluation and treatment of this life threatening condition. If the diagnosis of gallstone pancreatitis is confirmed and a stone is identified, sphincterotomy is clearly indicated.

To date, DS has been safely performed by this author in more than 2,000 patients. Table 6 illustrates the distribution of cases and the rates of success, while Table 7 identifies the significant complications associated with sphincterotomy. In all series, it has become obvious that the frequency of complications associated with sphincterotomy decreases proportionately with the experience of the endoscopist. Also of significance is that despite the increased mean age of 66 years for the patient population undergoing sphincterotomy, mortality has remained less than 0.5 percent. This is most significant, since

Table 5. Endoscopic papillotomy.

Indications
Choledocholithiasis
Cholangitis
Pancreatitis
Short stenosis or stricture
Tumor
Contraindications
Coagulopathy
Long stricture
Proximal disease

Table 6. Endoscopic papillotomy. Experience in 2079 procedures.

	Attempted	Performed	% Success
Common duct stones	1726	1690	97.9
Papillary stenosis	353	335	94.8
Total	2079	2025	97.4
Intact gall bladders	313 (15.5%)		
Age range	26–97		
Mean age	67.6		
Patients over 65	1413 (68%)		
History cholangitis	1123 (54%)		
Mean hospital stay	3.8 Days		

morbidity and mortality in surgical series of sphincterotomy and/or common duct exploration in this same population is considerably higher [19, 20].

The performance of sphincterotomy for the treatment of choledocholithiasis, especially in the patient who is status post cholecystectomy, is a primary indication for DS. However, controversy surrounds the performance of sphincterotomy in patients with gall bladders *in situ*. In my opinion, the performance of sphincterotomy and removal of common duct stones in patients with gall gladder *in situ* is advantageous, reducing operative morbidity and mortality and speeding recovery. This view is shared by many, and data supporting this approach is now available [21, 22].

Also, it is my opinion that cholangiography should be performed in patients presenting with cholestasis and/or jaundice and coexisting cholelithiasis prior to surgical exploration. Thus, if stones are found in the common bile duct, they can be removed after performance of a sphincterotomy and choledocholithotomy. The patient can subsequently undergo elective cholecystectomy either immediately after the endoscopic procedure or electively at a later date. This approach is not only safe and prudent but cost-effective. In addition, cholangiography preoperatively in this clinical situation is advantageous to the surgeon. Preoperative cholangiography has been shown to be more accurate in determining the presence of common duct stones than intra-operative cholangiography. Adoption of this approach thus enhances patient care.

Gallstone pancreatitis

Patients presenting with acute pancreatitis and gallstone disease should be carefully observed, monitored and stabilized. If the patient's clinical condition deteriorates, he/she should undergo immediate ERCP and sphincterotomy to relieve obstruction [23, 24]. Gallstone pancreatitis is caused by a stone impact-

Table 7. Complications of endoscopic papillotomy (N = 2025).

	No.	%
Bleeding*	31	
Cholangitis, fever	22	5.5
Pancreatitis	45	
Perforation, pain	13	
Emergency surgery	13	0.64
Deaths	2	0.099
*Transfusions	11	

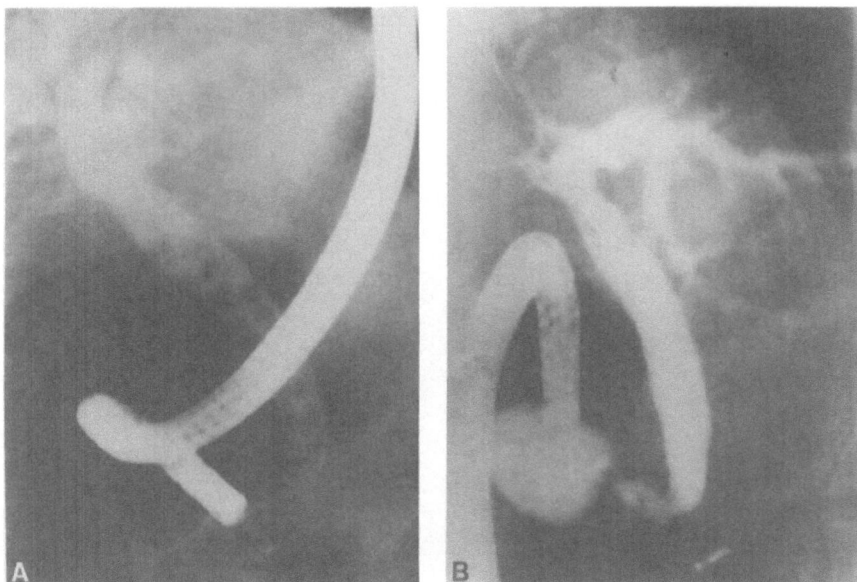

Fig. 5. A. ERCP demonstrating multiple stones in common bile duct. B. Post sphincterotomy ERCP after stones extracted.

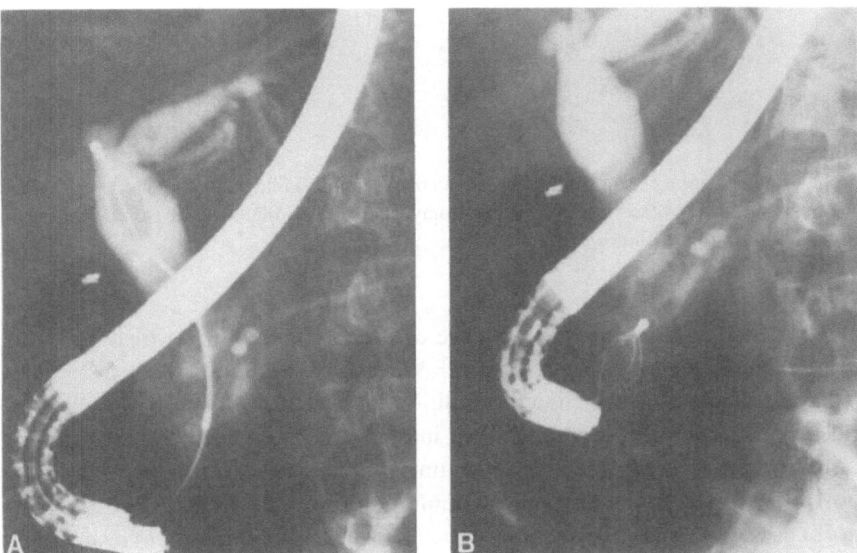

Fig. 6. A. ERCP demonstrating lucency in common hepatic duct. Basket has entrapped stone. B. Stone entrapped in basket being removed from common bile duct through sphincterotomy.

66

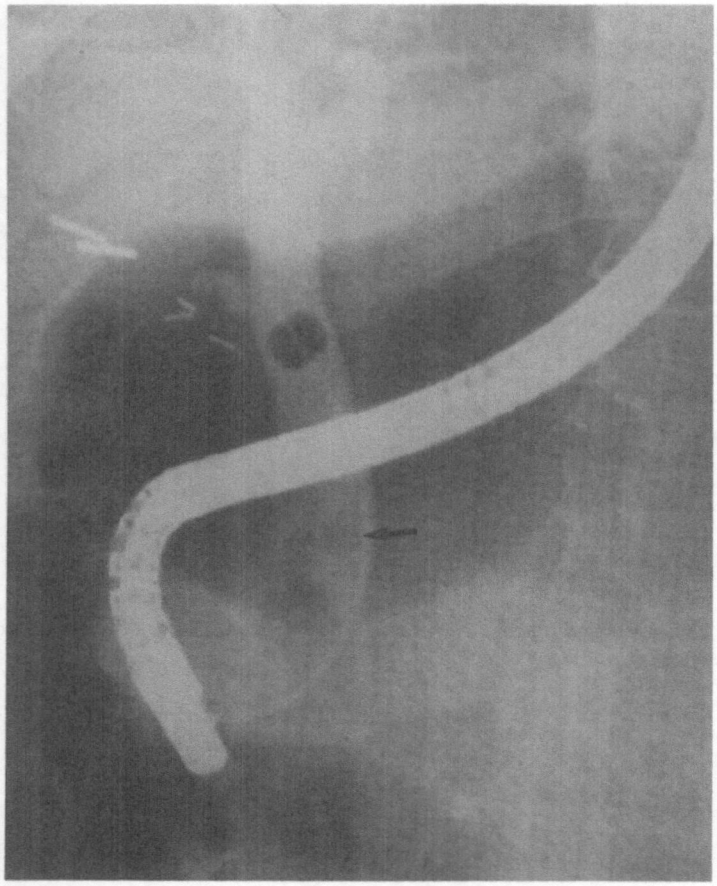

Fig. 7. Cholangiogram demonstrating lucency in distal common bile duct (arrow). An occlusion balloon has been advanced through sphincterotomy, and balloon inflated above stone. Withdrawal of balloon into duodenum will remove stone.

ing in the ampulla and obstructing the common channel into which both the bile duct and pancreatic duct drain [25]. When the obstructing stone dislodges, pancreatitis subsides, the clinical condition improves, and urgent intervention can be postponed. Following clinical improvement, subsequent cholangiography should be performed to determine the presence or absence of stones. Obviously, if a stone is present, it should be removed by sphincterotomy. In most cases, gallstone pancreatitis is transient, usually occurring as a single incident, and may not require immediate or urgent intervention. Following resolution of the pancreatitis and improvement of the patient's clinical condition, cholangiography should be performed, Figures 5 through 8 are cholangio-

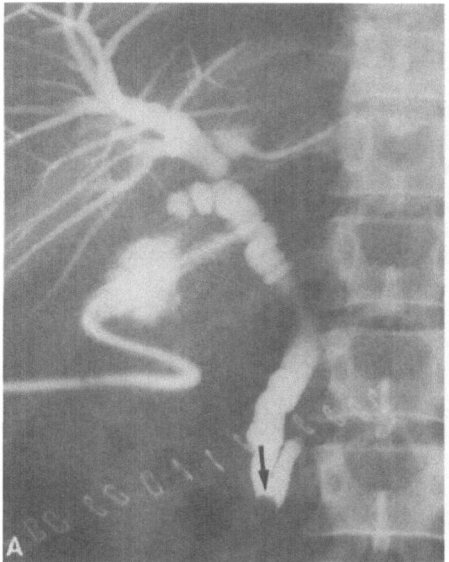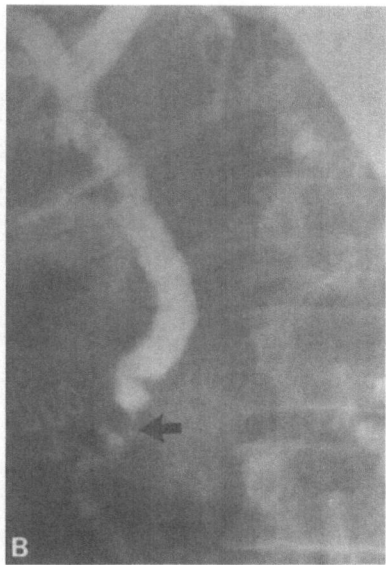

Fig. 8. A. T-tube cholangiogram showing stone in distal common bile duct obstructing flow of contrast. Reflux of contrast into pancreatic duct is seen. B. Post sphincterotomy cholangiogram which demonstrates flow of contrast into duodenum. Stone has been removed.

grams demonstrating common duct stones and the endoscopic extraction techniques. Figure 8 is an example of gallstone pancreatitis demonstrating a common channel.

Lithotripsy

The development of baskets strong enough to perform mechanical lithotripsy or stone crushing has enabled the endoscopist to remove most retained stones [26–28]. Our experience with mechanical lithotripsy is extensive, with an overall success rate of 73% for fracturing large stones. In my experience, the larger baskets, which are introduced through a large-channel endoscope, are more effective in entrapping the stones and subsequently crushing them (Fig. 9). Another technique for fracturing stones, Electrohydraulic Lithotripsy [EHL], has recently become available and is currently under evaluation (Fig. 10) [28–29]. EHL requires the insertion of a bipolar electrical probe into the bile duct which discharges a shock-wave directed against a large stone, fragmenting it. Although our experience is still limited in this collaborative experience, EHL appears to be 90% effective. The technique requires that the special probe be near to or in contact with the stone. The bile duct must be filled with liq-

68

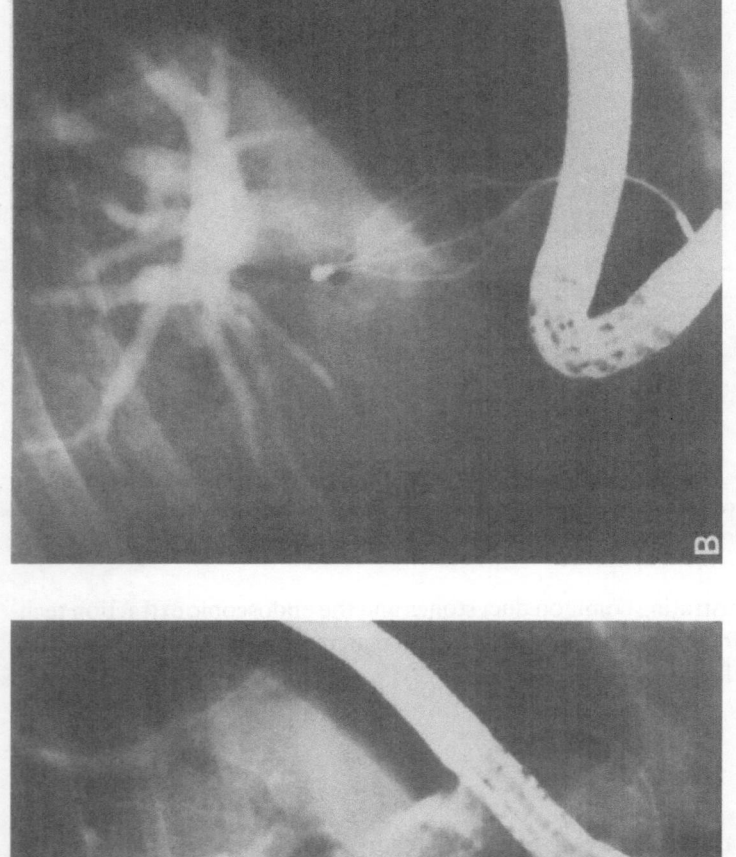

Fig. 9. Sequential mechanical lithotripsy. A. Large filling defect in mid common bile duct seen on ERCP. B. Large lithotripter basket entrapping stone.

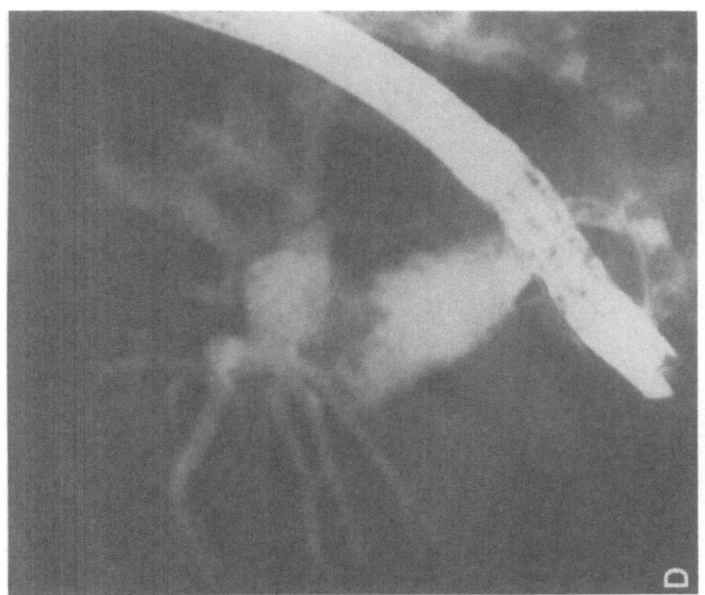

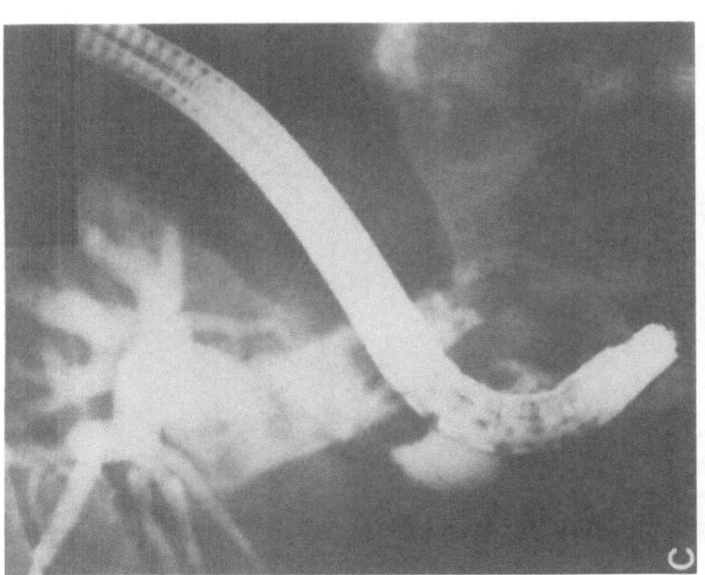

Fig. 9. C. Sequential mechanical lithotripsy. Stone fragments remaining in duct after lithotripsy. D. Large fragments removed from duct through sphincterotomy. Smaller particles should pass spontaneously through sphincterotomy.

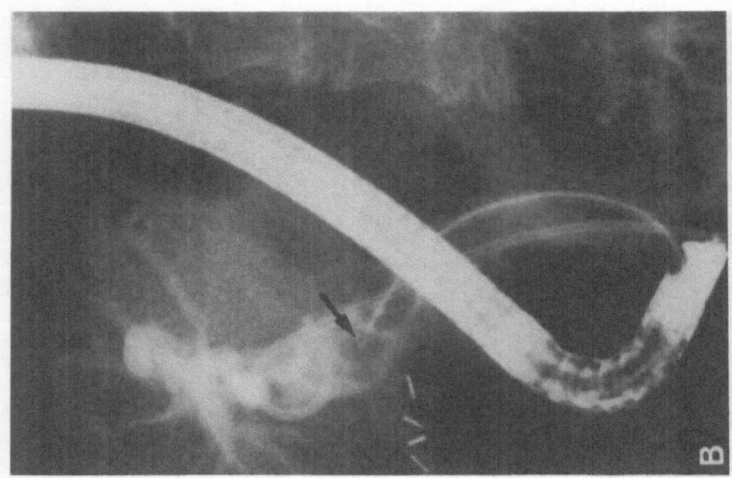

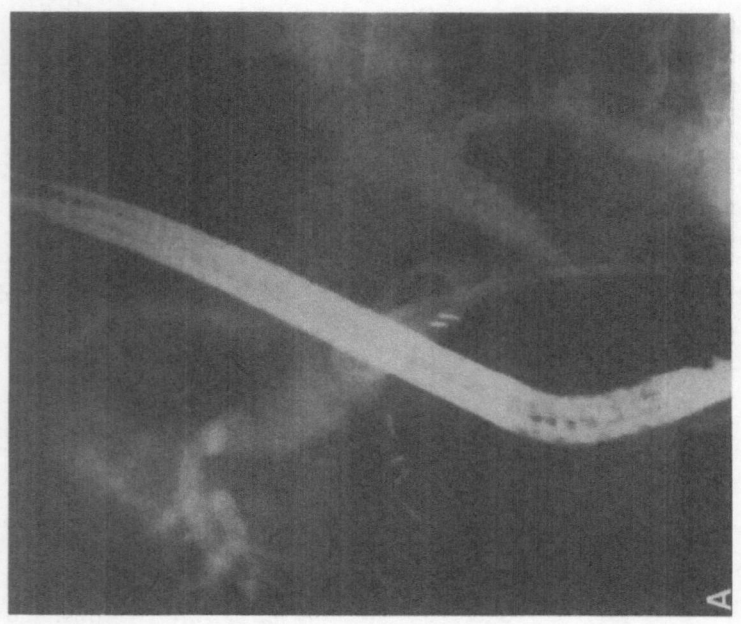

Fig. 10. A. Cholangiogram showing lucency and prosthesis which was placed earlier to prevent stone impaction. B. Electrohydraulic lithotripter probe contained in balloon (arrows) firing charge and fragmenting stone.

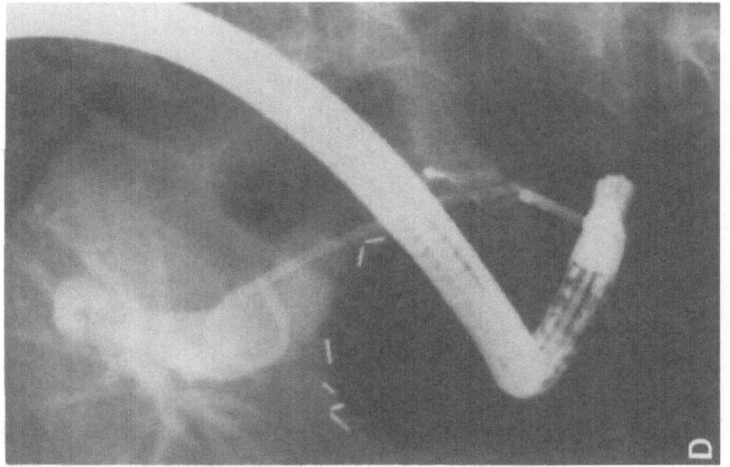

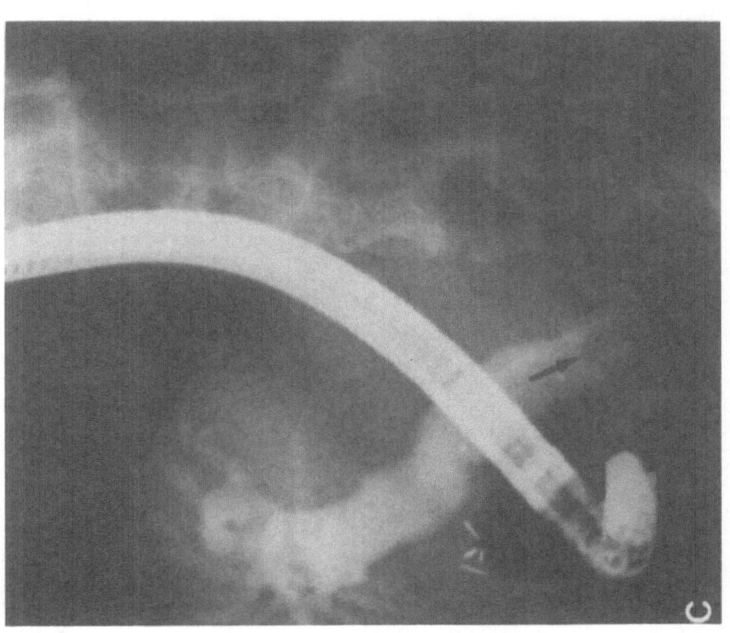

Fig. 10. C. No obvious lucencies in common duct except for fragment in distal duct (arrow). D. Basket with entrapped stone fragment being removed.

72

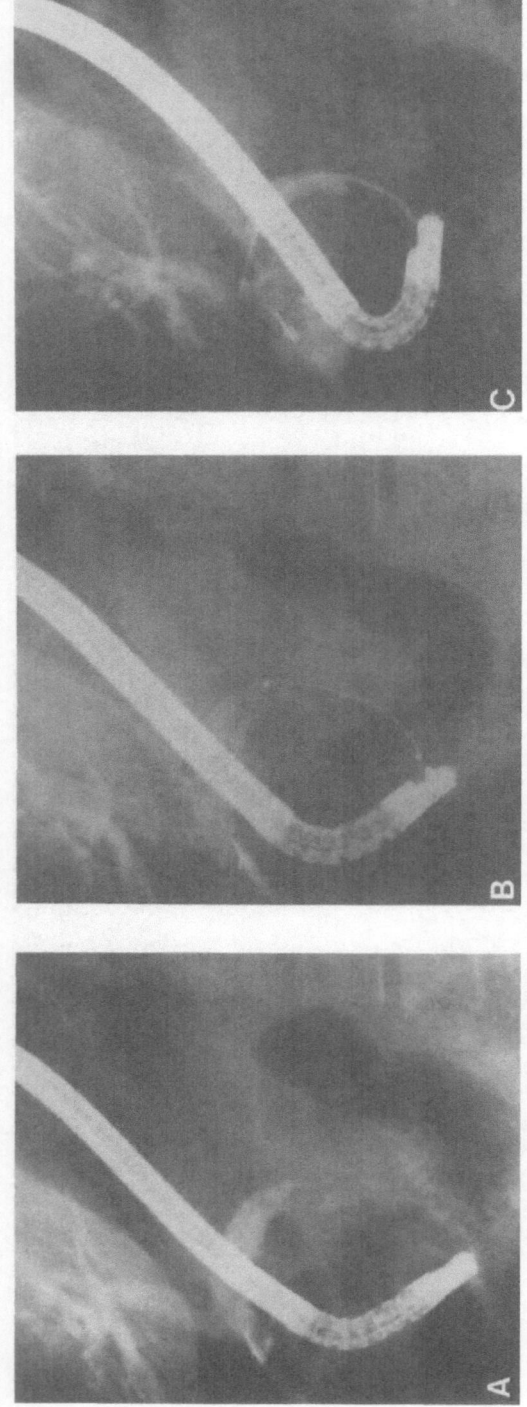

Fig. 11. A. 1 cm stone seen in distal common bile duct on ERCP cholangiogram. B. Balloon catheter inserted into duct over guide wire. Opaque markers delineate length and position of balloon. C. Electrohydraulic probe passed through dilated sphincter and positioned near stone for discharge and fragmentation.

uid, i.e., contrast and saline, which is activated by a shock-wave produced by a bipolar charge. Basic safety is established by placing the probe within a balloon catheter maintaining its central position, thus avoiding injury to the bile duct wall when the electrohydraulic probe is discharged. In patients in whom surgery is contraindicated and the risk of performing DS is too great, EHL can be utilized safely. Figure 11 illustrates such a case. This patient, who had a T-tube in place and in whom DS could not be performed, underwent balloon dilatation of the sphincter to facilitate introduction of the EHL probe. Following dilatation of the sphincter, the electrohydraulic probe was introduced, and the stones were fragmented and removed. This newer approach to the management of primary or retained common bile duct gallstones strengthens the position of endoscopy in the management of biliary tract disease.

Percutaneous endoscopic extraction of retained stones [PEERS]

The technique utilizing a choledochoscope which is introduced percutaneously through a T-tube tract is a safer alternative to the catheter technique [30–31]. The endoscope is advanced through a mature T-tube tract similarly to the catheter technique but accomplishes both a direct examination and extraction of common bile duct stones. The percutaneous basket extraction technique, as described by Burhenne and others, is successful and safe but requires prolonged exposure to fluoroscopy [32, 33]. The endoscopic technique (Fig. 12) requires less exposure to radiation because the endoscope is used for direct visualization and entrapment of stones reducing fluoroscopy requirements. PEERS is successful in extracting medium-sized stones and, because of the reduced fluoroscopy exposure, I recommend it in lieu of the percutaneous approach. In addition, biopsies can be obtained under direct visualization (Fig. 13) if mucosal lesions are identified.

If a flexible choledochoscope is not available, the percutaneous basket extraction technique is certainly an alternative. However, if neither technique is available or if conditions predicate alternative therapy, I prefer to perform a sphincterotomy and extract the stones from below, even in a patient with a T-tube in place. My reasoning for this more aggressive approach is based on the fact that if the sphincter is left intact after percutaneous stone manipulation, retained particles not retrieved by the extraction technique can and often produce biliary tract symptoms, i.e., cholangitis and cholestasis.

74

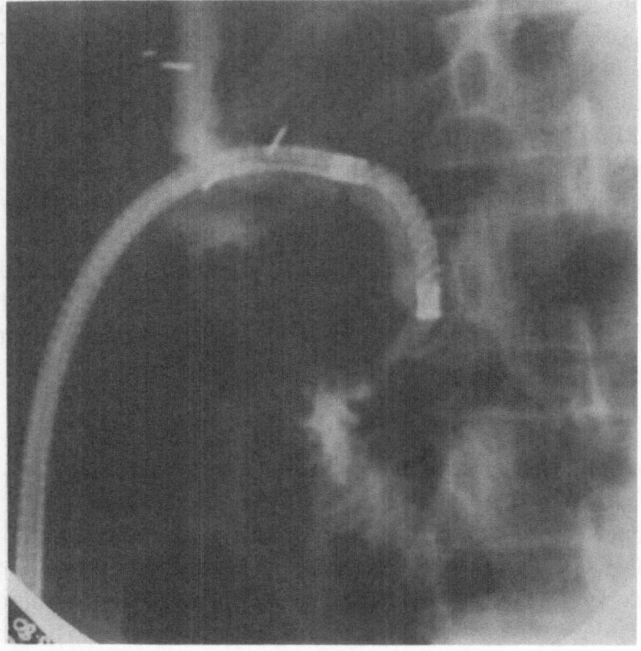

Fig. 12. Flexible choledocoscope introduced through mature T-tube tract into distal common bile duct.

Peroral choledochoscopy

Some patients who have undergone choledochoduodenostomy may present with recurrent episodes of cholangitis, jaundice, pancreatitis or cholestatis: The Sump Syndrome [34, 35]. To elucidate the cause of symptoms and to rule out the presence of stones, digestive particles or air in the biliary tree, I use a standard endoscope for direct entry and examination of the bile duct through the patent enterostomy [36]. In some patients, reflux of gastrointestinal contents into the common bile duct can and frequently does occur. In addition, air is usually present further confusing the picture. To be more accurate in establishing a diagnosis and confirming the presence of filling defects in the sump of a choledochoduodenostomy, I examine the bile duct directly by employing a standard forward-viewing endoscope which is advanced directly through the enterostomy. After entering the bile duct, filling defects can be positively ruled in or out (Figs. 14, 15). Air bubbles are identified as such, and stones or other filling defects are identified by their usual appearance. If stones are present, they can be extracted through the enterostomy, or, the sump can be drained by performing a DS. If an abnormal mucosal structure is present, a biopsy can be obtained under direct vision using this instrument.

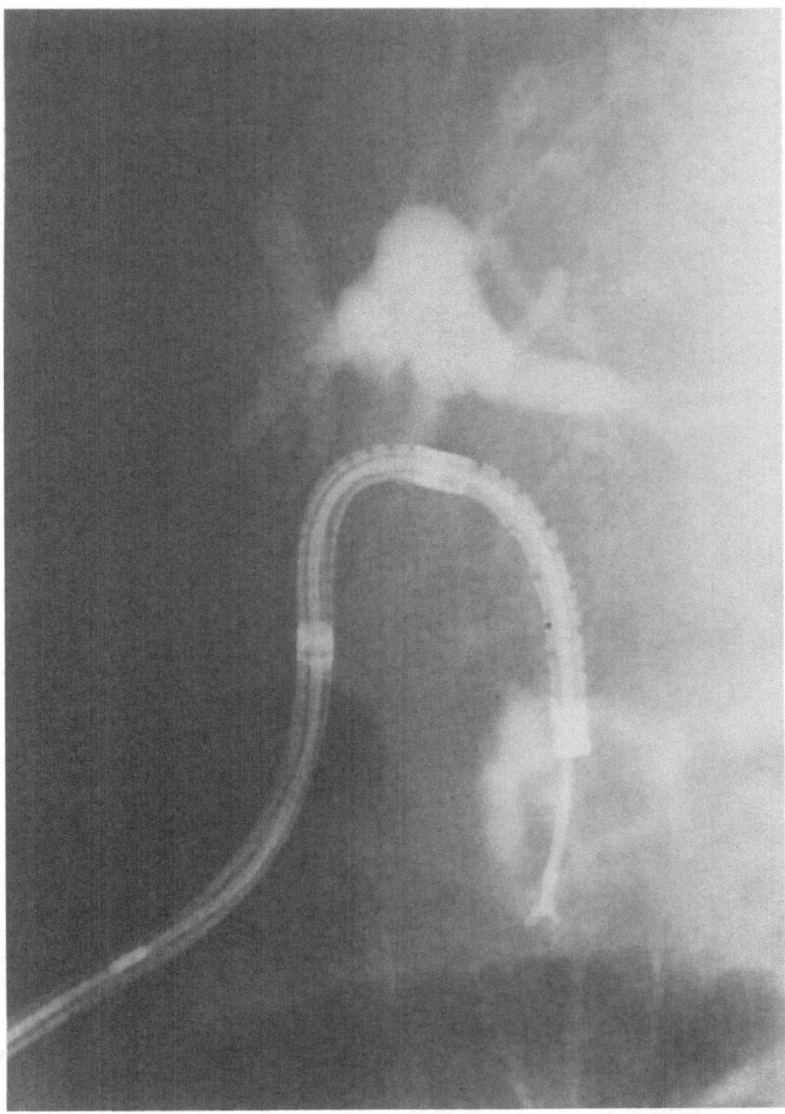

Fig. 13. Flexible choledochoscope advanced through T-tube tract into distal common bile duct. Biopsy forcep is seen extending from endoscope, blades open for biopsy.

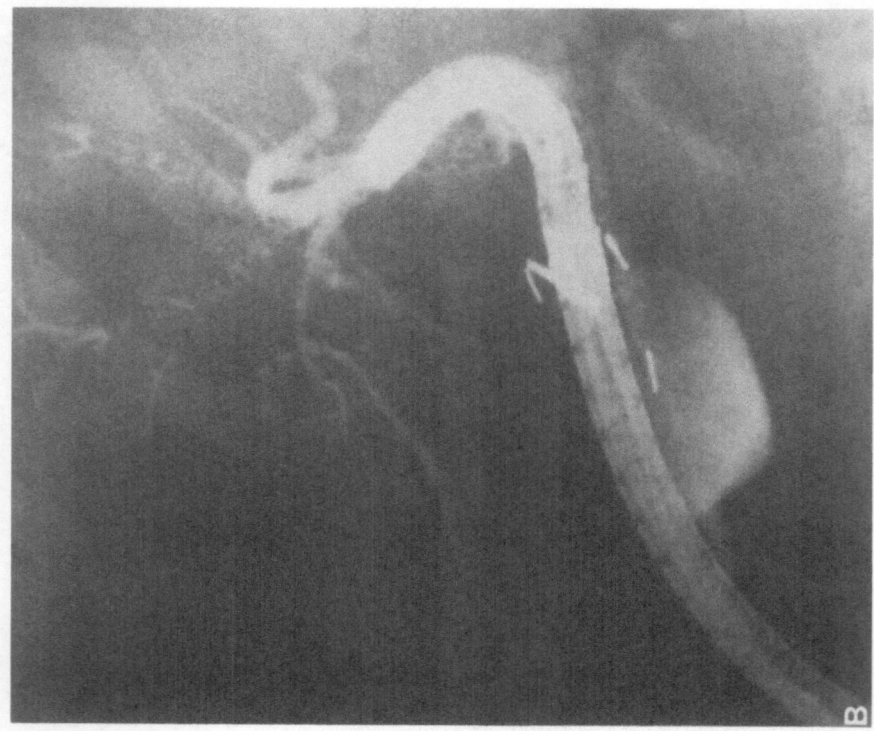

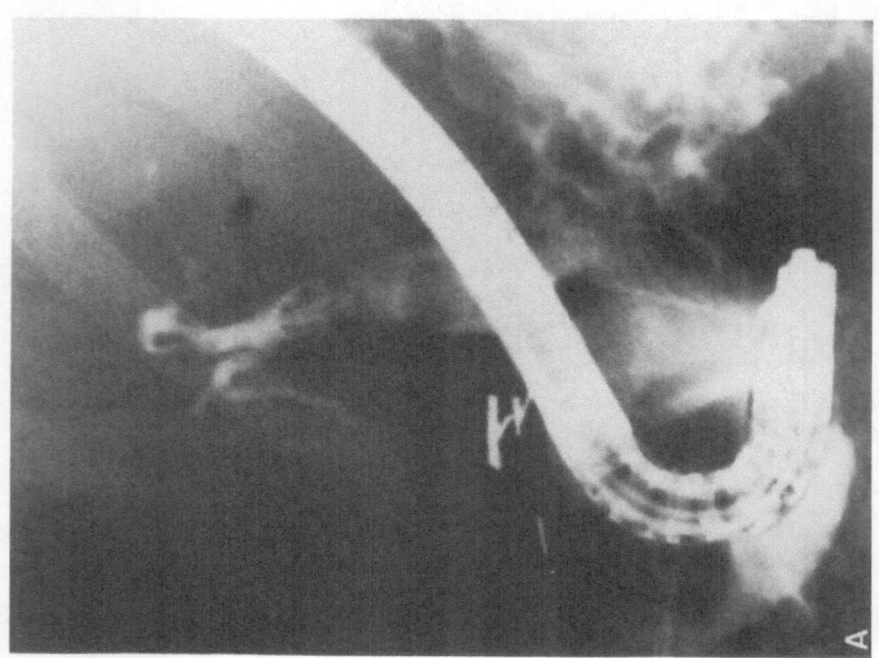

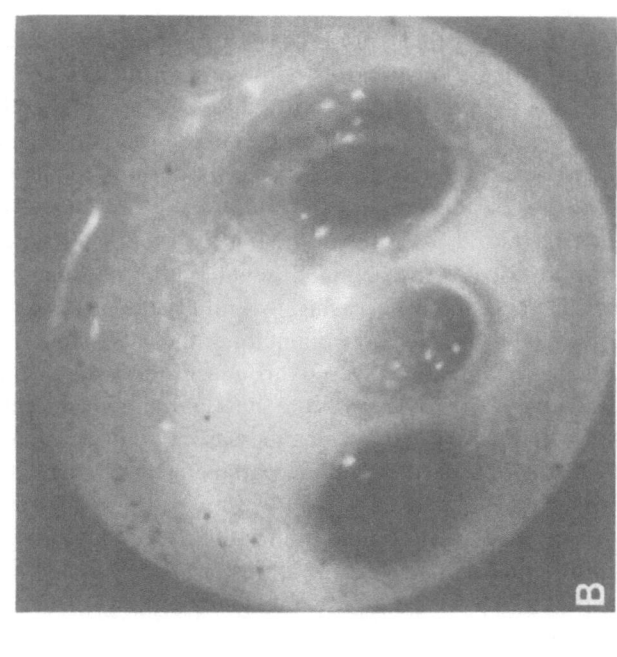

Fig. 14. A. Cholangiogram obtained at ERCP in patient with choledochoduodenostomy. Note multiple filling defects. B. Standard forward viewing endoscope advanced through choledochoduodenostomy into common hepatic duct.

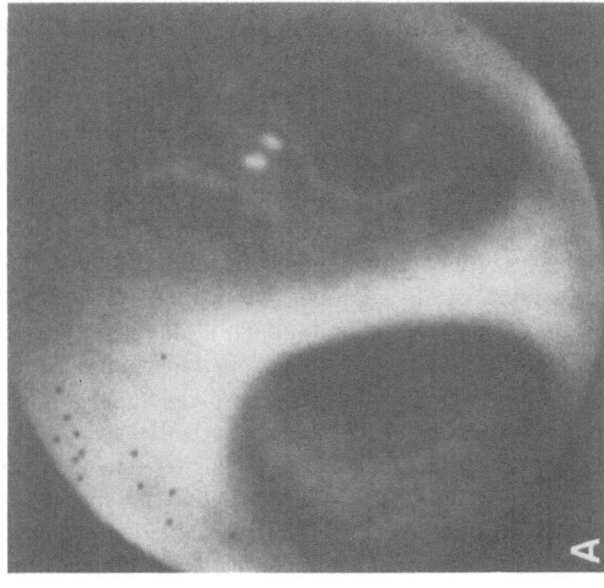

Fig. 15. A. Bifurcation of hepatic ducts seen with endoscope passed through choledochoduodenostomy. B. Endoscopic view of bifurcations of right hepatic duct.

Endoscopic hydrostatic dilatation [EHD]
(Balloon Cholangioplasty – Pancreaticoplasty)

Catheters with polyethylene balloons have been successfully used in the management and treatment of strictures of the biliary tree and pancreas [37–39]. Since the introduction of Gruntzig-type balloon catheters used for cardiovascular purposes, modifications have been made so that this technology can be utilized endoscopically. EHD has been successfully used to dilate strictures occurring at the site of a surgical choledochoduodenostomy as well as in the treatment of other acquired strictures of the biliary tree, i.e., strictures occurring secondary to injuries of the common hepatic and bile ducts. Successful dilatation has been accomplished using 4–12 mm balloons. The size of the balloon catheter is determined by the diameter of the endoscope channel. Larger balloons, i.e., 8–12 mm, are delivered through an endoscope which has a channel size of 4.2 mm. Early results indicate that this method is effective in dilating strictures of both the biliary tree and pancreas. In addition, this technique has been applied to strictures occurring in patients with other biliary tract disorders, i.e., sclerosing cholangitis (Fig. 16). In sclerosing cholangitis, dilatation of the dominant stricture in combination with a drug regimen are gaining more support in the primary management of this disorder [40].

Patients presenting with the postcholecystectomy syndrome, biliary dyskinesia or dysfunction of the sphincter of Oddi, have been treated with dilatation of this sphincter. The balloon catheters are advanced over guide wires and positioned in the ampulla, after which dilatation is carried out generating pressures of 4 to 6 atmospheres which are held for 30 seconds. This procedure is repeated 2 to 3 times. Most patients experience relief of symptoms following the dilatation, and nearly 60% experienced complete relief with no recurrences (Table 8). The remainder, 40% presented with recurrent symptoms 3 to 29 weeks later (mean = 22 weeks), although their symptoms were initially relieved after the dilatation procedure. At later presentation, a DS was performed. Eighty-five percent of those patients who underwent the second procedure experienced total relief of symptoms (follow-up of 39 months).

The most promising application for balloon-dilatation technology has been for the treatment of benign strictures of the biliary tree. Some patients who have sustained injury to the biliary tree, usually due to surgical trauma, may subsequently develop strictures of the bile ducts. Because these patients usually experienced complicated post-surgical courses, they were considered poor candidates for repeat surgery. Thus, alternative therapy, i.e., dilatation, has been applied in this situation (Fig. 17). In my experience, I have found that an inflammatory stricture is usually more difficult to negotiate with a catheter and guide wire than a malignant one because of the composition of the fibrous tissues. My rate of success in treating all benign strictures exceeds 85%. The suggestion that stenosis may recur following dilatation has prompted me to provide more permanent measures which include placing a large-caliber prosthesis through the dilated stricture to maintain the integrity of the lumen of the bile duct. 10 Fr and 12 Fr prostheses have been successfully placed in patients whose bile duct strictures have been dilated and follow-up surveys indicate that good results have been achieved for more than one year before an exchange becomes necessary. Prostheses have remained functional for a mean of 13 months, range, 3 months to 28 months. This approach to the management of benign strictures is gaining acceptance and other centers are currently utilizing this new technology with increasing success.

Transpapillary endoscopic endoprostheses

Nonsurgical decompression techniques for biliary obstruction has rapidly developed and gained general acceptance in the past six years [41–43]. Percutaneous insertion of internal-external drainage catheters has been used to provide palliation for both malignant and benign strictures affecting the biliary tree. These techniques are performed routinely when endoscopic treatment is unavailable or has failed. However, because more severe complications including cholangitis, sepsis, bleeding, and pneumothorax have occurred with long term management using external drains, the endoscopic approach is favored [44].

Table 8. Endoscopic hydrostatic dilatation (EHD) (N = 136).

Bile duct strictures:	36
Hepatic duct:	21
Bile duct:	15
Papillary stenosis/dyskinesia:	84
Pancreatic duct strictures:	16
Results	
Biliary tree	
Improved:	86 (72%)
Pancreatic ducts	
Improved:	10 (63%)
Complications (N = 39)	
Fever	16
Septicemia	1
Pancreatitis	22 (18%)
Mortality	0
Surgery	0

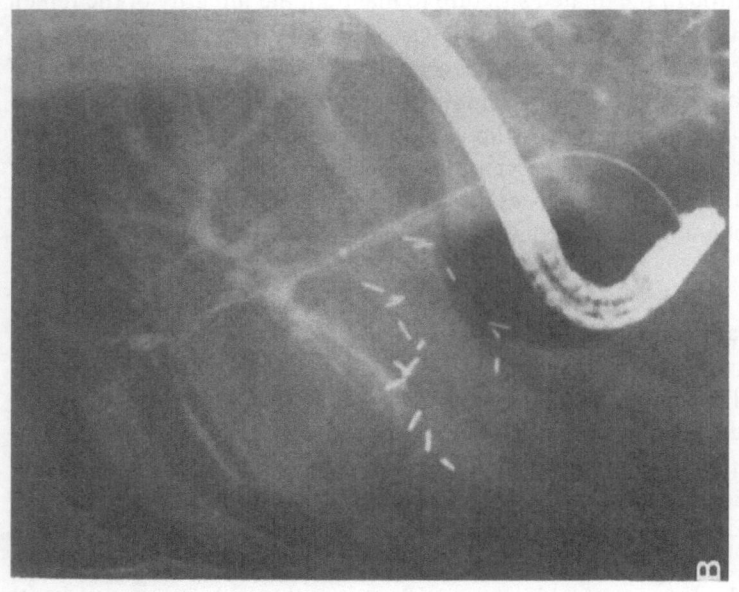

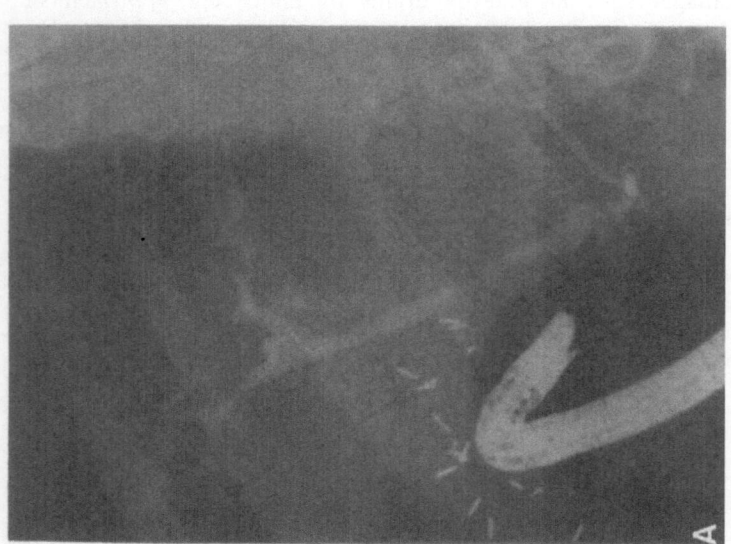

Fig. 16. A. Cholangiogram showing sclerosing cholangitis with dominant stricture of bile duct.
B. Balloon catheter advanced over guide wire.

81

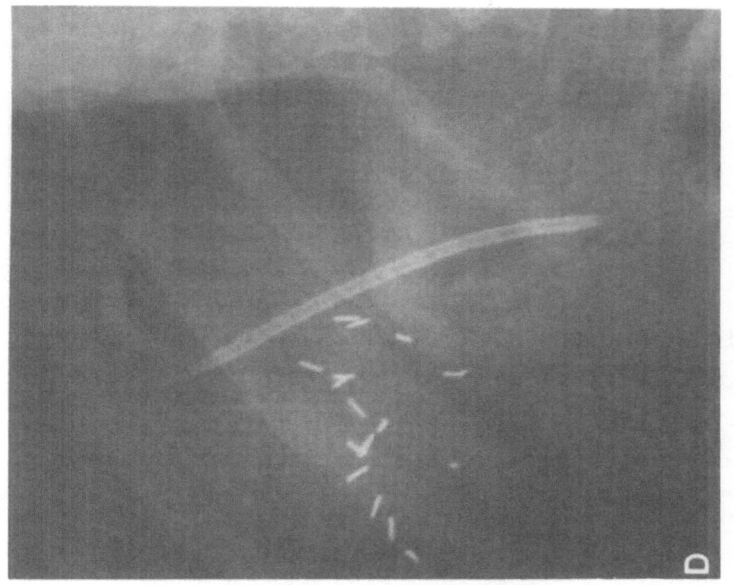

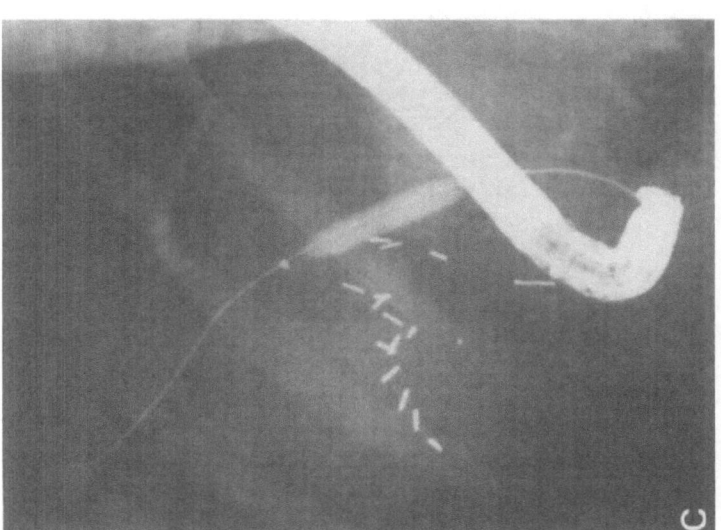

Fig. 16. C. Fully inflated balloon dilating strictures of bile duct. D. Large caliber prosthesis placed through strictures to maintain luminal integrity.

82

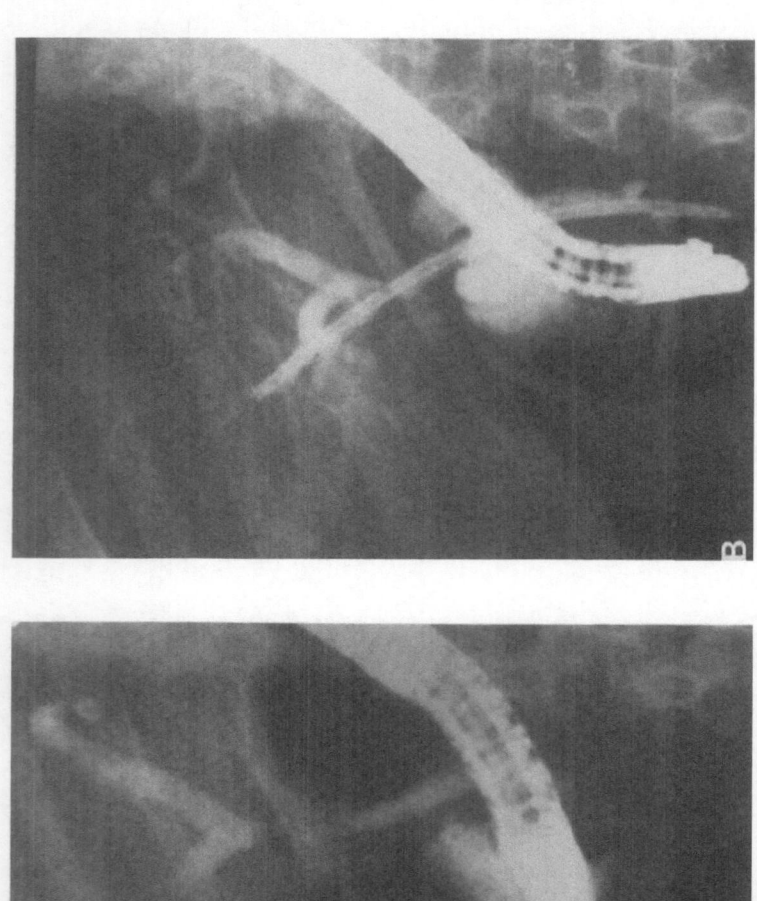

Fig. 17. A. Acquired stricture common hepatic duct with moderate proximal dilatation. Patient experienced recurrent episodes of cholangitis. B. Large prosthesis placed through stricture into right hepatic duct.

83

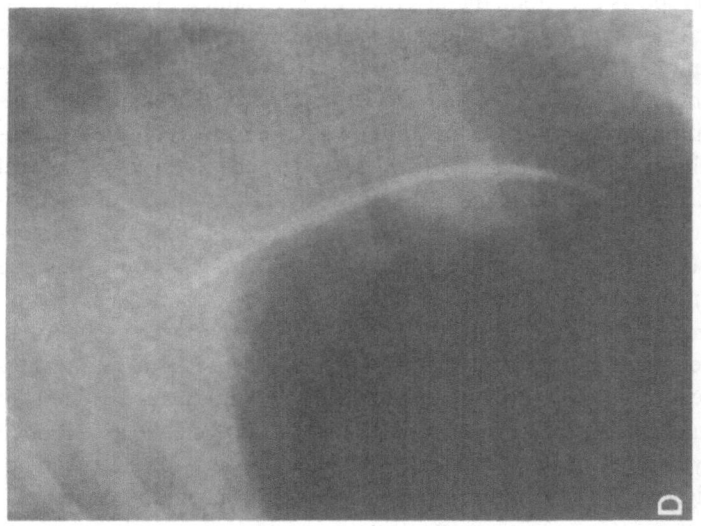

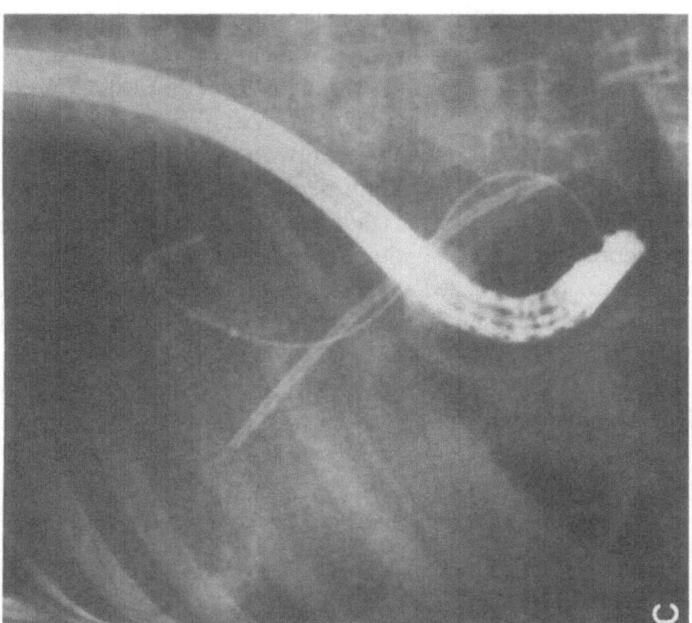

Fig. 17. C. With prosthesis in right hepatic duct, guide wire advanced into left hepatic duct, balloon dilatation carried out. D. Prostheses placed into both right and left hepatic ducts. Patient asymptomatic 15 months with normal chemistries.

Endoscopic decompression techniques using transpapillary duodenal drains began to develop shortly after the radiologic techniques were available [12–16]. Initial reports described the insertion of 5 Fr diameter prostheses and nasobiliary drains which were the largest that could be inserted because of channel restrictions of the endoscopes. However, these drains did provide decompression, but occlusion accompanied by recurrent jaundice and cholangitis occurred within three months. More effective drainage was provided by inserting more than one small drain. However, despite the presence of several small drains, occlusion still occurred within three to four months. Newer endoscopes with larger channel sizes which accommodated 7 Fr drains were introduced, and, subsequently, endoscopes with jumbo channels have become available permitting the insertion of prostheses as large as 10 and 12 Fr [45–48].

My experience includes the insertion of more than 600 endoprostheses of all sizes for the treatment of both benign and malignant disease. Table 9 indicates the specific locations of strictures treated with internal drainage. Strictures of the bifurcation of the bile ducts or of specific hepatic ducts can be approached endoscopically. However, the diameter of the prosthesis may be restricted because of the rigidity of the stricture in these locations. Secondary cholangitis usually occurs more frequently in patients with proximal lesions than in those with strictures of the common bile duct. A bifurcation tumor can be treated with: 1) one large prosthesis, which has been shown to provide drainage for both duct systems, or 2) placement of several prostheses which are selectively placed into each hepatic system. Figures 18 through 20 demonstrate different types of high grade strictures and illustrate the use of endoprostheses.

Endoscopic and/or transhepatic prostheses provide excellent alternative methods for palliation in patients with unresectable lesions [47–50]. Adjunctive chemotherapy or radiotherapy, if indicated, may be utilized during the course of decompression since the patient's clinical condition usually improves after the implementation of decompression therapy. Should adjunctive therapy not be included in the regimen, the patient is managed with palliation provided by endoprostheses.

Occlusion rates of prostheses are directly proportional to the internal diameter of the tubing. A smaller diameter prosthesis will obviously occlude earlier

Table 9. Distribution and location of obstructive biliary lesions.

Proximal hepatic duct – bifurcation		87
Distal bile duct		369
Pancreas	331	
Periampullary	38	
Ampulla of vater		17
Total		473

than a larger one. Data exists which indicates that a bacterial film forms on the internal surface of the prosthesis providing a surface on which debris and sludge may accumulate [51]. This evidence appears to be the leading explanation for the cause of occlusion. To date, no treatment is effective to prevent occlusion. In our institution, prophylactic antibiotics are usually begun before the insertion of a prosthesis, but there is no evidence that this prevents the formation of the microscopic bacterial film. Chenodeoxycholic acid has also been used in an attempt to reduce lithogenicity of bile and subsequent occlusion; however, occlusion is not attributed to cholesterol precipitation and stone formation. Thus, this latter form of prophylaxis has also been ineffective. A choloretic agent to increase the flow of bile may be tenable as a form of therapy to prevent early prosthetic occlusion. The logic behind this is that the increased flow of bile would prevent stasis, aggregation and occlusion.

The type of material used in making a prosthesis does not appear to affect occlusion rates. However, as reported in studies in which flow rates were measured *in vitro,* catheter configuration does affect flow rates and patency [52]. The fact that a straight prosthesis remains patent longer than one which has a pigtail or 'C' configuration or is tightly tapered has been supported by these studies. The reason for this, apparently, is that in forming a pigtail or 'C' or when tapering a catheter, the lumen of the catheter is restricted, thus reducing flow rate. Because the flow rate has been reduced in these altered catheters, occlusion occurs earlier. Therefore, a large-caliber, straight, 12Fr, prosthesis should remain patent and functional for more than six months [53].

The rate of success in inserting prostheses through benign and malignant strictures is approximately 90% in all series reported. This compares favorably to the insertion rate for percutaneous prostheses and, given the lower complication rate for endoscopic prostheses, the endoscopic drains are my choice for palliation and decompression of biliary obstruction. In unresectable lesions, the ideal approach to the diagnosis and management of the patient would be, as indicated in the earlier algorithm, cholangiogram followed by decompression. Subsequent to the insertion of an endoscopic or transhepatic prosthesis, staging for metastases should be carried out. If other ancillary tests indicate that the lesion has metastasized or is too large for resection, a large prosthesis should complete the therapeutic-palliative endeavor [54].

An interesting report from Neff *et al.* indicated that, in carcinoma of the pancreas, patient survival was directly related to the reduction of bilirubin levels following preoperative drainage procedures [55]. In one group of patients in their series the serum bilirubin level returned to normal or near normal following drainage, and the 30-day mortality for that group was only 10%. A second group demonstrated less than 50% reduction in bilirubin levels following drainage, and the 30-day mortality in that group exceeded 33%. The third

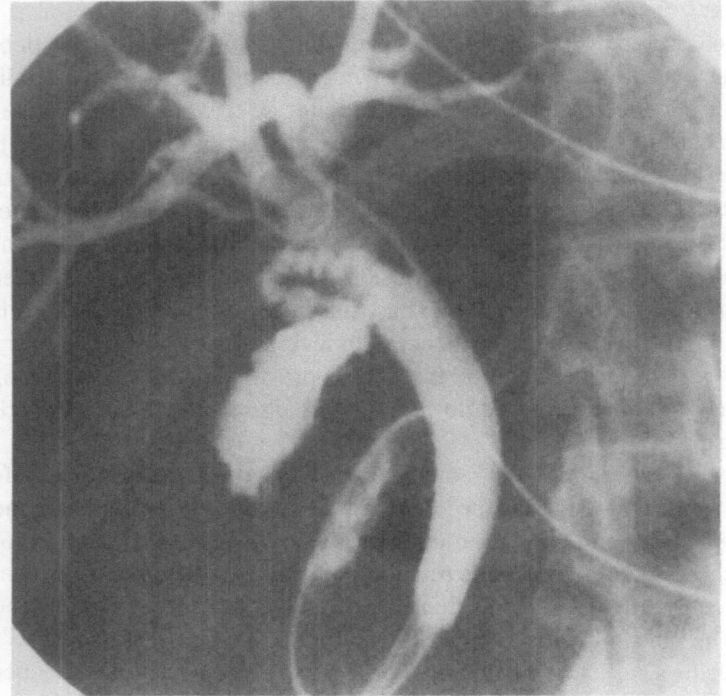

Fig. 18. Cholangiogram obtained through nasobiliary prosthesis. Note opacified pigtail in common hepatic duct.

group exhibited little or no reduction in bilirubin with preoperative drainage, and the 30-day mortality in that group was 88%. Even though preoperative decompression has been controversial, the data from Neff's study serves to separate favorable surgical groups. In general, patients with carcinoma of the pancreas who enjoyed the most favorable operative results were younger and healthier. These patients benefit from bypass surgery as opposed to alternative methods of palliation. The remaining two groups of patients in Neff's study were, in general, older, and poorly nourished. These patients revealed evidence of long-standing disease and were very ill at the time of surgery. These latter patients, then, are better candidates for nonsurgical decompression techniques since their survival is usually shorter, i.e., three to four months.

Radiotherapeutic endoprostheses

I have introduced a new approach to the treatment of patients with neoplasms of the biliary tree and pancreas which includes the insertion of Iridium 192 pro-

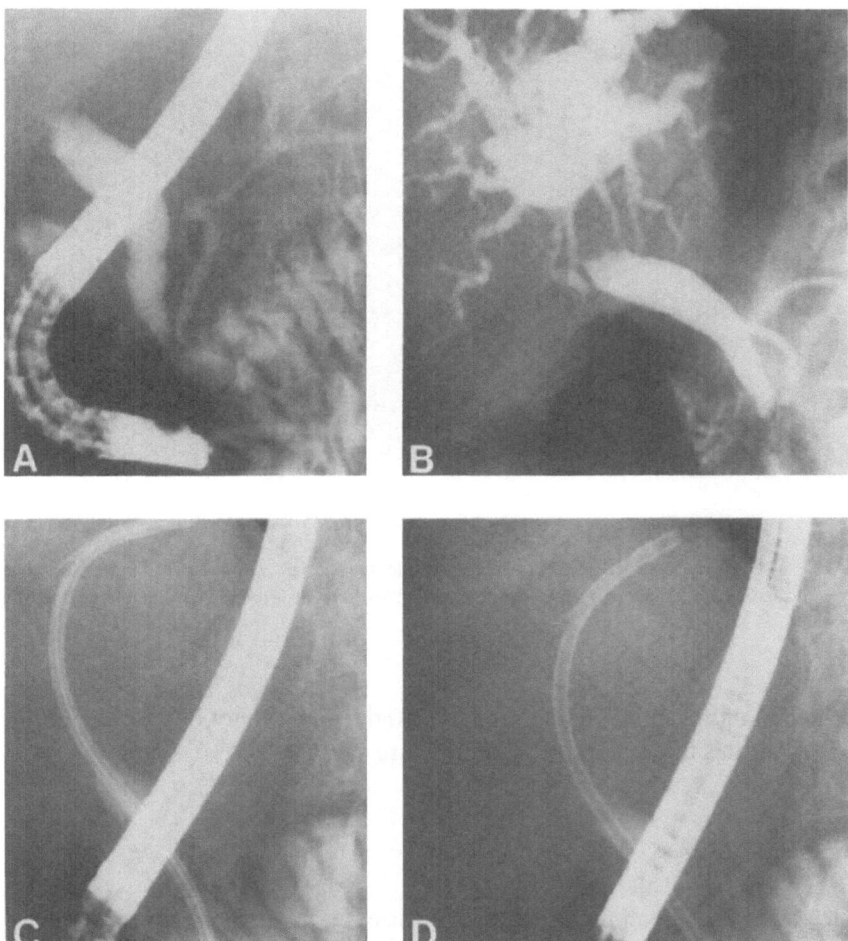

Fig. 19. A. High grade obstruction common hepatic duct noted on ERCP cholangiogram. Note normal pancreatic duct. B. High grade obstruction negotiated with guide wire, contrast injected demonstrating dilated proximal biliary tree. C. Large caliber prosthesis (12Fr) being advanced over guide wire through obstruction. D. Guide wire removed, prosthesis positioned. Note emptying of proximal biliary tree.

viding intraluminal irradiation to the tumor [56]. Once the Iridium loaded prosthesis is placed within the tumor, a maximum tumor dose of radiation can be delivered. We have had success in inserting these prostheses in patients with lesions of the bifurcation, common hepatic duct, common bile duct, pancreas and ampulla. Naturally, all of these patients were considered poor surgical risks and were specifically referred for endoscopic decompression and radiotherapy using this intraluminal technique. Since the procedure has been per-

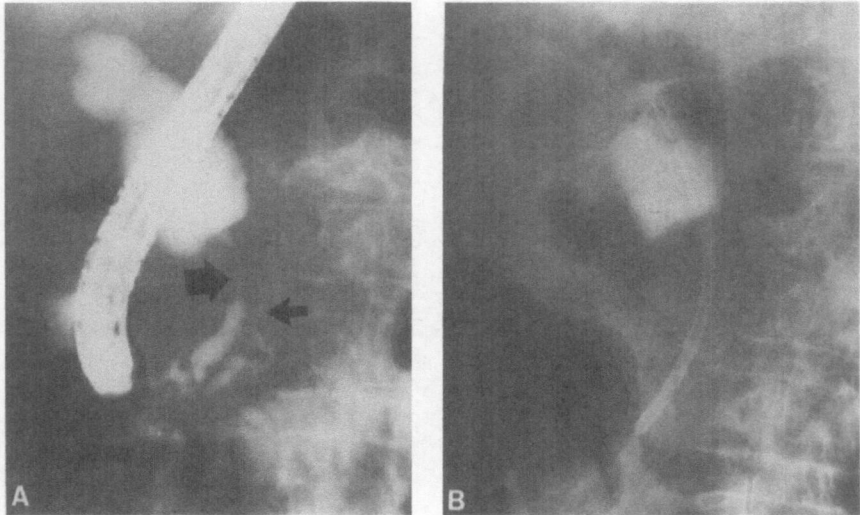

Fig. 20. A. High grade obstruction distal common bile duct (large arrow), corresponding to stricture pancreatic duct (small arrow). B. Large caliber prosthesis inserted into proximal bile duct for drainage.

formed in only a small number of patients, the data cannot be considered significant at this time, and further studies are suggested.

Pancreatic diseases

The endoscopic treatment of pancreatic diseases has gained more acceptance since early results appear favorable. I have offered treatment varying from balloon dilatation of the sphincter and/or stricture to insertion of prostheses. In both idiopathic pancreatitis and pancreatitis secondary to pancreas divisum, the results have been good using the patient as his/her own control. Good results from decompression provided by pancreatic endoprostheses have prompted me to recommend more permanent treatment, and I strongly recommend surgical treatment in patients who have good response to the drainage technique (Figs. 21, 22) [57, 58].

In summary, the endoscopic approach to the diagnosis and management of diseases of the biliary tree has made great advances since its introduction. From its origin as a pure diagnostic procedure, ERCP and its therapeutic technology has outpaced our imagination and is well on its way to exceeding all expectations. Newer technology is already under investigation. This includes: 1) the ultrasound-equipped endoscope for transmitting images from within the

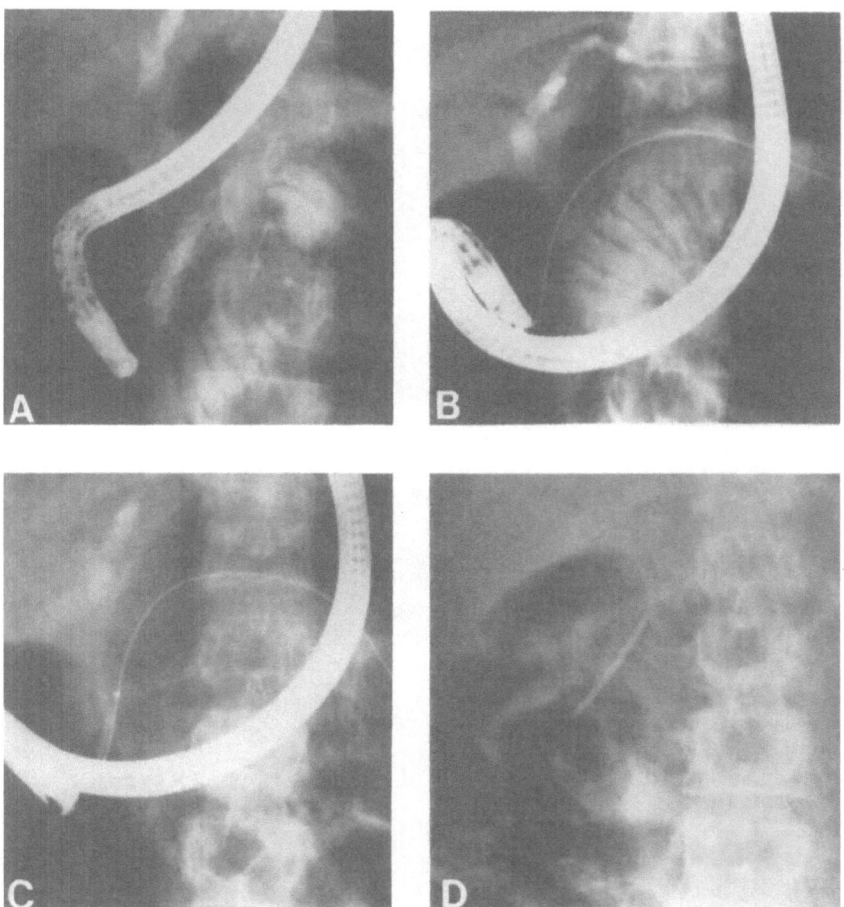

Fig. 21. A. Patient with pancreas divisum, post sphincterotomy of minor papilla draining dorsal duct in this congenital variant. Blush of contrast is due to overfilling of rudiment of ventral duct. B. Guide wire advanced through stenosed minor papilla sphincterotomy into body and tail of dorsal duct. C. Balloon dilator catheter distended in dorsal (minor) sphincter. D. Straight prosthesis placed into dorsal duct traversing stenosed sphincter.

abdominal cavity, and 2) laser therapy for the treatment of intraluminal lesions of the biliary tree and pancreas. We anxiously await the development of these advanced technologies and look forward to future technologic advances.

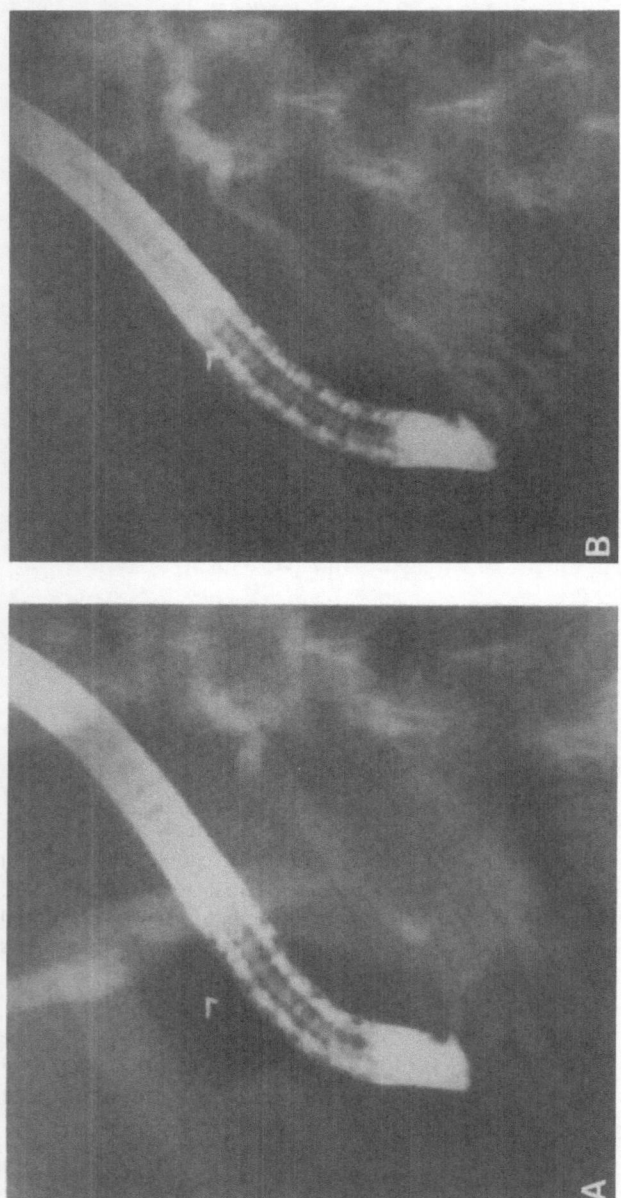

Fig. 22. A. Stricture distal common bile duct in patient with chronic pancreatitis. B. Stricture pancreatic duct in head. Proximal pancreatic duct dilated.

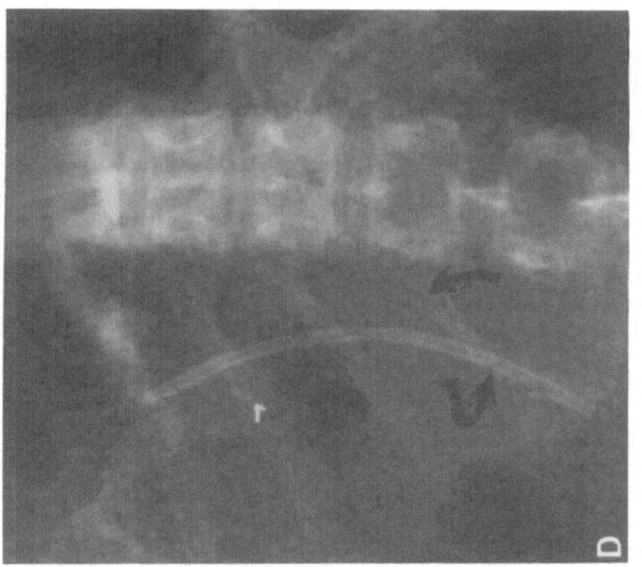

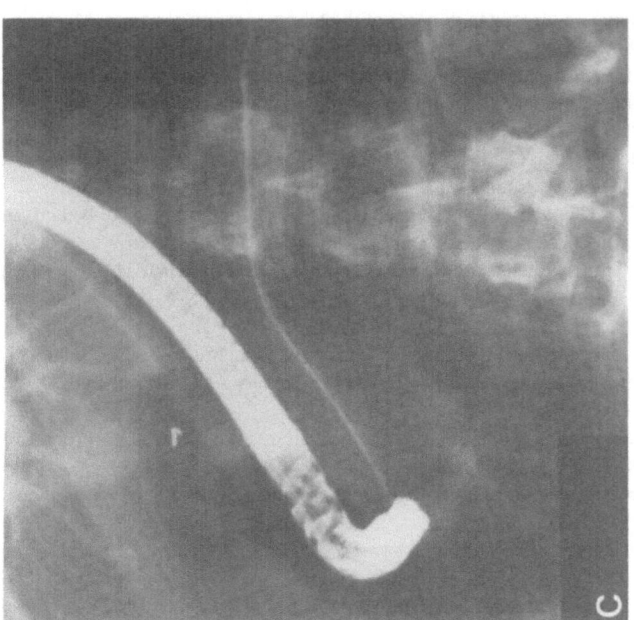

Fig. 22. C. Guide wire traversing stricture of main pancreatic duct. D. Large caliber prosthesis in bile duct for decompression. Prosthesis in pancreatic duct for decompression (arrows).

92

References

1. Oi I: Fiber duodenoscopy and endoscopic pancreatocholangiography. Gastrointest Endosc 17: 59–62, 1970
2. Cotton PB: Cannulation of the papilla of Vater by endoscopy and retrograde cholangio-pancreatography (ERCP). Gut 13: 1014–1025, 1972
3. Dickinson PB, Belsito AA, Cramer GG: Diagnostic value of endoscopic cholangiopancreatography. JAMA 225: 994–998, 1973
4. Stewart ET, Vennes JA, Geenen JE: Atlas or endoscopic retrograde cholangiopancreatography. St. Louis: CV Mosby 1977
5. Siegel JH: Endoscopic retrograde cholangiopancreatography (ERCP); present position, and papillotomy. NY State J Med 78: 583–591, 1978
6. Kawai K, Akasaka Y, Murakami K, et al.: Endoscopic sphincterotomy of the ampulla of Vater. Gastrointest Endosc 20: 148–151, 1974
7. Classen M, Safrany L: Endoscopic papillotomy and removal of gall stones. Br Med J 4: 371–374, 1975
8. Safrany L: Duodenoscopic sphincterotomy and gall stone removal. Gastroenterology 72: 338–343, 1977
9. Geenen JE, Hogan J, Shaffer RD, et al.: Endoscopic electrosurgical papillotomy and manometry in biliary tract disease. JAMA 237: 2075–2078, 1977
10. Siegel JH: ERCP update: diagnostic and therapeutic applications. Gastrointest Radiol 3: 311–318, 1978
11. Siegel JH: Endoscopic management of choledocholithiasis and papillary stenosis. Surg Gynecol Obstet 148: 747–752, 1979
12. Siegel JH: Interventional endoscopy in diseases of the biliary tree and pancreas. Mt. Sinai J Med 51: 535–542, 1984
13. Cotton PB, Burney PG, Mason RR: Transnasal bile duct catheterization after endoscopic sphincterotomy: method for biliary drainage, perfusion and sequential cholangiography. Gut 20: 285, 1979
14. Soehendra N, Reynders-Frederix V: Palliative bile duct drainage – a new endoscopic method of introducing a transpapillary drain. Endoscopy 12: 8, 1980
15. Siegel JH, Harding GT, Chateau F: Endoscopic decompression and drainage of benign and malignant biliary obstruction. Gastrointest Endosc 28: 79–82, 1982
16. Siegel JH, Yatto RP: Transduodenal endoscopic decompression of obstructed bile ducts. NY State J Med 83: 203–305, 1983
17. Cotton PB: Progress report, ERCP. Gut 18: 316–341, 1977
18. Siegel JH, Yatto RP: Approach to cholestasis – an update. Arch Int Med 142: 1877–1879, 1982
19. Siegel JH: Endoscopy and papillotomy in diseases of the biliary tract and pancreas. J Clin Gastroenterol 2: 337–347, 1980
20. Siegel JH: Endoscopic papillotomy in the treatment of biliary tract disease: 258 procedures and results. Dig Dis Sci 26: 1057–1064, 1981
21. Siegel JH: The intact gall bladder and duodenoscopic sphincterotomy; Safety in numbers. Gastrointest endosc 144, 1985
22. Cotton PB: 2–9 year follow up after sphincterotomy for stones in patients with gall bladders. Gastrointest Endosc 157, 1986
23. Safrany L, Cotton PB: A preliminary report, urgent duodenoscopic sphincterotomy for acute gallstone pancreatitis. Surgery 89: 424–8, 1981
24. Rosseland AR, Solhang JH: Early or delayed endoscopic papillotomy (EPT) in gallstone pancreatitis. Ann Surg 199: 165–167, 1984
25. Siegel JH, Tone P, Menikeim D: Gallstone pancreatitis: Pathogenesis and clinical forms – the

emerging role of endoscopic management. Am J Gastroenterol 81: 774–778, 1986
26. Riemann JF, Seuberth K, Demling L: Clinical application of a new mechanical lithotripter for common bile duct stones. Scan J Gastroenterol 17 (Suppl) 78: 378, 1982
27. Riemann JF, Demling L: Lithotripsy of bile duct stones. Endoscopy 15: 191, 1983
28. Siegel JH, Pullano W, Ramsey WH: Lithotripsy – to crush or explode? State of the art. Gastrointest Endosc 15: 191, 1983
29. Silvis SE, Siegel JH, Hughes R, Katon RM, Sievert CE, Sivak MV: Use of electrohydraulic lithotripsy to fracture common bile duct stones. Gastrointest Endosc (Abstr) 32: 155, 1986
30. Siegel JH, Sherman HI, Davis Jr RC: Modification of a bronchoscope for percutaneous choledochoscopy. Gastro-intest Endosc 27: 179–181, 1981
31. Berci G, Hamlin JA: A combined fluoroscopic and endoscopic approach for retrieval of retained stones through the T-tube tract. Surg Gynecol Obstet 153: 237–240, 1981
32. Burhenne HJ: The technique of biliary duct stone extraction. Radiology 113: 567, 1974
33. Mazzariello R: Review of 220 cases of residual biliary tract calculi treated without reoperation: an eight year study. Surgery 73: 299, 1973
34. Barkin MS, Silvis S, Greenwald R: Endoscopic therapy of the 'sump' syndrome. Dig Dis Sci 25: 597, 1980
35. Siegel JH: Duodenoscopic sphincterotomy in the treatment of the sump syndrome. Dig Dis Sci 26: 922, 1981
36. Siegel JH: Peroral choledochoscopy in the sump syndrome: use of a thin caliber endoscope to negotiate a choledochoduodenostomy. Gastrointest Endosc 28: 192–193, 1982
37. Siegel JH, Guelrud M: Endoscopic cholangio-pancreatoplasty: hydrostatic balloon dilatation in the bile duct and pancreas. Gastrointest Endosc 29: 99, 1983
38. Guelrud M, Siegel JH: Hypertensive pancreatic duct sphincter as a cause of pancreatitis; successful treatment with hydrostatic balloon dilatation. Dig Dis Sci 29: 225–231, 1984
39. Siegel JH, Yatto RP: Hydrostatic balloon catheters: A new dimension of therapeutic endoscopy. Endoscopy 16: 231–236, 1984
40. Siegel JH, Pullano W, Ramsey WH: Sclerosing cholangitis, benign bile duct strictures and biliary cutaneous/peritoneal fistulas: room at the top for endoscopic management. Gastrointest Endosc (Abstr) 32: 166, 1986
41. Nakayama T, Ikedo A, Okuda K: Percutaneous transhepatic drainage of the biliary tract: technique and results in 104 cases. Gastroenterology 74: 554, 1978
42. Perieras RV Jr, Rheingold OF, Hutson D, et al.: Relief of malignant obstructive jaundice by percutaneous insertion of a permanent prosthesis in the biliary tree, Ann Intern Med 89: 589, 1978
43. Ring EJ, Oleaga JA, Reinman DB, et al.: Therapeutic application of catheter cholangiography. Radiology 128: 333, 1978
44. Kreek MJ, Balint JA: Skinny needle cholangiography. Gastroenterology 78: 598–604, 1980
45. Siegel JH, Daniel SJ: Endoscopic and fluoroscopic transpapillary placement of a large caliber biliary endoprosthesis. Am J Gastroenterol 79: 461–5, 1984
46. Huibregtse K, Tytgat GN: Palliative treatment of obstructive jaundice by transpapillary introduction of large bore bile duct endoprosthesis. Gut 23: 371–375, 1982
47. Siegel JH: Improved biliary decompression using large caliber endoscopic prostheses. Gastrointest Endosc 30: 21–23, 1984
48. Huibregtse K, Katon RM, Coene PP, Tytgat GNJ: Endoscopic palliative treatment in pancreatic cancer. Gastrointest Endosc 32: 334–338, 1986
49. Burchanth F: A new endoprosthesis for non-operative intubation of the biliary tract in malignant obstructive jaundice. Surg Gynecol Obstet 146: 78, 1879
50. Ferrucci Jr JT, Mueller PR: Interventional radiology of the biliary tract. Gastroenterology 84: 974–985, 1982

94

51. Speer AG, Farrington H, Costerton JW, Cotton PB: The role of bacterial biofilm in clogging of biliary stents. Gastrointest Endosc (Abstr) 32: 156, 1986
52. Leung JWC, DelFavero G, Cotton PB: Endoscopic biliary prostheses: A comparison of materials. Gastrointest Endosc 31: 93–5, 1985
53. Siegel JH, Pullano W, Wright G, Halpern G: The ultimate large caliber endoprosthesis – 12 Fr: Poiseuille was right – bigger is better. Gastrointest Endosc (Abstr) 31: 158, 1985
54. Siegel JH, Snady H: The significance of endoscopically placed prostheses in the management of biliary obstruction due to carcinoma of the pancreas: Results of nonoperative decompression in 277 patients. Am J Gastroenterol 81: 634–641, 1986
55. Neff RA, Fankuchen EI, Cooperman AM, et al.: The radiological management of malignant biliary obstruction. Clin Radiol 34: 143–6, 1983
56. Siegel JH, Ramsey WH, Rosenbaum A, Halpern G, Nonkin R, Jacob H, Lichenstein J: A new double lumen therapeutic biliary prosthesis for direct endoscopic implantation of Iridium into malignant tumors. Am J Gastroengerol (Abstr) 81: 883, 1986
57. Siegel JH: Evaluation and treatment of acquired and congenital pancreatic disorders: Endoscopic dilatation and insertion of endoprostheses. Am J Gastroenterol (Abstr) 78: 696, 1983
58. Pullano W, Siegel JH, Ramsey WH, Cooperman A: Effectiveness of endoscopic drainage in patients with pancreas divisum: Endoscopic and surgical results in 31 patients. Am J Gastroenterol (Abstr) 81: 887, 1986

4. Bleeding problems in hepato-biliary patients

S.I. SCHWARTZ

Acute and chronic liver disease can be associated with significant hemostatic abnormalities that may contribute to an intraoperative and/or postoperative bleeding problem. The majority of patients with *acute* hepatitis do not have a marked abnormality in any of the hemostatic factors. By contrast, abnormal coagulation tests may be associated with subacute hepatitis but rarely is there consequent significant bleeding. *Fulminant* hepatitis may be associated with hemorrhagic symptoms due to a reduced level of Factor VII that has a short biologic half life of 5 hours. Also DIC may occur as a consequence of: 1) activation of blood coagulation by release of necrotic hepatic tissue into the circulation or, 2) impaired hepatic removal of activated clotting factors, or 3) decreased levels of antithrombin III. But the issue of DIC in fulminant hepatitis is not resolved and intravascular microthrombi are rarely found at autopsy.

The surgeon is more interested in bleeding disorders accompanying operative procedures in patients with chronic liver disease, i.e., cirrhosis. It is appropriate to consider the pathophysiology of the hemostatic abnormalities associated with chronic liver disease. Platelets may be reduced in number or be functionally abnormal. Many of the coagulation factors manufactured in the liver may be reduced. Included in this category are decreased fibrinogen, prothrombin, Factor V, VII, IX, X, XI, XII, and antithrombin III. There is a question as to whether Factor VIII is reduced. Fibrinolysins may be unchecked due to decreased hepatic production of fibrinolytic inhibitors or to delayed hepatic clearance of circulating plasminogen activators. Thus, during an operative procedure on a cirrhotic patient, any combination of thrombocytopenia, impaired coagulation, or augmented fibrinolysis may evolve.

Thrombocytopenia is frequently encountered in patients with cirrhosis as a consequence of the splenic pooling and sequestration associated with hypersplenism. There is little correlation between the platelet count and the extent of splenomegaly. Thrombocytopenia is usually not an important cause of bleeding in cirrhotic patients and as an isolated manifestation does not constitute an indication for splenectomy. Between 1/3 to 2/3 of thrombocytopenic patients subjected to a portal decompressive procedure will have a resultant return of the platelet count to normal. Isolated splenectomy in the cirrhotic patient is contraindicated because it precludes the potential for a distal or central splenorenal shunt. The thrombocytopenia may be caused by recent intake of alcohol. In many cirrhotic patients with thrombocytopenia the bleeding time remains normal. Also, abnormal platelet function related to a preponderance of smaller, less active platelets has been noted in these patients.

The liver is the sole source of plasma fibrinogen with a steady state synthetic rate of 1.7 to 5 grams per day. But there is a large reserve, and up to twenty-fold increases occur in patients with peripheral consumption. This explains why hypofibrinogenemia is uncommon in liver disease and in most disorders with increased fibrinogen destruction rates.

Recent studies indicate that cirrhosis may result in an acquired dysfibrinogenemia. An abnormal composition of carbohydrate side chains on the beta and gamma chains of fibrinogen results in abnormal fibrin polymerization and may reduce the clotability of blood in these patients.

A decrease of Vitamin K dependent coagulation factors II, VII, IX, and X, which is not explained by malabsorption of Vitamin K or by Coumarin therapy, suggests hepatic disease. Contrary to general belief, coagulation disturbances associated with impaired absorption of Vitamin K in patients with obstructive jaundice rarely occur. In many of these jaundiced patients, coagulation factor assays reveal increases in levels of fibrinogen, Factors V and VIII, but impaired fibrinolytic activity – a point that will be considered in the discussion of therapy of cirrhotic patients undergoing operations on the biliary tract.

There is experimental evidence that Factor VIII may be synthesized in the liver, but a significant amount is produced in other organs. The reduction of antithrombin III, an important coagulation inhibitor in patients with cirrhosis, may contribute to intravascular clotting. In the presence of portal hypertension, endotoxins absorbed from the intestine bypass the liver and enter the systemic circulation unaltered, and as such, may cause platelet aggregation and thrombin formation. The occurrence of intravascular thrombosis in cirrhotics is supported by a decreased half-life of fibrinogen, prothrombin, and plasminogen, and by the ability of heparin to correct these lowered levels.

Increased fibrinolytic activity in patients with cirrhosis may be caused by reduced production of fibrinolytic inhibitors or by impaired hepatic clearance of circulating plasminogen activators. Unfortunately, the tests of pathologic fibrinolysis are non-specific and the increase in FDP frequently encountered in cirrhotic patients may be caused by other mechanisms. Fibrinolytic activity in some tissues may be increased in response to ill-defined stimuli present in the upper gastrointestinal tract associated with bleeding from trauma (including surgical trauma) or necrosis of the mucosa or of blood vessels.

Superimposed on these relatively specific abnormalities, a consumptive co-agulopathy has been postulated as an additional mechanism for deranging the hemostatic process in patients with chronic liver disease. Evidence for this is derived from observations that hemorrhagic phenomena and decreased concentrations of clotting factors occur. Laboratory abnormalities, however, similar to those found in clear-cut cases of DIC are not a consistent feature of liver disease. So the issue of DIC remains unresolved.

Hemostatic problems have been associated with specific surgical procedures in cirrhotic patients. These include portosystemic shunts, hepatic resection, transplants, and peritoneovenous shunts. Portal decompressive procedures have been complicated by abnormal fibrinolysis. Grossi and associates demonstrated that low fibrinogen levels and marked spontaneous fibrinolytic activity were present in cirrhotic patients with serious clotting abnormalities that developed during shunt procedures. The fibrinolytic activity at times increased significantly intraoperatively and the increase paralleled the amount of blood replacement. In most instances, the diffuse bleeding could be stopped by the administration of an antifibrinolytic drug EACA (Amicar).

A variety of hemostatic abnormalities has been reported in cases of extensive liver resection, either for trauma, or for tumor. A major resection is generally associated with a transient decrease in Vitamin K dependent clotting factors, and an increase in fibrinogen concentration. There may be an increase in FDP suggesting intravascular coagulation.

In the case of orthotopic liver transplantation, an acute coagulopathy may develop during or immediately after the anhepatic state. This is probably related to the failure to remove activated clotting factors and fibrinolytic activators. The severity of the coagulopathy appears to be related to the state of preservation of the donor organ. With a well preserved liver, the coagulation abnormalities are rapidly normalized. Rejection is accompanied by activation of coagulation, increased FDP, and thrombocytopenia.

Reinfusion of ascitic fluid such as that which occurs with a peritoneovenous shunt may be associated with a prolonged PT and a decrease in plasma levels of factors V, VII, IX, and fibrinogen. DIC may evolve and progress to cause bleeding from existing varices.

A number of studies has attempted to define hemostatic defects in cirrhotic patients to determine patients at risk for bleeding during an operation. Currently there is no specific assay that is more reliable than routine screening tests. The preoperative screening should include platelet count, bleeding time to assess platelet function, and the prothrombin time and activated partial thromboplastin time to detect abnormalities in the coagulation mechanism. In the face of diffuse intraoperative bleeding, FDP and a fast euglobulin lysis time should be added to differentiate between DIC and excessive fibrinolysis. It must be emphasized, however, that the clot lysis time, and even plasminogen assays, are not specific for increased fibrinolysis because these tests can be altered by a reduction in fibrinogen and plasminogen synthesis respectively. Also, a modest increase in FDP is frequently encountered in patients with liver disease.

In 1981 I published the first paper drawing attention to the problem of excessive bleeding that accompanies biliary tract operations in cirrhotic patients [1]. At that time, an exhaustive review of the literature failed to uncover a single article that specifically dealt with the problem of bleeding during biliary tract surgery in the cirrhotic patient. We conducted a review of our institutional experience. The records of patients operated on at our hospital between 1965–1980 provided the source for the study. All the records that indicated simultaneous discharge codings for cirrhosis and cholecystectomy or for cirrhosis and operations on the extrahepatic biliary tract were reviewed. A total of 33 patients were considered: 21 who had cholecystectomy, 7 who had cholecystectomy during a shunting procedure, and 5 who underwent operations on the common duct. All were cirrhotic.

To provide comparative data, we reviewed the records of 100 randomly selected non-cirrhotic patients who had undergone cholecystectomy during the same period. Also the records of 50 randomly selected cirrhotic patients who had undergone shunting procedures for bleeding varices were examined as were 25 randomly selected non-cirrhotic patients who had undergone choledochotomy or reconstruction of the common duct.

In the non-cirrhotic patient, cholecystectomy was rarely associated with significant blood loss. The mean transfusion requirement was less than 15 ml; only one patient required a transfusion. On the other hand, in the 21 cirrhotic patients subjected to cholecystectomy, there was a mean transfusion of 3800 ml, with a range of 0–9000.

Nine patients with varying types of cirrhosis undergoing cholecystectomy had no excessive bleeding. Coagulation studies, platelet counts, and liver function tests demonstrated no significant abnormality, with the exception of one patient with biliary cirrhosis. Only one of these patients required a single unit transfusion. In this group there was one patient who received intraoperative intravenous infusion of vasopressin, and in another patient in the group the gallbladder was encased by a cirrhotic liver, and only that segment that was peritonealized was removed. The mucosa of the hepatic side was cauterized.

12 of the 21 patients with cirrhosis undergoing cholecystectomy had excessive bleeding, with greater than 1500 ml blood loss. The liver function tests were normal in four patients and the coagulation studies were normal in 5, with 2 minor abnormalities in the group of patients with 1500 ml transfusion. Five of the 12 patients required greater than 4 units of blood, i.e., between 8–16 units.

In this group was one alcoholic who had normal liver function tests and co-agulation studies and his gallbladder bed was oversewn during cholecystectomy. He required 2 units of blood intraoperatively, 6 units postoperatively, and at time of re-exploration the bleeding was diffuse and ultimately responded to the intraoperative infusion of vasopressin combined with EACA. Another patient in this group had undergone cholecystostomy without incident for acute cholecystitis one year prior to elective cholecystectomy. His subsequent cholecystectomy required a 9 unit transfusion. Also in this group was an alcoholic patient who had previously undergone a portacaval shunt, and at the time of cholecystectomy had normal portal pressure. That patient required $5^1/_2$ liters of blood.

The last two patients had massive transfusion requirements; both developed sepsis in the postoperative period related to infected hematomas, and they died.

In considering the results of cholecystectomy performed during a portal decompressive procedure, it was noted that when the mean transfusions for shunts alone were used as a basis, cholecystectomy did NOT add significantly to that requirement in 6–7 patients. One patient died postoperatively related to exsanguination from the gallbladder bed. That patient had significantly impaired liver function tests and a markedly reduced platelet count.

The third and perhaps most important group under consideration had operation for biliary obstruction in the face of cirrhosis. The mean transfusion requirement in our hospital for 50 randomly selected non-cirrhotic patients undergoing a similar operation was approximately 1 unit of blood. All 5 patients who were cirrhotic bled massively and died within 2 weeks of their operation. One patient had a simple exploration of the common duct and removal of calculi and died of uncontrollable bleeding. Four patients with secondary biliary cirrhosis (2 as a consequence of stricture from a previous anastomosis and 2 related to malignant processes in the gallbladder or intrahepatic ducts) died following operation on the common duct. Three of these patients unequivocally exsanguinated while the other two required large amounts of blood and died of sepsis. Thus, our review emphasized the fact that biliary tract operations in cirrhotic patients were associated with increased operative and early postoperative bleeding, and consequent increased morbidity and mortality.

The factors we thought could be indicted as contributory included the vascularity of the liver accompanied by scarring, hypertrophic nodularity, and increased intrahepatic arteriovenous shunting, portal hypertension and the consequent development of large collaterals, and the complex coagulopathy characteristic of many patients with liver disease.

Several articles have subsequently addressed this same issue with varying results and conclusions. In a series of 429 patients undergoing cholecystectomy, 43 patients had cirrhosis with a prothrombin time not more than $2^1/_2$ seconds above control and 12 patients with greater impairment. These were compared with 374 patients with normal liver function. Mortality was 1.1% in the control group, and 9.3% with less marked cirrhosis, and 83.3% in severe cirrhosis [2].

Thus, 10 out of the 12 severely cirrhotic patients died; 3 of these died of massive intraabdominal bleeding during the operation. Three others died of hepatic and renal failure, and four from sequential organ failure due to sepsis. Cirrhotic patients had a much greater blood and fresh frozen plasma requirement than did the control group. All 10 high risk patients who died had excessive bleeding during cholecystectomy. In this paper, it was suggested that the only liver function test other than the prothrombin time that was a valuable indicator of the postoperative course was determination of the albumin level.

In 1983 two articles appeared back-to-back, touching on the subject. Doberneck and associates [3] reported on the morbidity and mortality after operation in non-bleeding cirrhotic patients in an attempt to identify factors that portend a grave prognosis. Mortality rates were significantly increased by emergency operation, a gastrointestinal related operation, ascites, or bilirubin concentration greater than 3.5, or prothrombin time greater than 2 seconds, a partial thromboplastin greater than 2 seconds, and an alkaline phosphatase concentration greater than 70 units, and an operative blood loss greater than 1000 ml. They did not specifically address the problem of bleeding in cirrhotic patients, but of the 102 patients reviewed, 24 required greater than 2 units of blood during an operative procedure.

The article by Castaing et al. [4] discussing the surgical management of gallstones in cirrhotic patients, agreed with our finding that simultaneous surgical treatment of gallstones does not increase the operative risk at the time of a shunt procedure. But the authors preferred cholecystolithotomy rather than cholecystectomy.

Two articles have recently appeared on hepatic resection for hepatocellular carcinoma associated with liver cirrhosis. Kinami and associates [5] reported an operative mortality rate of 12% in the small tumor group, and 17% in the large tumor group. Two of the 35 patients died of intraabdominal bleeding, and three of liver failure.

Presenting the Western Experience, Bismuth and associates [6] considered 35 patients with cirrhosis and hepatocellular carcinoma with a 14% mortality. Interestingly, bleeding did not seem to be a major factor. No patient survived five years.

The management of hemostatic failure in patients with liver disease undergoing an operation must be tailored to the specific clinical circumstance. Therapy is generally based on fresh frozen plasma to correct coagulation defects. Actually, fresh frozen plasma contains all the coagulation factors and inhibitors present in blood and does represent the most suitable agent for the correction of multiple defects found in liver disease. It does suffer from the fact that large amounts of plasma may be required to correct the coagulation defects, particularly defective Factor VII. Prothrombin complex concentrates are available and contain high concentrations of Factor II, VII, IX, and X. But there is a great risk that they may transmit hepatitis.

Associated with the administration of concentrates of coagulation factors, there is an increase in the incidence of thrombosis, and perhaps even DIC because these factors are not cleared adequately by the liver. Also, the low levels of antithrombin III may come into play. The risk may be less for recently modified concentrates that have been reported to have lower levels of activated clotting factors. The concomitant administration of small amounts of fresh frozen plasma to increase the levels of antithrombin III at the time that concentrates are administered may diminish the risk. The risk is sufficient enough, however, that the concentrates should be limited if at all possible.

Platelet therapy must be selective. The use of platelet concentrates in cirrhotic patients with hypersplenism is likely to be ineffective, even in the presence of severe thrombocytopenia because the platelets are removed from the circulation by the enlarged spleen.

The use of heparin in liver disease has been proposed because of the suggestion that DIC sometimes complicates liver disease but there is no convincing evidence that heparin is of value in these patients, and because of its anticoagulant effect, it can be potentially dangerous. A recent controlled study failed to show any benefit of the use of heparin, and therefore it is no longer recommended. The use of low-dose subcutaneous heparin has been advocated in patients with cirrhosis undergoing resection in order to obviate the possibility of deep venous thrombosis or DIC, but once again, no firm clinical evidence is available.

A difficult situation is presented by the patient with severe liver disease, intraoperative bleeding, thrombocytopenia, hypofibrinogenemia, and increased fibrin degradation products who also demonstrates clinical signs suggestive of organ ischemia. In these patients, treatment with heparin will exaggerate the bleeding, even if there is concomitant transfusion therapy of platelets and fibrinogen. In these patients, even in the absence of evidence of fibrinolysis, there may be benefit from the use of fibrinolytic inhibitors to stabilize fragile hemostatic plugs in regions of local bleeding, such as gastric mucosal ulcers, bleeding varices, and bleeding from intraperitoneal vessels disturbed by the surgical procedure. The administration of synthetic fibrinolytic inhibitors such as EACA (Amicar), may have a place in the management of gastrointestinal bleeding in which local fibrinolysis may be important and in managing the pre- and postoperative blood loss in cirrhotic patients undergoing shunt surgery or other procedures.

102

In our experience, EACA has played an important role in the control of bleeding in two specific instances of cirrhotic patients undergoing cholecystectomy in whom the bleeding was profound until the anti-fibrinolytic agent was administered.

The indications for elective cholecystectomy in cirrhotic patients should be more restrictive and if an operation is mandated, increased intraoperative blood loss should be anticipated. Suturing of the peritoneum overlying the gallbladder bed may reduce the bleeding from that area, and the operative approach of mucoclasis, originally described by Pribram has proved effective. In this procedure, the cystic artery and duct are ligated, the gallbladder excision is limited to the extrahepatic peritonealized portion, and the mucosal surfaces are then cauterized.

The importance of portal hypertension is attested to by the finding that when a cholecystectomy is performed as part of a shunting procedure there is usually no excessive bleeding. But we have noted that bleeding can occur in the face of normal pressure. Intravenous vasopressin has proved useful in reducing bleeding during shunting procedures, and this should be extrapolated to biliary surgery. Many years ago, Dr. Sedgwick, of the Lahey Clinic, said that when contemplating a duct reconstruction in a patient with biliary cirrhosis and portal hypertension, one should do a preemptive central splenorenal shunt, followed by a concomitant duct reconstruction to reduce the incidence of bleeding.

The final issue relates to the use of EACA, and on our experience, evidence of increased fibrinolysis was demonstrated in two patients, and EACA, which blocked the activation of plasminogen to form plasmin, caused almost immediate cessation of bleeding.

The surgeon who operates on a cirrhotic patient should be appreciative of the potential hemostatic defects, the tests to define these defects, and should have a plan for treatment of any untoward bleeding that may ensue.

References

1. Schwartz SI: Biliary tract surgery and cirrhosis: A critical combination. Surgery 90: 577–583, 1981
2. Aranha GV, Sontag SJ, Greenlee HB: Cholcystectomy in cirrhotic patients: a formidable operation. Am J Surg 143: 55–60, 1982
3. Doberneck RC, Sterling Jr WA, Allison DC: Morbidity and mortality after operation in nonbleeding cirrhotic patients. Am J Surg 146: 306–309, 1983
4. Castaing D, Houssin D, Lemoine J, Bismuth H: Surgical management of gallstones in cirrhotic patients. Am J Surg 146: 310–313, 1983
5. Kinami Y, Takashima S, Miyazaki I: Heaptic resection for hepatocellular carcinoma associated with liver cirrhosis. World J Surg 10: 294–301, 1986
6. Bismuth H, Houssin D, Ornowski J, Meriggi F: Liver resection in cirrhotic patients: A western experience. World J Surg 10: 311–317, 1986

5. Septic problems in hepato-pancreatico-biliary (HPB) surgery

M.C.A. PUNTIS and R.L. SIMMONS

Infection of the liver

The liver has, in common with the lungs, a specialised population of resident phagocytic cells. These two large organs also share the property of each being exposed to a particular source of potentially infecting pathogens. The lungs are exposed to air borne micro-organisms, whereas the liver is the first line of defence for gut borne micro-organisms escaping into the portal circulation. If micro organisms taken up by the phagocytes are not thereby destroyed then their continuing accumulation will go on to produce local infections.

The liver can be the seat of infections caused by a wide range of different pathogens, all causing individual problems of recognition, diagnosis and treatment. We will dwell in this chapter on infections presenting problems in management in current surgical practice but, others will be mentioned for completeness at the end of this section.

Pyogenic liver abscess

In 1936 Ochsner, De Bakey and Murray gave an account of the current management of liver abscess with an analysis of their series of 47 cases [1]. Since that time there have been substantial changes, not only in the diagnostic techniques and treatment as would be expected, over almost 50 years, but also in the apparent nature of the condition [2]. The age of the patient and the underlying aetiology and also the response of the patient's host defence system to the infection all seem to have changed. Thus the entire clinical picture of pyogenic liver abscess has changed for reasons all of which are not yet fully explained [3].

The clinical picture. 50 years ago liver abscess was a disease of young people due to pylophlebitis often following appendicitis. The clinical picture was that of a clear cut septic process. The patient was toxic with a wildly swinging pyrexia and rigors [1]. There was pain in the right upper quadrant of the abdomen and tender hepatomegaly clinched the diagnosis. Nowadays, hepatic abscess occurs more often in elderly people, in two recent series the average age of presentation was 60 years [4, 5]. In 50–60% of these cases the underlying cause was biliary obstruction by either stone or tumour. Systemic bacteraemia from whatever origin can also cause infection in the liver. This is more likely in regions of the liver that are damaged or ischaemic [6]. In young adults abdominal trauma is now an increasingly common cause of hepatic infections and abscesses [7]. Liver abscess is rare in children there only being about 100 cases reported in the literature [8].

Pyogenic liver abscesses can be divided into two types [9]. Type 1: multiple abscesses throughout the liver which represent between 50 and 70% of cases [5]. These abscesses may be either microscopic or macroscopic [7]. Type 2: solitary abscesses, often situated in the right lobe. The patient with a solitary abscess often presents with a long history and rather vague symptoms. Pain, nocternal sweating, vomiting, anorexia, malaise and weight loss being the usual picture [10]. Some patients have symptoms strongly suggestive of pulmonary disease [7]. The clinical signs may not clearly point to a specific pathology and the diagnosis is usually made by the astute clinician requesting an ultrasound, (US) hepatic scintiscan or computed tomography scan of the liver.

Multiple abscesses often develop in the presence of an obstructed infected biliary tract. The clinical course is much more acute, a clearly septic patient presents with jaundice, pyrexia and a tender liver. Hepatic imagining is of less use in patients with microscopic abscesses as the individual abscesses escape the resolving power of present imaging techniques.

Aetiology. Bacteria can spread to the liver by several routes. The portal of infection has a bearing on the nature and course of the subsequent abscess or abscesses.

Arterial spread. Bacteria arriving in the liver as part of a generalised bacteraemia will result in multiple small abscesses throughout both lobes. Damaged or diseased liver probably presents a more favourable site for bacterial growth, abscesses occur in necrotic tumours [6] and damaged regions following trauma which may be either penetrating or non penetrating. Blunt liver trauma can often be the focus for formation of an abscess in septic patients [7]. The susceptible regions of the liver will often have stagnant pools of blood and bile and hence have reduced Kupffer cell populations. It might be that the local oxygen tissue tensions favours certain bacteria, four out of the five abscesses resulting from non penetrating trauma in Rubin's series were infected with anaerobes [7].

Portal spread. This was once the commonest route for bacteria to reach the liver. In Pitt's recent series of patients, only 14% had portal spread of infection [5]. This change is probably due to more efficient treatment of the predisposing conditions, appendicitis and diverticulitis. Liver abscess is surprisingly rare in inflammatory bowel disease [11].

Bacteria arriving via the portal route cause large, often single abscesses which might develop from a cluster of smaller abscesses merging into each other. A solitary abscess is usually found in the right lobe. The traditional view [12] is that the portal blood is streamed, the splenic blood going to the left lobe and the intestinal blood to the right lobe. This asymmetry of distribution may however be simply due to the right lobe being larger and its true cause remains speculative. One possible explanation from animal work is that the host defence mechanisms are not uniformly efficient throughout the liver [13].

Biliary spread. This is now the commonest cause of pyogenic liver abscesses. 41% of patients in Pitt's 1975 series [5] resulting from an obstructed, infected biliary system. Why the stagnant bile becomes infected only in a proportion of patients with obstructive jaundice is not clear, but once the infection is established the increasing pressure of suppuration results in the infection breaking into the liver. Both lobes of the liver are affected resulting in multiple small abscesses. As liver tissue is progressively destroyed, the vessel walls will be breached and bacteria may pass into the circulation with a marked worsening of the patient's condition.

Direct spread. Infection may spread into the liver substance from, for example, a sub-hepatic abscess which will then form a solitary abscess in the adjacent liver. In cases of penetrating liver trauma, foreign bodies and bacteria can be driven deep into the liver substances and perpetuate infections.

Cryptogenic. In most series the cause of some abscesses is given as cryptogenic, 18% in Pitt's series [5]. This is because the available diagnostic techniques are not sufficiently sensitive to elucidate the cause at present. Wallack [14], for example, reports bilateral pyogenic hepatic abscesses from completely quiescent and asymptomatic diverticular disease. Where only careful pathological examination demonstrated bacteria in the portal vein. Lee and Black [15] propose that hepatic abscesses originate in hepatic infarcts becoming colonised by anaerobic bacteria.

Diagnosis of pyogenic liver abscess. Pyogenic liver abscesses do not have a standardised clinical presentation. Table 1 shows the percentage frequency of different symptoms in several series. Similarly the pattern of signs is shown in Table 2. Thus liver abscess should figure in the differential diagnosis of any patient with pyrexia and left upper quadrant pain. Chronicity of symptoms does not preclude the diagnosis. The mean duration of symptoms in Buckman's series was 8 weeks (range 1 to 16) [6]. Clearly, the diagnosis cannot reliably be made clinically. Haematological and biochemical investigations are non-specific. Many seriously ill patients will be anaemic. Many patients with pyogenic abscesses have very high white blood cell counts, around 20,000 per cu. mm. However, a normal white blood count does not preclude the diagnosis. In Balasegaram's series 50% of the fatal cases did not have a leucocytosis [16]. Liver function tests are often disturbed with a raised bilirubin, alkaline phosphatase and transaminases. There is often hypoalbuminaemia.

Some means of imaging the liver must be used to confirm the diagnosis. Plain x-rays of the chest or abdomen may confirm the presence of hepatomegaly but do not have great diagnostic specificity. Changes in the right lung base may be seen if a peripherally situated hepatic abscess is inflaming the diaphragm. Technetium colloid liver scans can demonstrate filling defects in the liver with a resolution of less than 2 cm, but can provide no information as to the nature of the filling defects. Various other scans using galium or indium have been described, but have not become universally accepted. Ultrasonography by a skilled operator is useful and can provide some further information about the filling defect, differentiating between solid and fluid filled lesions and detecting the presence of any intra-cavity debris. The bile ducts may also be imaged and measured, the level of any obstruction can be assessed by

Table 1. Symptoms of pyogenic hepatic abscess. Figures are the percentage of patients with each symptom.

Author	Rubin	Balasegaram	Conter
Ref No	7	16	29
No of patients	53	125	42
Symptoms			
Fever	87	98	88
Chills	38	30	79
Anorexia	38	65	48
Nausea/vomiting	28	68	31
Weakness/malaise	30	33	79
Weight loss	25	74	50
Dyspnoea	13		
Cough	11	19	
Pleurisy	9		
Haemoptysis	4	6	
Night sweats	11	15	
Pruritus			17
Diarrhoea		20	12
Abdominal pain			64

ultrasound and the presence of stones detected if they are of sufficient size. Any enlargement of the pancreas consistent with a tumour may also be seen.

The investigation of choice however, is computed tomography. Modern apparatus has a resolution of 5 mm allowing very small abscesses to be detected. Also a good deal of information about the nature of the space occupying lesions in the liver may be deduced from quantifying the x-ray absorption of the lesions.

Provided hydatid disease has been excluded by appropriate seriology it is safe to sample the contents of liver abscesses by percutaneous fine needle puncture under either ultrasound or CT control. This allows not only the infecting organisms and its antibiotic sensitivity to be determined but the abscess may also be drained.

Angiography has been advocated in the past by some workers, but for diagnostic purposes CT is less invasive and more useful. If however, hepatic resection is indicated as a therapeutic measure, then angiography is necessary.

Treatment. Liver abscess has 100% mortality if untreated [1]. Adequate treat-

Table 2. Signs of pyogenic liver abscess. Figures are the percentage of patients presenting with each sign.

Author	Rubin	Balasegaram	Conter
Ref No	7	16	29
No of patients	53	125	42
Signs			
Hepatomegaly	51	89	26
Tenderness in the			
upper right quadrant	47	97.2	50
Jaundice	23	11	36
Abdominal distension	21	24	
Right pleural effusion	11	36	21
Friction rub over			
liver or right	4		
lower chest			
Rales right lung	8		
Elevated right diaphragm	9		
Ascites	6	29	
Erythema & swelling			
of abdominal wall	2		
Oedema of legs		13	
Shock		3	26
Splenomegaly		23	
Mass			17

ment consists of antibiotics and drainage, even so some patients treated aggressively in this fashion will still die. The use of antibiotics alone or just drainage has virtually the same prognosis as no treatment. Pitt and Zuidema report 37 deaths out of 38 patients treated in a limited way because of other medical reasons [5].

There are two approaches available for draining hepatic abscesses: surgical drainage, and closed percutaneous drainage under CT or US control. These are complimentary methods each having its own strengths and weaknesses. Percutaneous drainage avoids the stress of general anaesthesia and laparotomy. It should, however, only be contemplated where surgeon and radiologist can confer and manage the patient jointly, so that in the event of complications such as peritonitis immediate surgery can be undertaken.

After the location of all the loculi in the abscess have been defined by contrast enhanced CT the best and shortest route or routes to the most dependent part of the abscess or abscesses can be planned to minimise the risk of contamination. It is desirable for the abscess to be punctured without traversing the peritoneum, pleura or other uninfected structure, although Manko [17] reported successfully draining a subphrenic abscess by passing the catheter through a polycystic liver. Under local anaesthesia using fluroscopy, or if necessary ultrasound, a needle is used to puncture and sample the abscess cavity. A specimen of pus is sent for culture and sensitivity determinations. A guide wire is passed into the cavity through the needle which is then removed, the drainage catheter is then passed over this guide wire. If necessary tract dilators may be used to enable catheters as large as 24 French gauge to be placed within the cavity. Which can then be lavaged and contrast studies performed; the catheter is placed on continuous suction [18]. If a patient does not improve within 24–48 hours then the presence of further undrained loculi must be assumed and open surgical drainage considered after attempting further imaging.

A primary surgical approach is appropriate when other surgical procedures are needed such as decompression of the biliary tract. In the past it has been taught that abscesses should be drained extra-peritoneally. This is no longer the case since the introduction of potent antibiotics; for although antibiotics cannot adequately penetrate the thick membrane of the abscess, they can prevent spread of the infection to virgin territory. Adequate tissue levels must be obtained before surgery and then continued for 3 months at least. The position of drains at operation, should be direct and to the most dependent part. Various types of sump and irrigating drainage systems have been described. Sauer for example [19] describes a sump system using red rubber drains. It is difficult to compare the overall effectiveness of percutaneous and surgical drainage because their indications are different and no prospective randomised study has been undertaken. In a series of 13 patients reported by

Gerzof [20] and treated by percutaneous drainage, two patients had major complications and two patients requires subsequent open drainage. These figures are comparable with other reported series. Johnson [21] reports that percutaneous drainage patients have a shorter hospital stay. Percutaneous drainage is advocated for very ill and immuno-compromised patients [22].

Following drainage the progress of abscesses can be followed by serial sinograms. Antibiotics must be continued even after the abscess is apparently gone and for at least three months. The final choice of antibiotic will depend on the result of sensitivity testing on samples of the pus. Prior to this a rational choice of antibiotic should be made to cover the likely pathogens. There is no single antibiotic effective against the whole range of bacteria that have been isolated from liver abscesses. A potent cephalosporin such as ceftazidime in combination with an aminoglycoside or acyl-ureido-penicillin is a good starting point.

Many authors have compared the outcome of their earlier cases with their more recent patients, and find that mortality is diminishing and this is attributed to improved diagnosis by imaging techniques, potent antibiotics and advances in anaesthesia and intensive care [20, 23]. The success rates reported for each technique reflect the skill exercised in selecting patients for each treatment, or combination of percutaneous and later surgical drainage. The best overall results will come from units where there is close collaboration between radiologists and surgeons.

Other liver infections. The clinical pattern of hepatitis and progressive liver damage with hepatitis A virus and especially the more dangerous hepatitis B virus is well known [24]. The course of the disease in some HBsAg positive patients is made worse by co-infection or super-infection with the Delta agent [25, 26]. Appropriate serology should be performed in all patients suspected of carrying hepatitis B virus because of the risk of infection to medical and nursing personnel. Other viruses such as cytomegalovirus can cause hepatitis although their effects on other organs usually cause greater clinical concern.

Granulomatous infections of the liver can be seen in Brucellosis [27]. The liver can be involved secondarily as part of more wide spread infective conditions. For example, actinomycosis, candidiasis and TB. Bacterial hepatitis has been described, it presents as a pyrexia of unknown origin and is diagnosed by histology and culture of a liver biopsy [28].

Protozoal infections of the liver are not uncommon malaria and leishmaniasis are well known in tropical parts of the world. The most important infection in this group, however, is the hepatic amoebic abscess. This has previously been uncommon in the Western World. Rubin reports 6% of amoebic abscesses in his series in 1974 [7] whereas Conter and co-workers found that 50% of liver abscesses in their unit between 1968 and 1983 were ameobic in origin [29]. They attribute this increase to greater mobility of people into and out of endemic areas (Mexico in the case of these authors). Balasegaram in contrast writing from Kuala Lumpur in Malasia has a 15 year series of 125 patients with pyogenic abscess and 317 with amoebic abscess.

Entamoeba histolytica is found in human faeces in its cystic form. After ingestion of contaminated material the cysts pass into the intestine where they are digested and 4 metacystic trophozoites are released. These grow in the crypts of liberkuhn causing dysenteric symptoms. After a while the trophozoites migrate to the bowel lumen adopt the cystic form and are passed. A colony of ameboe can grow and inflame the caecum and terminal ileum. They may then ulcerate and enter the portal circulation and reach the liver causing an abscess. An amoebic abscess presents with a similar clinical picture to a pyogenic abscess. Serological tests will help to confirm the diagnosis of ameobiasis. CT and ultrasound may be used to determine the location and number of abscesses. Ameobic abscesses may be treated solely with ameobicides (metronidazole) although some patients will require drainage if they fail to respond adequadetely. 15% in Conter's series required drainage [29].

In Balasegaram's very large series [16] the mortality for ameobic abscesses was 5% compared with 32.8% for pyogenic abscesses.

Various worms can affect the liver. This is a considerable problem in the Orient, Clonorchis being exceptionally common cause of jaundice there. Ascaris and schistosomiasis can also involve the liver. Infection with echinococcus is perhaps the most troublesome helminthic infection of the liver in the Western World, Middle East and Australia [30]. There are several ongoing projects to detect and control this disease [31, 32].

Pancreatic abscess

Pancreatic abscesses are rare [33]. Pseudocysts developing after acute pancreatitis can become infected resulting in a pancreatic abscess. This may be managed in the same general way as a hepatic abscess. That is, by systemic antibiotics and localisation of the abscess by CT or US [34] and then percutaneous drainage [35]. Similar antibiotics as recommended for liver abscesses may be used, that is ceftazidime in combination with an aminoglycoside or mezlocillin. Alternatively it can be treated by open operation and packing [36] which is reported to have a better prognosis than closed drainage [37]. Stone [38] has compared different treatments in a 20 year experience of 57 cases and finds open drainage and daily pack changes following subtotal pancreatectomy has the best survival (20 out of 20 patients in this group survived). Some features have been identified with a poor prognosis: bacteraemia, residual abscess, multiple organ systems failure and polymicrobial growth on culture of the abscess [39].

Biliary infections

Human bile is sterile in healthy individuals without biliary pathology [40, 41]. However when stones are present in the gall bladder episodes of acute cholecystitis can occur. These are usually inflamatory only at first and secondarily infection supervenes. If the neck of the infected gall bladder is blocked for a prolonged period then an empyema results. If the bile ducts are blocked by stone, tumour or benign stricture obstructive jaundice ensues. The stagnant column of bile above the obstruction can become infected and cholangitis develops – a dangerous condition requiring urgent effective treatment. The obstructed biliary system can become infected spontaneously or as a sequelae of percutaneous transhepatic biliary drainage. We will confine ourselves in this section to considering how infective complications of operations can be prevented and how established infection can be managed.

Prevention of infective complications in cholecystectomy. Cholecystectomy is the commonest major abdominal operation in both the U.K. and U.S.A., about 500,000 per annum in the U.S.A. [42]. The commonest post-operative complications are infective including minor wound infections, intraabdominal abscesses, cholangitis and septicaemia. Overall post-operative infections have been calculated to cause on average 4 days extra hospital stay per patient [43]. Much work has been expended on trying to define which patients are at greatest risk of developing postoperative infections, so that appropriate preventative steps can be taken. There is a good correlation between the presence of micro-organisms in the bile at the time of operation and subsequent infective complications [44, 45]. An immediate gram stain of bile during the operation has, however, not been shown to be of use as a prognostic factor and bactibilia can only be reliably demonstrated by culture of the bile [44]. This takes too long to be of any predictive value.

The reported incidence of infected bile at operation, depends on the type of patients studied and figures between 8–42% are recorded [46]. A study of U.K. patients having elective cholecystectomy found that 30% of these patients have infected bile [47]. The problem now is to try and identify preoperatively those patients who are likely to have infected bile. Several factors when assessed in isolation have been shown to be associated with bactibilia: age, level of plasma bilirubin, obstruction by stones, number of stones in the bile duct, recent episode of cholecystitis, but when the appropriate multivariant analysis is done (for these are not truly independent variables) only age remains a significant risk factor for having infected bile [48]. In another study using cluster analysis of many preoperative and postoperative variables, 8 have been identified as associated with a high risk of having biliary organisms: jaundice at operation, recent rigors, emergency operation or within 4 weeks of admission, age over 70, previous biliary operation, common bile duct obstruction and stones in the bile duct [49]. The nature of the underlying pathological process is also significant. Keighley found only 11% of young patients with gall bladder stones to have infected bile whereas 100% of patients with common bile duct stones were infected [47].

Exploration of the bile ducts is well established as being associated with a greater incidence of morbidity and mortality than simple cholecystectomy [50]. When the bile duct is explored supra-duodenally it has been the practice of most surgeons to drain the duct in the same way, either with a temporary T-tube or a more permanent choledochoduodenostomy, sphincteroplasty or sphincterotomy. There are some recent studies showing that a simple chole-dochoduodenostomy for exploration of the duct need not be closed around a T-tube and that immediate closure has a lower incidence of post-operative infection [51, 52]. In a further retrospective study it has been shown that choledochoduodenostomy has a lower infection rate and morbidity than T-tube drainage [53]. In a large retrospective study with long follow-up (median follow-up 47 months) the incidence of infected complications has been found to be the same for the 3 techniques of permanent bile drainage [54] although it must be remembered that patients will have been selected for each type of treatment for various undisclosed reasons.

From these data we can conclude that a high proportion of patients, especially elderly or jaundiced patients, all patients having the duct explored and any patient having an emergency or second biliary operation should receive some sort of antibiotic prophylaxis against subsequent infective complications [55]. Some authors advocate giving antibiotics to all patients having biliary surgery [56].

Bacteriology of the bile. Several authors have reported on the types of bacteria that can be isolated from the biliary tract in various pathological conditions. Data from some of these patients is summarised in Table 3. It can be seen that *E. coli* and *klebsiella* species are the most prevalent pathogens in bile. The likelihood of finding anaerobes in bile cultures will depend on the efficiency of the bacteriological culture methods used, some earlier studies might have underestimated the incidence of anaerobic infection [57].

Faecal streptococci have been considered a biliary organism of low pathogenicity. It is however important when it causes septicaemia. Blenkhorn and co-workers [58] found that 23% of postoperative bacteraemias of intra-abdominal origin were caused by faecal streptococci.

Bacteria may find access to the bile by several routes. By the systemic circulation, by the portal circulation, via the lymphatics or by direct ascent from the duodenum. The first route is not thought to be common as bacteria are most frequently of intestinal origin rather than from a distant septic site.

The portal blood is often sterile in the presence of biliary infection. Lymphatic spread is a possibility but the walls of the vessels contain fewer organisms than the lumen [59]. Upward migration from the duodenum is the most likely route. This would explain the particular flora found [60] and why infected bile is less common with distal malignant obstruction of the bile ducts [46].

Anaerobic bacteria in particular can deconjugate bile acids which leads to a general decrease in the concentration of bile acids in bile and a consequent decrease in cholesterol solubility with subsequent stone formation. Furthermore the bilirubin released as it is deconjugated can form insoluble calcium bilirubinate which forms the basis of all non-pigment stones [59, 61]. The mechanism helps to perpetuate the relationship between gall-stones and infection.

Choice of antibiotic. The ideal prophylactic antibiotics will achieve a high blood level and rapid tissue penetration during the surgical manipulation of

Table 3. Percentage of bile specimens containing each organism.

Author	Armstrong	Gallagher	Keighley
Ref No	48	44	46
No of patients	86	31	43
Organism			
Aerobic			
Gram positive			
Strep faecalis	10.5	9.7	9
Haemolytic strep	2.3		2.3
Strep viridians	2.3	6.5	4.5
Staph aureus	1	12.9	7.1
Staph albus			2.3
Gram negative			
E. coli	48.8	58.1	23
Klebsiella spp	19.8	35.5	16
Entrobacter spp	3.5		7.0
Proteus spp	4.8		4.7
Pseudomonas spp	5.8		4.7
Salmonella spp	1.2		
Seratia spp	3.5		
Actinobacter spp	2.4		2.3
Anaerobic			
Gram positive			
Clostridium spp	12.8	6.5	9
Anaerobic strep	4.8		4.7
Gram negative			
Bacteroides spp	4.8	3.2	

the duct and must be active against the usual pathogens. Although many antibiotics in common use achieve high bile concentrations in normal patients this is not the case with an obstructed biliary system. Cephalosporins such as cefuroxime are popular for prophylaxis but they have only one quarter of the activity of penicillin G against faecal Streptococci [62]. For this reason one of the acyl-ureidopenicillins such as Mezlocillin or Piperacillin is recommended by some authors [62, 64]. These are active against streptococci, pseudomonas and anaerobes. They also achieve high blood levels. A single dose with induction is usually adequate in all but the most compromised patient, that is one who is deeply jaundiced or immuno-suppressed. Stone [65] has found that prolonged administration of antibiotics can cause the emergence of resistent strains.

An alternative approach to sepsis prophylaxis in the high risk patients having bile duct exploration is peritoneal lavage with a topical antibiotic solution (Neomycin and Polymixin), this alone has been found to be as good as lavage together with systemic broad spectrum antibiotics. The numbers however, are small in this study [66]. In a larger series, Lord and co-workers have shown that irrigation with an antibiotic solution is better than irrigation with just normal saline. The control group had a 3% wound infection rate in 63 biliary operations whereas the treatment group had no infections. This study includes 200 patients altogether having other intestinal operations and the wound infection rate is similarly much improved by the antibiotic lavage solution in these patients [67].

At one time it was thought that percutaneous transhepatic drainage of bile would be beneficial in patients with obstructive jaundice to reduce the serum bilirubin levels prior to operation. This however has not proved to be the case and the number of septic complications with this pre-treatment proved to be excessive there is also evidence that it would be necessary to decompress the biliary tree for at least six weeks in order to reverse the intracellular damage that is done by biliary obstruction.

Cholangitis. The importance of cholangitis in the aetiology of pyogenic hepatic abscess has already been mentioned. Cholangitis typically presents with Charcot's triad of swinging fever with rigors, recurrent abdominal pain and fluctuating jaundice. In more severe cases Reynolds pentad will be encountered, that is Charcot's triad with shock and mental obtundation. This condition has a high mortality (up to 45%) even in specialised hepato-biliary units [68, 69].

The primary treatment of patients presenting with cholangitis is with suitable antibiotics in adequate dosage. Dooley and Co-workers recommend mezlocillin or cefotaxime plus gentamicin and metrodinazole [70]. Many patients will improve on this regime and Pitt [71] recommends withholding surgery when possible, until the sepsis is under control. Those patients who show no response in 48 to 72 hours should undergo urgent operation and the small proportion of patients presenting with septic shock [2.7% in Pitt's series] underwent immediate operation to decompress the biliary system, these patients had suppurative cholangitis. As an alternative to surgical decompression and in very sick patients endoscopic methods are now available. Endoscopic sphincterotomy has been reported to be successful in 88% of patients with recurrent pyogenic cholangitis [72]. Major complication rate in this series was 7.5% with 1.5% mortality. The majority of these, however, occurred in the early part of the series. If prolonged drainage and access to the biliary tree is required transnasal biliary drains may be inserted endoscopically [73].

Percutaneous transhepatic biliary drainage initially appeared to be a very useful technique for pre-operative biliary drainage [74]. It subsequently became apparent that this technique was attended by an unacceptably high infection rate [75], associated with a high postoperative rate of septic complications [76]. A new type of drainage catheter has however been described [77] which incorporates a non-return valve and an antiseptic barrier. It is reported to reduce septic episodes.

Little and his co-workers have defined risk profiles for morbidity and mortality in cholangitis. The primary determinants for morbidity were bile duct trauma and liver damage and for mortality, bile duct trauma, liver damage, pancreatitis and age. Findings such as these will of course be influenced by the referral pattern in individual centres and such analyses will need to be repeated elsewhere [68].

References

1. Ochsner A, DeBakey M, Murray S: Pyogenic abscess of the liver II. An analysis of 47 cases with review of the literature. Am J Surg 40: 292–319, 1938
2. Anon: Editorial. Pyogenic liver abscesses Br Med J 280: 1155–1156, 1980
3. Palmer ED: The changing manifestations of pyogenic liver abscess JAMA 231: 192, 1975
4. Bertel CK, Van Heerden JA, Sheedy PF: Treatment of pyogenic hepatic bascess. Surgical v percutaneous drainage. Arch Surg 121: 554–558, 1986
5. Pitt HA, Zuidema GD: Factors influencing mortality in the treatment of pyogenic hepatic abscess. Surg Gynecol & Obstet 140: 228–34, 1975
6. Buckman TG, Zuidema GD: The role of computerized tomographic scanning in the surgical management of pyogenic hepatic abscess. Surg Gynaecol & Obstet 153: 1–9, 1981
7. Rubin RH, Swartz MN, Malt R: Hepatic abscess: changes in clinical, bacteriologic and therapeutic aspects. Am J Med 57: 601–10, 1974
8. Tam PKH, Saing H, Lau JTK: Three successfully treated cases of non amoebic liver abscess. Arch Dis Child 58: 828–9, 1983
9. Butler JJ, McCarthy TJ: Pyogenic liver abscess. Gut 10: 389–399, 1969
10. Editorial: Pyogenic liver abscess – continuing problem of management. Lancet 1: 1170–1711, 1976
11. Crass JR: Liver abscess as a complication of regional enteritis. Interventional considerations. Am J Gastroenterol 78: 747–749, 1983

12. Rothenberg RE, Linder W: The single pyogenic liver abscess: a study of 24 cases. Surg Gynecol & Obstet 39: 31–40, 1934
13. Tanaka N: Biliary Sepsis. PhD Thesis 1985, Lund, Sweden
14. Wallack MK, Brown AS, Austrian R, Fitt WT: Pyogenic liver abscess secondary to asymptomatic sigmoid diverticulitis. Ann Surg 184: 241–243, 1976
15. Lee JF, Black GE: The changing clinical pattern of hepatic abscess. Archiv Surg 104: 465–470, 1972
16. Balasegaram M: Management of hepatic abscess. Curr Probl in Surg 185: 282–340, 1981
17. Manco LG: Percutaneous drainage of a left subphrenic abscess through a polycystic liver. J Clin Ultrasound 12: 222–224, 1984
18. Mandel SR, Boyd D, Jaques PF, Mandell V, Staab EV: Drainage of hepatic intra-abdominal and mediastinal abscesses guided by computerized axial tomography. Am J Surg 145: 120–125, 1983
19. Sauer PF: The red rubber sump. Surg Gynecol & Obstet 162: 183, 1986
20. Gerzof SG, Johnson WC, Robbins AH. Nabseth DC: Intra hepatic pyogenic abscesses: treatment by percutaneous drainage. Am J Surg 149: 487–494, 1985
21. Johnson WC, Gerzof SG, Robbins AH, Nabseth DC: Treatment of abdominal abscess. Comparative evaluation of operative drainage versus percutaneous catheter drainage guided by computed tomography or ultrasound. Ann Surg 194: 510–520, 1981
22. Skibber JM, Lotze MT, Garra B, Fauci A: Successful management of hepatic abscesses by percutaneous catheter drainage in chronic granulomatous disease. Surgery 99: 626–629, 1986
23. Silver S, Weinstein A, Cooperman A: Changes in the pathogenesis and detection of intrahepatic abscess. Am J Surg 137: 608–610, 1979
24. Koff RS, Galambos J: Viral hepatitis. In: Schiff L and Schiff ER (eds) Diseases of the Liver. J B Lippincott Company, Philadelphia, Toronto, 1982
25. Moestrup T, Hansson BG, Widell A, Nordenfeld E: Clinical aspects of delta infection. Br Med J 286: 87–90, 1983
26. Rizetto M, Verme G: Delta hepatitis – present status. J Hepatol 1: 187–193, 1985
27. Nagalotimath SJ, Darbar RD, Jogalekar MD: Granulomatous hepatitis in brucellosis. J Ind Med Assoc 72 (1): 1–4, 1979
28. Weinstein L: Bacterial hepatitis: a case report of an unrecognised cause of fever of unknown origin. N Engl J Med 299: 1052–1054, 1978
29. Conter RL, Pitt HA, Tompkins RK, Longmire WP: Differentiation of pyogenic from ameobic hepatic abscess. Surg Gynecol & Obstet 162: 114–120, 1986
30. Hau T: Infections of the liver and spleen. In: RL Simmons and RJ Howard (eds) Surgical Infectious Diseases. Appleton-Century-Crofts, New York
31. Craig PS, Zeyhle E, Romig T: Hydatid disease: research and control in Turkana II. The role of immunological techniques for the diagnosis of hydatid disease. Trans Roy Soc Trop Med Hygiene 80: 183–92, 1986
32. Pitt HA, Korzelius J, Tompkins RK: Management of hepatic Echinococcus in Southern California. Am J Surg 152: 110–115, 1986
33. Goodale RL, Dressel TD: Infections of the pancreas. In: Simmons RL and Howard RJ (eds) Surgical Infectious Diseases. Appleton-Century-Crofts, New York
34. Crass RA, Meyer AA, Jeffrey RB, Federle MP, Grendall JH, Wing VW, Trunkey DD: Pancreatic abscess: impact of computerized tomography in early diagnosis and surgery. Am J Surg 150: 127–131, 1985
35. Gerzoff SG, Johnson WC, Robbins AH, Spechler SJ, Nabseth DC: Percutaneous drainage of infected pancreatic pseudocysts. Arch Surg 119: 888–893, 1984
36. Bradley EL, Fulenwider JT: Open treatment of pancreatic abscess. Surg Gynecol & Obstet 159: 509–513, 1984

37. Pemberton JH, Becker JM, Dogois RR, Nagorney DM, Ilstrup D, Remine WH: Controlled open lesser sac drainage for pancreastic abscess. Ann Surg 203: 600–604, 1986
38. Stone HH, Strom PR, Mullins RJ: Pancreatic abscess management by subtotal resection and packing. World J Surg 8: 340–345, 1984
39. Malangoni MA, Shallcros JC, Seiler JG, Richardson JD, Polk HC: Factors contributing to fatal outcome after treatment of pancreatic abscess. Ann Surg 203: 605–613, 1986
40. Csendes A, Fernadey M, Unbec P: Bacteriology of the gall bladder bile in normal subjects. Am J Surg 129: 629–631, 1975
41. Scott AJ: Progress report: bacteria and diseases of the biliary tract. Gut 12: 487–492, 1977
42. Henry ML, Carey LC: Complications of cholecystectomy. Surg Clin of North America 63: 1191– 1204, 1983
43. Keighley MRB, Graham NG: Infective complications of choledochotomy with T-tube drainage. Br J Surg 58: 764–768, 1971
44. Gallagher P, Ostick G, Jones D, Schofield PF, Tweedle DEF: Intraoperative microscopy of bile – is it useful? Br J Surg 69: 473–474, 1982
45. Vogt DF, Hermann RE: Choledochoduodenoscopy, Choledochojejunestomy or sphincteroplasty for biliary and pancreatic disease. Ann Surg 193: 161–168, 1981
46. Keighley MRB: In: Blumgart LH (ed) The Biliary Tract. Churchill Livingstone, London, 1982
47. Keighley MRB: Micro organisms in the bile. Ann Roy Coll Surg Eng 54: 329–334, 1977
48. Armstrong CP, Dixon JM, Duffy SW, Elton RA, Taylor TV, Davies GC: Choledochotomy and sepsis in benign biliary disease. J Roy Coll Surg Edin 32: 343–347, 1985
49. Keighley MRB, Flim R, Alexander-Williams J: Multivariate analysis of clinical and operative findings involved with biliary sepsis. Br J Surg 63: 528–531, 1976
50. Cruse PJE: Incidence of wound infections on general surgery services. Surg Clin of North America 55: 1269–1275, 1975
51. Payne RA, Woods WGA: Primary suture or T-tube drainage after choledochotomy. Ann Roy Coll Surg Eng 68: 196–198, 1986
52. Lygidakis NJ: Choledochotomy for biliary lithiasis: T-tube drainage or primary closure. Am J Surg 146: 254–256, 1983
53. Lygidakis NJ: Infective complications after choledochotomy. J Roy Coll Surg Edin 27: 233–237, 1982
54. Worthley CS: Exploration of the common bile duct for benign conditions: an analysis of 413 patients. Aust N.Z. J Surg 52: 478–483, 1982
55. Gierscksky K-E: Antimicrobial prophylaxis in biliary and gastrointestinal surgery. Scand J Gastroenterol (Suppl) 85: 104–110, 1983
56. Elke R, Widmer M, Trippel M, Gruber UF: Mezlocillin single-dose prophylaxis in biliary tract surgery. Eur Surg Res 15: 297–301, 1983
57. Brook I, Altman RP: The significance of anaerobic bacteria in biliary tract infection after hepatic portoenterostomy for biliary atresia Surgery 95: 281–283, 1984
58. Blenkharn JI, Blumgart LH: Streptococcal bacteria and hepatobiliary operations. Surg Gynecol & Obstet 160: 139–141, 1985
59. Lotveit T: Bacterial infection of the liver and biliary tree. Scand J Gastroenterol (Suppl) 85: 104–110, 1983
60. Barnham M: The gut is a source of the haemolytic streptococci causing infection in surgery of the intestine and biliary tracts. J of Infection 6: 129–139, 1983
61. Thornton JR, Heaton KW: Do colonic bacteria contribute to cholesterol gallstone formation? Effects of lactulose on bile. BMJ 282: 1018–1020, 1981
62. Kaye D: Enterococci: biological and epidemiological characteristics and *in vitro* susceptibility. Arch Int Med 142: 2006–2009, 1982

63. Dooley JS, Gooding A, Hamilton-Miller JMT, Brumfitt W, Sherlock S: The biliary excretion and pharmacokinetics of Mezlocillin in jaundiced patients with external bile drainage. Liver 3: 201–206, 1983

64. Morris DL, Mojaddedi ZJ, Burdon DW, Keighley MRB: Clinical and microbiological evaluation of Piparacillin in elective biliary surgery. J Hosp Inf 4: 159–164, 1983

65. Stone HH, Haney BB, Kolb LD, Geheber CE, Hooper CA: Prophylactic and preventative antibiotic therapy: timing, duration and economics. Ann Surg 189: 691–699, 1979

66. Pitt HA, Postier RG, Gadacz TR, Cameron JL: The role of topical antibiotics in 'high risk' biliary surgery. Surgery 91: 518–524, 1982

67. Lord JW, LaRaje RD, Diliana M, Gordon MT: Prophylactic antibiotic wound irrigation in gastric, biliary and colonic surgery. Am J Surg 145: 209–212, 1983

68. Little JM, Cunningham P: Obstructive jaundice in a referral unit: surgical practice and risk factors. Aust N Z J Surg 55: 427–432, 1985

69. O'Connor MJ, Schwartz ML, McQuarrie DG, Sumner HW: Acute bacterial cholangitis: an analysis of clinical manifestations. Arch Surg 117: 437–441, 1982

70. Dooley JS, Hamilton-Miller JMT, Brumfitt W, Sherlock S: Antibiotics in the treatment of biliary infection. Gut 25: 988–998, 1984

71. Pitt HA, Postier RG, Cameron JL: Consequences of peroperative cholangitis and its treatment on the outcome of operation for choledocholithiasis. Surgery 94: 447–452, 1983

72. Lam SK: A study of endoscopic sphincterotomy in recurrent pyogenic cholangitis. Br J Surg 71: 262–266, 1984

73. Kozarek RA: Transnasal pancreaticobiliary drains. Indications and Insertion Technique. Am J Surg 146: 250–253, 1983

74. Molnar W, Stockum AE: Relief of obstructive jaundice through a percutaneous transhepatic catheter – a new therapeutic method. AJR 122: 356–357, 1974

75. McPherson GAD, Benjamin IS, Habib NA, Bowley NB, Blumgart LH: Percutaneous transhepatic drainage in obstructive jaundice: advantages and problems. Br J Surg 69: 261–264, 1982

76. Randall PE, Hutchinson GH: Wound infection after biliary tract surgery. Br J Clin Prac 34: 200–202, 1980

77. Blenkharn JI, McPherson GAD, Blumgart LH: Septic complications of percutaneous transhepatic biliary drainage. Evaluation of a new closed drainage system. Am J Surg 147: 318–321, 1984

6. Abdominal drains in surgery of the liver, pancreas and biliary system

O.T. TERPSTRA, M.C.A. PUNTIS, E.I. GALPERIN and T. HOLMIN

Introduction

The use of drains in abdominal surgery has been and still is an area of much debate. Aside from the economical aspects – 5 million surgical drains annually used in the United States [1] – are unresolved problems of efficacy and potentially harmful side-effects. Tradition and surgical bias too often dictate the use of drains instead of scientific data based upon experimental studies and clinical trials. However, a drain is a foreign body that carries an inherent morbidity of its own. Intraperitoneal drains are commonly used for one of the following indications: therapeutically, to drain localized fluid collections in the abdomen, like abcesses, or prophylactically, to be warned of and to drain fluid collections anticipated after biliary hepatic or pancreatic surgery. While there is hardly any controversy on the use of drains for peritoneal abcesses, the prophylactic use of drains is more debatable. Another prophylactic indication for peritoneal drainage was thought to be the presence of diffuse peritonitis. Yates in 1905 already demonstrated that intraperitoneal drains were sealed off six hours after placing [2]. These findings were later confirmed by Agrama and co-workers. They demonstrated that drains inserted into the peritoneal cavity of dogs failed to show the presence of colored fluid injected intraperitoneally, one to seven days after placing. On autopsy all tubes of different material and design were surrounded and occluded by omentum [3]. Although it is commonly believed that clotting causes obstruction of drains, Zacharski et al. found that tissue fragments are responsible and little fibrin was evident in the tubes [4].

Drainage can be divided into two systems: 1) passive drains, functioning by overflow and influenced by pressure differentials, occasionally assisted by gravity, and 2) active drains, working by an external source of suction, either by continuous suction, open to the air like in sump drains or by closed suction (Hemovac®, Drevac®). Commonly used types of passive drains are made of rubber or silastic and of the penrose or corrugated type.

From a mechanical point of view the abdomen is a fluid-filled container with flexible walls. In the erect position the normal upper abdominal pressure is subatmospheric (-5 to -8 cm H_2O). Intraabdominal pressure increases temporarily when exposed to atmospheric pressure during surgery or when fluid collections form, but it is questionable whether the routine use of passive drains after upper abdominal surgery should be advocated [1].

The harmful effects of intraperitoneal drains by acting as a conduit for bacteria coming in rather than for fluid coming out, were investigated by Cerise and co-workers. When bacteria were applied on the skin around the drain, left in the upper abdomen, after splenectomy one out of every five animals had a positive culture from the splenic bed 24 hours later, increasing to positive cultures in more than half of the animals after three days of drainage [5]. More data on the negative effects of intraperitoneal drains will be discussed in the section on drainage after biliary surgery.

Peritoneal defence mechanisms

The presence of bacteria contaminating the peritoneal cavity initiates a series of reactions to either remove the bacterial load from the peritoneal cavity or isolate it within a limited region. In man these natural defence mechanisms are rarely adequate to deal with substantial contamination and the mortality from untreated peritonitis is therefore high [6].

There are three principle components of the peritoneal defence system.
1. Removal by lymphatics
2. Phagocytosis
3. Sequestration by adhesions.

Lymphatic absorption

The mesothelium lining the peritoneal cavity is a thin layer of cells lying on a vascular matrix. Over the diaphragm however, the cells are modified, for it is in this area that the lymphatic drainage of the peritoneum is located. Lymphatics spread out centrifugally on the abdominal side of the diaphragm. They are covered by the mesothelial cell but in many places there are defects or 'stomata' occurring at the junction between two or three cells. These pores overlie lymphatic channels. In this way, only the lymphatic endothelium and a very attenuated basal lamina separate the peritoneal cavity from the lumen of the lymphatic. The movement of the diaphragm with respiration alters the size of the stomata. This coupled with the pressure difference between the abdomen and the thorax results in a continual passage of fluid and suspended particles, such as bacteria, from the peritoneum into the lymphatics and thence away from the abdomen. The rest of the mesothelium lining of the peritoneal cavity is capable of absorbing only fluid, all particulate matter is taken up by the sub-diaphragmatic lymphatics and this forms a 'first line' in the peritoneal defences [7]. Bacteria implanted into the peritoneal cavity have subsequently been found in the lungs and general circulation within minutes in experimental animals. This mechanism is probably very satisfactory for removing small numbers of contaminating bacteria but in the event of massive contamination, such dissemination of the infection to the rest of the body is detrimental [8]. It is interesting that the neuromuscular reflexes seen in peritonitis – shallow respiration, muscular rigidity of the abdominal wall and paralytic ileus will all stop movement of intra-peritoneal fluid and diminish diaphragmatic lymphatic clearance of bacteria.

The peritoneal inflammatory response

If the lymphatic clearance is inadequate, then an inflammatory response ensues [9]. This is initiated by several agents including irritants in released gastrointestinal contents following perforation and activated complement components produced by the action of bacterial lipopolysaccharides on complement components. These agents increase the permeability of the vascular tissue lining of the peritoneal cavity and fluid pours into the peritoneal space. This fluid has the effect of diluting any toxic substances and will bring with it polymorphonuclear cells. These cells will migrate towards the contamination in the peritoneal cavity down the chemotactic gradients formed by the inflammatory process. The neutrophil phagocytes will remove and destroy many bacteria. Phagocytosis is improved after opsonisation of the bacteria, by either specific or non-specific opsonins. Sometimes after the neutrophil influx into the peritoneal cavity, macrophages begin to arrive [6]. These will again be moving along chemotactic gradients. The macrophages have 3 broad overlapping functions, phagocytosis, secretion and immune function. Macrophages may be activated by contact with several agents including interferon, endotoxin, complement or lymphokines. Their phagocytic capacity is then greatly enhanced. Macrophage killing of bacteria is by the internal secretion of lytic enzymes and oxidative free radicals [10]. Some of these toxic products may spill over from cells and damage surrounding tissue [11].

Macrophages secrete many active substances: lysozyme, interferon, prostaglandins, lymphokines and many others which will in turn modulate their own activity and that of other elements of the inflammatory reaction [12]. Macrophages secrete interleukin 1 (IL-1) and are also important in processing of antigens for presentation to T-lymphocytes [13].

Adhesions

Fibrinogen is found in the peritoneal fluid in peritonitis. This will be converted to fibrin by thrombin and this newly produced fibrin will cause adhesions to form between adjacent loops of bowel and the omentum. This mechanism will help to localise infection. In the normal peritoneal cavity, fibrin would be rapidly broken down by plasmin but the generation of this substance is defective in peritonitis [14]. The formation of adhesions around infection has a detrimental effect in that it prevents the ready access of phagocytic cells to the bacteria [15].

Host peritoneal defence mechanisms may prove to be ineffective in completely ridding the organism of contamination for many reasons. Substances such as haemoglobin and bile [16] have an adverse effect on phagocytic function. The generalised effects of trauma will also have an inhibiting effect [17]. Uncontrolled peritoneal infection will often proceed to cause generalised effects in the organism, especially on the pulmonary and cardiovascular system [18].

Treatment

The mainstay of therapy for peritonitis has been surgical intervention to remove toxic substances and to remedy the cause of the contamination, such as a perforated peptic ulcer. There are however, many new and exciting approaches to enhancing the host defence mechanisms such as the use of immuno-modulators to modify macrophage function [19] and the passive transfer of hyper-immune gammaglobulin or spleen cells [20]. Fibronectin has also been used clinically in severely septic patients [21].

Drainage in biliary surgery

Traditionally drains after cholecystectomy are used to be warned of accumulation of bile leaking from small ducts entering through the wall of the gall bladder or to be warned of hemorrhage. In a survey among the surgical clinics in Sweden 87% of the responding centers used a drain in cholecystectomy routinely, while after exploration of the common bile duct drainage of the abdominal cavity was carried out in all centers [22]. However, cholecystectomy without drainage was already practiced in 1913 as stated by Spivak and referred to as 'ideal cholecystectomy' [23]. The effectiveness of removing fluid from the abdominal cavity was rather low as demonstrated in dog experiments: after injection of a certain amount of liquid into the abdominal cavity, 40% of it is drained with a penrose drain, 39% with a rubber tube and 58% with a sump drain [24]. This is confirmed by Borgström and Truedson who measured the mean volume of fluid drained after cholecystectomy for acute cholecystitis: on the day of operation the average amount was 68 ml and 51 ml on the first postoperative day. After operation for chronic cholecystitis the values were 71 ml and 35 ml, respectively [22].

Five prospective, controlled trials on the use of drains in elective cholecystectomy have been reported. In only one of these studies an adverse effect, i.e. a transient rise in serum bilirubin, was found in patients without intraperitoneal drains [25]. The other studies either failed to demonstrate any advantage of draining [26] or showed a higher morbidity in patients who had a drain [27–29]. Undrained patients had a shorter hospital stay, less and shorter duration of postoperative fever and less wound complications. Drains appear to add to patient discomfort and consequently to their inability to cough, producing atelectasis and fever. Besides the problem of the drain acting as an entry for bacteria, as discussed earlier, another adverse effect of an intraperitoneal drain is the possibility that the drain, as a foreign body, stimulates the formation of fluid, or that a space is maintained where fluid can collect since apposition of tissue surfaces is prevented by the drain. In fact Elboim *et al.* found that in 24% of patients who had undergone cholecystectomy a subhepatic fluid collection could be demonstrated 2 to 4 days after the operation [30]. Only in two patients this had clinical importance. Asymptomatic fluid collections were more common after emergency operations and when drains were used; 30.9% of the patients with drains had an ultrasound detectable fluid collection against nil in the undrained group. From these data it can be concluded that in uncomplicated cholecystectomies drainage is unnecessary and perhaps even harmful. As mentioned earlier drainage of the common bile duct after exploration of the biliary system is routinely used in most centers. Data from prospective controlled studies as for drainage in cholecystectomy are lacking until now, but it is questionable whether the common bile duct should be routinely drained by a T-tube when an atraumatic technique of exploration is used, the bile duct wall is not inflamed and gross infection is absent.

Pancreatic drainage

Pancreatic surgery is mainly based on the usage of drains. There is no classification of pancreatic drainage at present. Pancreatic drainage can be divided into two groups: parapancreatic drainage and pancreatic duct drainage (Fig. 1). Parapancreatic drainage is used
1. to diminish enzyme intoxication in patients with acute pancreatitis. The drain tube can be introduced either through laparotomy or under laparoscopic control.

124

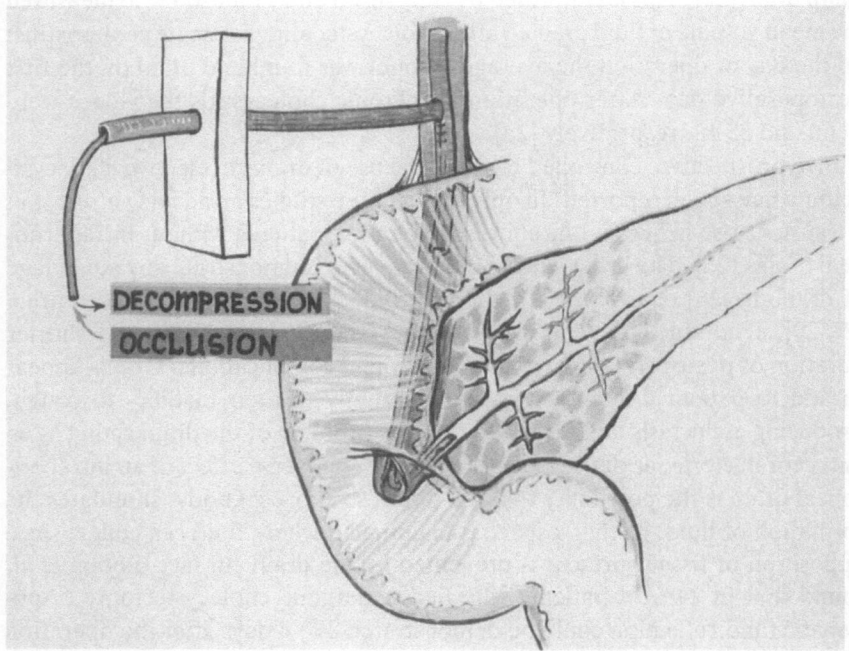

Fig. 1. Pancreatic duct drainage.

2. to drain in case of pancreatic necrosis and its purulent complications: abscesses, phlegmona in the area of pancreas, bursa omentalis and retro-peritoneal space. Exterioration of the tube can be performed through abdominal wall or backwards through lumbar incision.
3. as a signal drainage after pancreatic resection or other manipulations on the gland. This drainage can prevent further spreading of inflammation when developed.

Pancreatic duct drainage can be used as follows: 1) for decompression of the duct after pancreatic resection, wirsungotomy and for safety of pancreaticojejunostomy, 2) for long-term splintage of longitudinal pancreaticojejunostomy in chronic pancreatitis (Fig. 2), and 3) for injection of an occlusive mass in the pancreatic duct in patients with acute necrotic pancreatitis. Drains can be inserted either during the operation or endoscopically. In ten patients with chronic pancreatitis we performed a longitudinal pancreaticojejunostomy (Puestow's operation) using the transpancreatic stent. Both ends of the stent were exteriorized so that it could be washed and replaced when necessary. The drain must be left in place for 1–2 years and prevents the narrowing of the anastomosis. We hope that this procedure can improve the results of Pues-tow's operation. Our experiments in dogs show that occlusion of the pancreat-

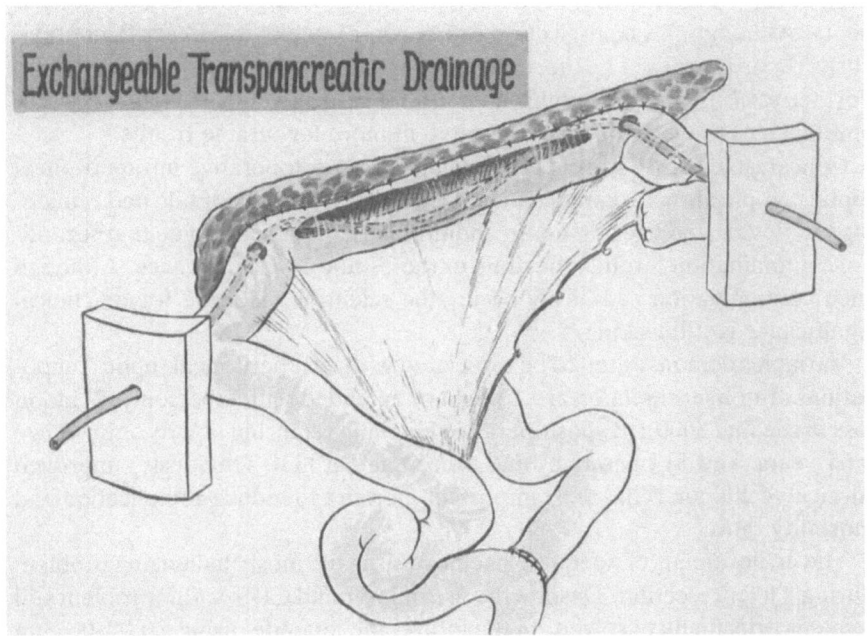

Fig. 2. Method of drainage after longitudinal pancreaticojejunostomy.

ic duct can stop the development of acute pancreatitis induced by the injection of bile into the pancreatic duct. Those experiments started our clinical tests. We introduced a drain tube into the pancreatic duct in patients with acute necrotic pancreatitis for duct decompression. If the inflammation stops, the procedure is over; if the inflammation goes on and hemorrhagic necrotic pancreatitis develops we inject cyanoacrilate composition 'contrablock' into the same drain to occlude completely the pancreatic duct. This procedure gave good results in 3 patients. I believe that in future with the development of endoscopic techniques, pancreatic drainage will be more necessary and useful than now. It is unlikely that in the future pancreatic surgery will be able to do away with drainage.

Drainage after hepatic resection

At the present time, the application of drains or not after liver resections is hardly a controversial problem. Most surgeons regularly use drains, at least after major liver resections, and many well-founded reasons for such a policy are prevalent. Despite the use of drains in 145 out of 149 (97.3%) liver resections, intraperitoneal septic complications occurred in 19 (12.8%) patients. Although this complication rate is considerable, it is lower than previously reported rates (22/108 or 20.4% and 23/138 or 16.7% according to Fortner *et al.* [31] and Thompson *et al.* [32] respectively). It is unlikely that omittance of drains would have resulted in more favourable results.

Conceivable causes for the high frequency of postoperative intraperitoneal septic complications are inadequate haemostasis, leakage of bile and remaining but devitalized liver tissue. In addition, a few surgeons argue that secondary contamination through the drain or the T-tube is of significance. Although such contamination can easily occur, the scientific evidence for its clinical significance is still lacking.

Variables demonstrated to be associated with intraperitoneal septic complications after liver resection are: 1) right or extended right lobectomy, 2) blood loss exceeding 3000 g, 3) postoperative bleeding requiring laparotomy, 4) age >65 years, and 5) operative time exceeding 5 h [33]. Obviously, improved surgical technique is the most important measure to reduce complication and mortality rates.

The achievement of adequate haemostasis is the most challenging problem during a liver resection. Despite the use of laser and CUSA, this problem still remains principally unsolved. In the future, the jet knife, using a 0.08–0.1 mm thin beam of water under high pressure, seems to be a more effective and a considerably cheaper alternative. Furthermore, studies in experimental animals have demonstrated that preservation of the sympathetic liver nerves results in a 75% decrease in blood loss from the resection surface after small, standardized liver resection [34]. If this data is applicable to the human situation, it should be important to avoid division of the sympathetic nerves running to the remaining liver parenchyma.

In summary, an improved surgical technique and an increased understanding of the role of the liver nerves may hopefully contribute to the possibilities to perform major liver surgery without drainage.

References

1. Moss JP: Historical and current perspectives on surgical drainage. Surg Gynecol Obstet 152: 517–527, 1981
2. Yates JL: An experimental study of the local effects of peritoneal drainage. Surg Gynecol Obstet 1: 473–479, 1905
3. Agrama HM, Blackwood JM, Brown CS, *et al.*: Functional longevity of intraperitoneal drains. An experimental evaluation. Am J Surg 132: 418–421, 1976
4. Zacharski LR, Colt J, Mayor MB, *et al.*: Mechanism of obstruction of closed-wound suction tubing. Arch Surg 114: 614–615, 1979
5. Cerise EJ, Pierce WA, Diamond DL: Abdominal drains: Their role as a source of infection following splenectomy. Ann Surg 171: 764–769, 1970

6. Hau T, Ahrenholz DH, Simons RL: Secondary bacterial peritonitis: the biologic basis of treatment. Current Problems in Surgery XVI: 1–65, 1979

7. Lill SR, Parsons RH, Buhac I: Permeability of the diaphragm and fluid resorption from the peritoneal cavity in the rat. Gastroenterology 76: 997–1001, 1979

8. Dumone AE, Maas WK, Iliescu H, Shin RD: Increased survival from peritonitis after blockade of transdiaphragmatic absorption of bacteria. Surg Gynecol Obstet 162: 248–252, 1986

9. Simmons RL, Ahrenholz DH: Pathology of peritonitis: a review. J Antimicrobiol Chemotherapy 7: (Suppl A) 29–36, 1981

10. Hashimoto S, Nomoto K, Matsuzaki T, Yokokura T, Mutai M: Oxygen radical production by peritoneal macrophages and kupffer cells elicited with Lactobacillus casei. Infection and Immunity 44.1: 61–67, 1984

11. Simon RH, Scoggin CH, Patterson D: Hydrogen peroxide causes the fatal injury to human fibroblasts exposed to oxygen radicals. J Biol Chem 256: 7181–7186, 1981

12. Tanner AR, Arthur MJP, Wright R: Macrophage activation, chronic inflammation and gastrointestinal disease. Gut 25: 750–783, 1984

13. Uranue ER: The regulatory role of macrophages in antigenic stimulation. Part two: symbiotic relationship between lymphocytes and macrophages. Advances in Immunology 31: 1–136, 1981

14. Moore KL, Bang NU, Broadie TA, Mattler LE, Marks CA: Peritoneal fibrinolysis: evidence for the efficiency of the tissue-type plasminogen activator. J Lab Clin Med 101: 921–929, 1983

15. Rotstein OD, Pruett TL, Simmons RL: Fibrin in peritonitis V. Fibrin inhibits phagocytic killing of Escherichia coli by human polymorphonuclear leukocytes. Ann Surg 203: 413–419, 1986

16. Freischlag J, Backstrom B, Kelly D, Busuttil RW: Blood and peritoneal neutrophil (PMN) adherence in rabbits: the effects of hemoglobin, peritoneal fluid and infection. J Surg Res 38: 635–640, 1985

17. Saba T: Effects of surgical trauma on the clearance and localization of blood-borne particulate matter. Surgery 71: 675–685, 1972

18. Richardson JD, De Camp MM, Garrison RN, Fry DE: Pulmonary infection complicating intra-abdominal sepsis. Ann Surg 195.6: 732–738, 1982

19. Tam PE, Hinsdill RD: Evaluation of immunomodulatory chemicals: alterations of macrophage function in vitro. Toxicology and Applied Pharmacology 76: 183–194, 1984

20. Onderdonk AB, Shapiro ME, Finberg RW, Zaleznik DF, Kasper DL: Use of a model of intraabdominal sepsis for studies of the pathogenecity of Bacteroides fragilis. Rev Inf Dis 6: (Suppl 1) S91–S95, 1984

21. Stevens LE, Clemmer TP, Laub RM, Miya F, Robbins L: Fibronectin in severe sepsis. Surg Gynecol Obstet 162: 222–228, 1986

22. Borgström S, Truedson H: Intraperitoneal drain in cholelithiasis operations. Acta Chir Scand (Suppl) 475: 1–23, 1977

23. Spivak JL: The surgical technique of abdominal operations. 4th ed. Springfield, Ill. CC Thomas 463, 1946

24. Hanna E: Efficiency of peritoneal drainage. Surg Gynecol Obstet 131: 983, 1970

25. Edlund G, Gedda S, Linden W van der: Intraperitoneal drains and nasogastric tubes in elective cholecystectomy. A controlled clinical trial. Am J Surg 137: 775–779, 1979

26. Gordon AB, Bates T, Fiddian RV: A controlled trial of drainage after cholecystectomy. Br J Surg 63: 278–282, 1976

27. Maull KI, Daugherty ME, Shearer GR, et al.: Cholecystectomy: to drain or not to drain. A randomized prospective study of 200 patients. J Surg Res 24: 259–263, 1978

28. Farha GJ, Chang FC, Matthews EH: Drainage in elective cholecystectomy. Am J Surg 142: 678–680, 1981

128

29. Budd DC, Cochran RC, Fouty Jr WJ: Cholecystectomy with and without drainage. A randomized prospective study of 300 patients. Am J Surg 143: 307–309, 1982
30. Elboim CM, Goldman L, Hann L, Palestrant AM, Silen W: Significance of post-cholecystectomy subhepatic fluid collections. Ann Surg 198: 137–141, 1983
31. Yanaya K, Kanematsu T, Takenaka K, Sugimachi K: Intraperitoneal septic complications after hepatectomy. Ann Surg 203: 148–152, 1986
32. Fortner JG, Kim DK, Maclean BJ, et al.: Major hepatic resection for neoplasia: personal experience in 108 patients. Ann Surg 188: 363–371, 1978
33. Thompson HH, Tompkins RK, Longmire Jr WP: Major hepatic resection. A 25-year experience. Ann Surg 197: 375–388, 1983
34. Kullendorff C-M, Zoucas E, Lindfeldt J, Holmin T: Excessive blood loss after standardized liver resection in rats with a denervated liver. World J Surg 8: 123–128, 1984

7. Trauma to the liver, pancreas and porta hepatis: aggressive and conservative management

J.M. LITTLE

Liver trauma

Background [1–13]

Each country has its own pattern of trauma and its own problems, and injuries encountered in civil practice differ from those of war. The mortality of knife and low velocity bullet wounds remains low – probably less than 5%. The wounds produced by shotguns and high velocity bullets are more commonly fatal, while blunt injury still carries a mortality of about 20% and has done so for 20 years or more. Nevertheless, there have been a number of real advances in the transport, reception, investigation and management of liver injuries and there is evidence that those who reach hospital now are more severely injured than those treated 10 years ago [13].

Investigations

Good quality organ imaging is readily available in most large hospitals. It remains more important, however, to suspect that the liver may be injured than it is to order imaging tests. A penetrating injury will generally be obvious, but the presence of multiple blunt injuries sustained in a motor vehicle accident may distract the clinician from recognising life threatening visceral damage. Unexplained shock must never be allowed to persist without considering the possibility of liver trauma.

There are very few investigations that must be available before a shocked patient is offered definitive treatment. Peritoneal lavage is helpful, particularly when the patient is unconscious or uncooperative and the clinical history and examination are unreliable. Lavage has a high degree of accuracy in pointing to visceral trauma, and probably outperforms organ imaging [14]. It may be contraindicated when many previous laparotomies have been carried out and when the patient is very young. It is unneccessary when a laparotomy is demanded on clinical grounds. The lavage technique and the interpretation of results have been well described by Simpson and Turner [15].

A coagulation screen should always be run when liver trauma is found or suspected. Coagulopathy (defined as more than 1.5 times prolongation of partial thromboplastin time and/or thrombin time, and/or platelet count less than 75,000 per cubic mm) has been shown by Little, Fernandes and Tait [13] to be a marker of fatal outcome. Its presence may dictate a more conservative approach at the time of surgery, perhaps with the use of temporary packing. Organ imaging is useful in patients with equivocal physical signs who are haemodynamically stable. The patient who is transferred with stable blood pressure from another hospital with a history of hypotension at the roadside or at the first hospital may be usefully investigated by scintiscanning, ultrasound or computerised tomography (CT). These tests are generally useful in only 20% of civil injuries in Australia [13].

Angiography has an even smaller place, although it is indispensable in the diagnosis of haemobilia. Furthermore, controlled embolisation of the damaged artery at the time of angiography provides the best treatment of traumatic haemobilia, replacing hepatic resection and hepatic artery ligation [16–18].

Biliary scanning with HIDA derivatives has recently been found useful for diagnosing biliary tract injury and biliary leaks after surgery for trauma [19]. Its place in management has yet to be defined. It will clearly seldom be used as a first-line investigation.

Problems of blunt injury

The great majority of injuries in many North American series is made up of penetrating injuries – either stab wounds or low velocity gunshots [2–7]. In areas of civil violence, penetrating injuries are common. Information from war zones is harder to obtain, and a clear picture of the mortality of war wounds to the liver is not currently available. A good account of the management of civilian bullet wounds has been given by Pachter and colleagues [20].

For surgeons in the majority of Western Countries, the major problem is blunt injury, usually resulting from motor vehicle accidents [1–13]. Sports injuries, industrial injuries and falls make up a varying percentage. From country to country and series to series, the mortality for blunt injuries is remarkably uniform at about 20%. About half these deaths are unrelated to the liver injury, and are caused predominantly by brain damage [8, 13]. Papers reporting better results seldom contain a stratification of patients according to severity of injury. A plea is entered for a consensus to be reached on a method of stratification [3, 13], so that valid comparisons can be made between the achievements of one institution and another.

About 80% of injuries can be managed by relatively simple means. In children, conservative management has achieved great success. Diagnosis is made either by ultrasound or CT, and subsequent management is determined by clinical observation and the results of repeated organ images. This subject has been well covered by Cooney [21]. An injury which has stopped bleeding at laparotomy can be safely left alone. A superficial crack or split can be left without drainage, but a deep cleft in the liver can be gently assessed with a finger and drained with a sump drain. Unless this is done, bile accumulation with pain, fever and infection are possible.

The temptation to insert deep liver stitches should be resisted. Closed cavities within the depths of the liver are likely to form, with subsequent haemobilia. Direct suture haemostasis, debridement of devitalised liver and adequate drainage provide a better regime of management than attempts to restore the liver contour.

Despite good agreement on the basics of injury management, several areas of controversy persist. These include 1) the place of hepatic resection, 2) hepatic artery ligation, 3) provision of bile duct drainage, 4) the management of hepatic venous injury, 5) the place of conservative management, and 6) the use of packing in management.

Hepatic resection

Formal hepatic resection carries a high mortality in the management of acute liver trauma [4]. This is hardly surprising, given the severity of associated injuries and the frequency of coagulation abnormalities. Debriding resection which removes liver tissue by developing the line of major splits is associated with a much lower mortality. Whichever technique is used, there must be a good reason to remove liver tissue. Sometimes dead liver can only be removed by cutting across live tissue. Removal of a liver lobe (usually the right) may offer the only access to an injury of the inferior vena cava of the major hepatic veins. Deep venous bleeding from the liver substance is sometimes (although rarely) accessible only after removal of liver tissue.

Exposure for this type of major surgery can be obtained by thoracic extension of a laparotomy through the sixth or seventh intercostal space [5]. Incisions made lower than this limit access to the dome of the right lobe and the vital area of entry of the hepatic veins into the vena cava. Access to the right atrium is excellent through this approach. Alternatively, excellent exposure can be gained by median sternotomy extension of a laparotomy incision. The morbidity of the sternotomy may be lower than that of the thoracoabdominal incision.

Whatever the approach and whatever the indications, the mortality associated with major removal of hepatic tissue remains at about 20% [4, 8], a reflection of the severity of injury which demands such radical surgery. The procedure is, however, relatively rarely indicated, and recent reports suggest that only about 10%–15% of patients with blunt injuries will need liver resection [4, 5, 13].

Hepatic artery ligation

The demonstration that hepatic artery ligation was well tolerated by humans was soon followed by a wave of enthusiasm for its use in hepatic trauma [3]. Surgeons who rarely saw major liver injuries began to believe that artery ligation was the answer to all their problems. In fact, most really difficult bleeding comes from the hepatic venous system and will not be controlled by arterial ligation. Only deep arterial bleeding will be controlled, and the technique seems to be applicable to about 3%–5% of all cases [2, 8, 13]. Selective ligation of the branch to the bleeding lobe is probably preferable to ligation of the proper hepatic artery. Occasionally, spreading necrosis of the hypoxic liver occurs, and death results. The few cases we have seen have occurred in patients with gross liver injury who have been severely shocked at one or more stages of their clinical course.

Hepatic artery embolisation will usually control post-traumatic haemobilia [16–18]. The major contraindication to its use would seem to be intra- or perihepatic sepsis [18]. Reviews of this subject are available in Sandblom and colleagues [17], Curet and colleagues [16] and Richardson and colleagues [18].

Biliary drainage

Biliary drainage was originally proposed as a way of preventing bile leakage after deep liver injury. Physiologically, bile duct drainage cannot lower peripheral bile ductular pressure and cannot prevent bile extravasation. Further, Lucas and Walt [22] have shown that bile duct drainage has been associated with an unduly high incidence of gastroduodenal haemorrhage, local sepsis and main duct leakage. T-tube drainage of the common duct has therefore fallen from favour. Cholecystostomy drainage has not been found to have the same complication rate, and may still have a place under certain circumstances. When a major, deep injury has been dealt with and there is a possibility of late haemobilia, the placement of a cholecystostomy tube is unlikely to do harm and may provide an early warning of bleeding into the biliary tree [8].

Venous injury

Injury to the main hepatic veins and the retrohepatic vena cava still carries a mortality of 50%–75% [23, 24]. In those countries where penetrating injury is common, through-and-through injuries of the inferior vena cava are seen. Where blunt injury is the rule, anterior tears due to avulsion of one of the main hepatic veins (usually the right) is more usual. Blood loss in either injury is likely to be massive, and mortality is correspondingly high. Different techniques are applicable to the management of the different types of injury.

Through-and-through injuries can only be managed by one or other form of vascular isolation of the liver. The technique described by Schrock and colleagues [23] has been widely used. Right atrial cannulation of the inferior vena cava and clamping of the portal triad allow right lobectomy and direct caval repair. Even in the most expert hands, the mortality is high (13 of 18 cases in the series of Kudsk, Sheldon and Lim [24]).

Avulsion injuries of the hepatic veins occur within the liver or at the insertion of the veins into the vena cava. The former can at times be managed by extending rents in the liver to gain access to the region of venous damage [25]. Partial avulsion of segments VII and VIII with tearing of the upper branch of the right hepatic vein is reasonably common in Australian experience. This injury can be dealt with by debriding resection of parts of segment VII and VIII and directly suturing the point of venous tearing. When the main right hepatic vein is avulsed from the vena cava, rapid right lobectomy and direct caval repair allows the salvage of some patients (5 of 13 patients in our own experience). It is clear that major venous injury remains an unsolved problem in the acute phase of liver injury.

Conservative management

The success of non-operative management in children is unquestioned [21]. Its applicability to adults has been more slowly recognised [26–30]. Organ imaging has allowed the accurate identification of injuries in haemodynamically stable adults. The area of damage can be followed by repeated imaging. If resolution occurs (as is usual), there is no indication for surgery. An enlarging collection may require angiography and/or endoscopic retrograde cholangiography to elucidate its nature. Appropriate surgery, arterial occlusion or percutaneous drainage can then be used. It must be stressed that conservative management does not represent an easy way to manage liver trauma. Each patient requires close monitoring, frequently in an intensive care ward. There must be excellent organ imaging facilities. Above all, there must be surgical services available to deal with complications at short notice. Subcapsular and intrahepatic haematomas may still rupture, posing demanding surgical problems that will tax the expertise of the most experienced hepatic surgeon.

Recent studies [13] suggest that 25%–30% of adult patients sustaining blunt injury can be managed without surgery. The increasing interest in non-operative management reflects the impact of good organ imaging, which diagnoses liver injury that would once have been missed and managed without operation anyway. While it is laudable to avoid operation when possible, it is most unlikely that conservatism will change the intrinsic mortality of liver injury. Death from 'unneccessary' laparotomy amongst these patients has been shown to be rare [13].

Packing

Packing of the liver was once a standard method of management of liver trauma. It fell into disfavour during the Second World War largely because of the vigorous opposition of Madding [31], who felt that packing led to more sepsis, poor drainage and more liver necrosis. There has been a revival in interest in recent years because the technique will allow temporary control of otherwise uncontrollable bleeding, particularly when coagulopathy is present and when a major liver injury is encountered in a hospital not equipped to deal with it [32–34].

When packing is employed, laparotomy sponges are generally used, and are packed around the liver, not into the depths of rents and tears. As many sponges should be used as are needed to control the bleeding; this may mean that 10–12 sponges are inserted. Transfer of the patient to a centre equipped to deal definitively with the injury should proceed as soon as the patient is stable. The period of control of bleeding should be used to administer coagulation factors and platelets to correct the coagulopathy.

When many packs are used in this way, problems arise with venous obstruction and possibly with pressure necrosis of the liver. We have observed venous engorgement of the lower half of the body, and tachycardia, low renal output and high fever are common. It is thus evident that packs should be removed as soon as blood coagulation has improved. They should be removed in the operating theatres by a surgeon prepared to proceed with definitive treatment [13, 34]. Gross liver swelling is common, and may make the liver bulky, friable and very difficult to handle. Nevertheless, Little and colleagues have recently reported the survival of 4 of 6 patients treated by packing in their hospital when all other methods of haemostasis had failed, and of 6 of 7 patients transferred to their care with massive liver injury from metropolitan or country hospitals.

Postoperative management [35]

Patients with severe liver injuries should be managed after operation in an Intensive Care Unit. Most will need respirator support, since respiratory distress syndrome is common. Major injury and shock cause widespread centrilobular necrosis of liver tissue, with varying degrees of hepatic functional impairment.

Coagulation disturbances may persist or become more severe, and infusions of factors II, VII, IX and X together with platelets may be needed for many days. Serum albumin falls, but is usually easily replaced. Total parenteral nutrition is commonly used, and vitamin K supplements are routinely added.

A resistant and dangerous hypoglycaemia may develop after major liver injury. While this is seldom seen after elective resection for tumour, it is common after surgery for major trauma. It can develop rapidly and produce fatal brain damage. Glucose infusions should be maintained at all times until liver function has recovered. TPN solutions will provide adequate glucose to support blood levels, but until TPN has started it is vital to ensure that intravenous dextrose runs continuously.

Pancreatic trauma

Epidemiology

Pancreatic injury is not common, being seen most often in those parts of the world where penetrating injury from knife and gunshot wounds are frequent. North American reports dominate the recent literature [36–43], and there has been considerable experience with the problem in Northern Ireland [44]. Reports from other countries tend to emphasize the importance of blunt trauma [45–47], usually secondary to motor vehicle accidents. The seat belt is well recognised as an injuring agent [46], the lap section of the belt compressing the pancreas against the spine in sudden deceleration injuries.

The intimate anatomical relationship between the duodenum and pancreas implies that the duodenum will commonly be damaged by trauma that affects the pancreas. Concurrent duodenal trauma has a profound impact on the outcome of injury, and it is necessary to consider both organs together.

Stratification of severity

It is well recognised that pancreatic duct disruption, massive parenchymal damage and associated duodenal injury are all important local factors determining the outcome of pancreatic trauma [36, 41]. Diagnosis of ductal damage is so important that Berni and colleagues [39] have advocated intraoperative pancreatography as a routine part of the assessment of severe pancreatic injury.

Various stratification systems are available which rank the severity of pancreatic trauma. None are entirely satisfactory because all rely on surgical judgement of the depth of pancreatic disruption and on the subjective impression of how 'massive' the trauma is.

The system proposed by Lucas [48] is perhaps the most widely used. Class I injuries of the pancreas are represented by capsular tears or contusions; those of the duodenum by serosal lacerations or intramural haematomas. Class II pancreatic injuries are those with disruption or laceration of the body or tail with duct damage; class II duodenal injuries are those in which the duodenum has been perforated. In class III pancreatic injury, there is severe disruption of the head and/or body of the gland; class III duodenal injuries are class I or II with associated pancreatic trauma of class I-III. Class IV injuries are severe combined pancreatic and duodenal disruptions, pancreatic trauma, rather than that of combined injuries. Although it is more unwieldy, Lucas's stratification system has much to recommend it.

Treatment repertoire

There is still no totally reliable diagnostic test which whill diagnose pancreatic injury. Elevation of serum amylase may occur in about 70% of blunt injuries, but in a lower proportion of penetrating wounds [37–45]. Exploration of major penetrating wounds should include mobilisation of the pancreatic head and wide opening of the lesser sac for thorough examination of the pancreas. Upper abdominal retroperitoneal haematoma should prompt complete exploration of the pancreas. If there is doubt about the presence of ductal damage, intraoperative pancreatography is helpful [39].

There is much difference of opinion in the literature on the subject of the surgical treatment of pancreaticoduodenal injuries, suggesting that the optimal methods have yet to be defined. A recent trend towards conservative surgery is evident. Splenic conservation is seen as worthwhile [49] since it avoids the infective risks of splenectomy. A significant incidence of diabetes follows extensive pancreatic resection (more than 80% of the gland) [36], and methods of pancreatic conservation have found favour in the last few years [40, 42, 43]. A helpful summary of current thinking is to be found in the paper by Wynn and colleagues [42].

There is general agreement that Class I pancreatic and duodenal injuries can be well managed by drainage alone [36, 38, 40, 42, 43]. Class II pancreatic injuries, with duct disruption in the body or tail of the gland can be managed by distal pancreatectomy or by Roux loop drainage of the distal segment of the gland or both proximal and distal segments. Jones [43], however, has pointed to the high morbidity associated with the Roux loop, and has recently reported that the technique is no longer used in his own hospital. It may still find a place from time to time when 80% or more of the gland would need resection because of a pancreatic laceration to the right of the superior mesenteric vessels. Class II duodenal injuries with complete localised perforation are well managed by serosal patching, employing either an intact loop or a Roux loop to cover the defect.

In complex class III and IV injuries of the duodenum and pancreas, subtotal pancreatic resection (neck, body and tail) or pancreaticoduodenectomy (partial or total) may be necessary, but the mortality is very high. For this reason, there has been a recent surge of interest in duodenal diverticulization [50] and the simpler technique of pyloric exclusion and gastrojejunostomy [51] which does not require gastric resection. These techniques concentrate on diverting gastric contents from the duodenum, permitting healing of damaged duodenum. Satisfactory results have been reported by groups using these more conservative methods [38, 40, 42, 43].

A technique of onlay patching with the open end of a Roux loop was reported by Campbell and Kennedy [44] as a means of managing some major combined injuries of the pancreas and duodenum. Jones [43] has reported a very high morbidity with onlay loops and has abandoned their use.

Pancreatic fistula, bleeding and sepsis are all common complications after pancreaticoduodenal trauma. The prolonged and complex postoperative course is probably best supported by total parenteral nutrition [42, 49] or enteral feeding by catheter jejunostomy [40].

Mortality

The mortality from combined pancreaticoduodenal injuries remains about 20%. The mortality of pancreatic injury alone or duodenal injury alone is low. Unfortunately, other injuries are common in association with pancreaticoduodenal trauma. Cogbill and colleagues [38] reported associated intraabdominal injuries in 98% of their patients with pancreatic trauma. Retroperitoneal vascular injury, in particular, poses technical and physiological problems that may be insurmountable. Major vascular injury may be seen in 25% of pancreatic injuries [38].

In the report from Wynn and colleagues [42], there was no mortality among patients sustaining class I pancreatic or duodenal injuries. 8% of those sustaining class II pancreatic injuries died as did 20% of those with class II duodenal injuries. The mortality was 16% for class III pancreatic injuries and 20% for class III duodenal trauma. All patients sustaining class IV trauma died.

Injuries to the porta hepatis

Epidemiology

Injuries to the structures in the porta hepatis are rare. About 90% are caused by penetrating trauma in North American series [52, 53]. The gall bladder was found to have been injured in 3% of laparotomies for trauma in one series [54].

The gall bladder is injured at least three times as often as the other portal structures [53, 54]. Injuries to the porta hepatis are nearly always associated with trauma to other organs. Sheldon and colleagues [52] noted a mean of 3.6 other organ injuries in each one of their series of patients.

Anatomical classification

The gall bladder, hepatic artery, bile ducts and portal vein may be injured individually or in combination. Portal vein injury is associated with the highest mortality [52], while duct injury is associated with a high morbidity, particularly if it is missed at the original laparotomy. Ivatury and colleagues [53] stress the importance of exploration of haematomas around the bile duct.

Treatment repertoire

Injury to the gall bladder is usually relatively easy to manage. Simple lacerations can be repaired; more complex damage can be managed by cholecystectomy [53, 54].

Hepatic artery injuries should be repaired if possible by vascular suture or graft. If this proves impossible, ligation appears to be safe [52].

Bile duct injuries need to be identified and repaired at once if long-term morbidity is to be avoided. Gartman and others [55] have advocated the use of HIDA scanning for the investigation of complex liver injuries in order to detect biliary damage. Accurate repair of tangential lacerations over a T-tube will usually suffice [53, 54]. Choledochoenterostomy will be required for more complex injuries.

Tangential lacerations to the portal vein should be repaired by accurate suture, using standard techniques of vascular isolation. More extensive injuries, such as those caused by bullet wounds, should ideally be managed by vascular grafting, using autogenous material such as splenic vein [52]. Sheldon and colleagues [52] make the point, however, that other vascular injuries may make the physiological and anatomical situations so unfavourable that compromises must be made and portal vein ligation considered if the hepatic artery is intact. Ligation is associated with some risk of portal hypertension, and is considered to demand second look procedures to check that gut ischaemia does not develop.

Results of management

Injuries to the porta hepatis carry a very high mortality. Sheldon and colleagues [52] reported that 35% of their patients died. They excluded gall bladder injuries – the most favourable and the commonest of such injuries – from consideration. Ivatury and others [53] considered only injuries to the biliary tree, including the gall bladder, and reported a mortality of 22%. These high death rates reflect the frequency of other injuries, particularly major vascular damage, and emphasise the need for vascular skills among surgeons who may have to deal with this kind of trauma.

References

1. Thomas DG, Wright JE: Ruptured liver. Aust N Z J Surg 37: 338–44, 1968
2. Lucas CE, Ledgerwood AM: Prospective evaluation of hemostatic techniques for liver injuries. J Trauma 16: 442–51, 1976
3. Flint LM, Mays ET, Aaron WS, Fulton RL, Polk HC: Selectivity in the management of hepatic trauma. Ann Surg 185: 613–18, 1977
4. Levin A, Gover P, Nance FC: Surgical restraint in the management of hepatic injury: a review of Charity Hospital experience. J Trauma 18: 399–404, 1978
5. Walt AJ: The mythology of hepatic trauma- or Babel revisited. Am J Surg 135: 12–18, 1978
6. Aldrete JS, Halpern NB, Ward S, Wright JO: Factors determining the mortality and morbidity in hepatic injuries: analysis of 108 cases. Ann Surg 189: 466–474, 1979
7. Elerding SC, Moore EE: Recent experience with trauma of the liver. Surg Gynec Obstet 150: 853–55, 1980
8. Little JM, Fleischer G: Liver injuries in Sydney: a 20 year experience. Aust N Z J Surg 50: 495–502, 1980
9. Hasselgren PO, Almersjo O, Gustavsson B, Seeman T: Trauma to the liver during a ten-year period. With special reference to the morbidity and mortality after blunt trauma and stab wounds. Acta Chir Scand 147: 387–93, 1981
10. Carmona RH, Lim RC, Clark GC: Morbidity and mortality in hepatic trauma: a 5 year study. Am J Surg 144: 88–94, 1982
11. Thomas EJ: Major liver trauma. Canad J Surg 26: 27–30, 1983
12. Hanna SS, Maheshwari Y, Harrison AW, Taylor GA, Miller HAB, Maggisano R: Blunt liver trauma at the Sunnybrook Regional Trauma Unit. Canad J Surg 28: 220–23, 1985
13. Little JM, Fernandes A, Tait N: Liver trauma. Aust N Z J Surg 56: 613–20, 1986
14. Marx JA, Moore EE, Jorden RC, Eule J: Limitations of computed tomography in the evaluation of acute abdominal trauma: a prospective comparison with diagnostic peritoneal lavage. J Trauma 25: 933–37, 1985
15. Simpson RL, Turner VF: Diagnostic, percutaneous peritoneal lavage in blunt abdominal trauma: rationale, technique and results. Aust N Z J Surg 56: 103–108, 1986
16. Curet P, Baumer R, Roche A, Grellet J, Mercadier M: Hepatic hemobilia of traumatic or iatrogenic origin: recent advances in diagnosis and therapy, review of the literature from 1976 to 1981. World J Surg 8: 2–8, 1984
17. Sandblom P, Saegesser F, Mirkovitch V: Hepatic hemobilia: hemorrhage from the intrahepatic biliary tract, a review. World J Surg 8: 41–50, 1984
18. Richardson A, Simmons K, Gutmann J, Little JM: Hepatic haemobilia: non-operative management in eight cases. Aust N Z J Surg 55: 447–52, 1985
19. Gartman DM, Zeman RK, Cahow CE, Baker CC: An evaluation of hepatobiliary scanning in complex liver trauma. J Trauma 25: 887–91, 1985
20. Pachter HL, Spencer FC, Hofstetter SR, Coppa GF: Experience with the finger fracture technique to achieve intra-hepatic hemostasis in 75 patients with severe injuries to the liver. Ann Surg 197: 771–78, 1983

21. Cooney DR: Splenic and hepatic trauma in children. Surg Clin N Amer 61: 1165–80, 1981
22. Lucas CE, Walt AJ: Critical decisions in liver trauma. Arch Surg 101: 277–83, 1970
23. Schrock T, Blaisdell FW, Mathewson Jr C: Management of blunt trauma to the liver and hepatic veins. Arch Surg 96: 698–704, 1968
24. Kudsk KA, Sheldon GF, Lim Jr RC: Atrial-caval shunting (ACS) after trauma. J Trauma 22; 81–5, 1982
25. Hanna WA, Wisheart JD: Management of hilar injury to the liver. J Roy Coll Surg Edinb 14: 328–32, 1964
26. Cheatham JE, Smith EI, Tunell WP, Elkins RC: Non operative management of subcapsular hematomas of the liver. Amer J Surg 140: 852–7, 1980
27. Geis WP, Schulz KA, Giacchino JL, Freeark RJ: The fate of unruptured intrahepatic hematomas. Surgery 90: 689–97, 1981
28. Lutzker LG, Chun KJ: Radionuclide imaging in the nonsurgical treatment of liver and spleen trauma. J Trauma 21: 382–7, 1981
29. Athey GN, Rahman SU: Hepatic hematoma following blunt injury: non-operative management. Injury 13: 302–306, 1982
30. Meyer HA, Crass RA, Lim RC, Jeffrey RB, Federle MP, Trunkey DD: Selective nonoperative management of blunt liver injury using computed tomography. Arch Surg 120: 550–4, 1985
31. Madding GF, Kennedy PA: Trauma to the liver. 2nd edition WB Saunders Co, Philadelphia, London, Toronto, 1971, p 85
32. Feliciano DV, Mattox KL, Jordan Jr GL: Intra abdominal packing for control of hepatic hemorrhage; a reappraisal. J Trauma 21: 285–90, 1981
33. Calne RY, McMaster P, Pentlow BD: The treatment of major liver trauma by primary packing with transfer of the patient for definitive treatment. Brit J Surg 66: 338–39, 1979
34. Svoboda JA, Peter ET, Dang CV, Parks SN, Ellyson JM: Severe liver trauma in the face of coagulopathy: the case for temporary packing and early re-exploration. Amer J Surg 144: 717–21, 1982
35. Lim RC, Giuliano AE, Trunkey DD: Postoperative treatment of patients after liver resection for trauma. Arch Surg 112: 429–35, 1977
36. Karl HW, Chandler JG: Mortality and morbidity of pancreatic injury. Amer J Surg 134: 549–54, 1977
37. Jones RC: Management of pancreatic trauma. Ann Surg 187: 555–64, 1978
38. Cogbill TH, Moore EE, Kashuk JL: Changing trends in the management of pancreatic trauma. Arch Surg 117: 722–8, 1982
39. Berni GA, Bandyk DF, Oreskovich MR, Carrico CJ: Role of intraoperative pancreatography in patients with injury to the pancreas. Amer J Surg 143: 602–05, 1982
40. Moore JB, Moore EE: Changing trends in the management of combined pancreatoduodenal injuries. World J Surg 8: 791–7, 1984
41. Smego DR, Richardson D, Flint LM: Determinants of outcome in pancreatic trauma. J Trauma 25: 771–6, 1985
42. Wynn M, Hill DM, Miller DR, Waxman K, Eisner ME, Gazzaniga AB: Management of pancreatic and duodenal trauma. Amer J Surg 150: 327–32, 1985
43. Jones RC: Management of pancreatic trauma. Amer J Surg 150: 698–704, 1985
44. Campbell R, Kennedy T: The management of pancreatic and pancreaticoduodenal injuries Br J Surg 67: 845–50, 1980
45. Heyse-Moore GH: Blunt pancreatic and pancreaticoduodenal trauma. Br J Surg 63: 226–8, 1976
46. Balasegaram M: Surgical management of pancreatic trauma, in Current Problems. In: Surgery XVI, Year Book Medical Publishers. Chicago, 1979

47. Lempinen M: Management of major abdominal trauma: pancreas. In: Carter D, Polk Jr HC (eds) Trauma. Butterworths, London, Boston, Sydney, Wellington, Durban, Toronto, 1981, pp 117–128

48. Lucas CE: Diagnosis and treatment of pancreatic and duodenal injuries. Surg Clin N Amer 57: 49–65, 1977

49. Robey E, Mullen JT, Schwab CW: Blunt transection of the pancreas treated by distal pancreatectomy, splenic salvage and hyperalimentation. Four cases and a review of the literature. Ann Surg 196: 695–699, 1982

50. Berne CJ, Donovan AJ, White HJ, Yellin RE: Duodenal 'diverticulization' for duodenal and pancreatic injury. Amer J Surg 127: 503–7, 1974

51. Vaughan GD, Frazier OH, Graham DY, Mattox KL, Petmecky FF, Jordan GL: The use of pyloric exclusion in the management of severe duodenal injuries. Amer J Surg 134: 785–90, 1977

52. Sheldon GF, Lim RC, Yee ES, Petersen SR: Management of injuries to the porta hepatis. Ann Surg 202: 539–45, 1985

53. Ivatury RR, Rohman M, Nallathambi M, Rao PM, Gunduz Y, Stahl WM: The morbidity of injuries to the extra-hepatic biliary system. J Trauma 25: 967–73, 1985

54. Posner MC, Moore EE: Extrahepatic biliary tract injury: operative management plan. J Trauma 25: 833–7, 1985

55. Gartman DM, Zeman RK, Cahow CE, Baker CC: The value of hepatobiliary scanning in complex liver trauma. J Trauma 25: 887–91, 1985

8. Does the ultrasonic dissector improve the quality of hepato-pancreatico-biliary (HPB) surgery?

W.J.B. HODGSON, M. KEMENY, J. SCHEELE and K.G. TRANBERG

The ultrasonic dissector was first used experimentally in 1978 and found to be useful in the animal model in hepatic resections and splenic transections. It was also interesting in pancreatic aspiration [1]. It was disappointing when tried in the fibrotic pancreas in the patient but it was a different story in hepatic surgery and in 1979 the first clinical paper was published [2].

In order to answer the question as to whether or not the ultrasonic dissector improves the quality of HPB surgery, it is first necessary to define the state of the art prior to the introduction of this device and then to attempt to show the place of the ultrasonic dissector and compare it with its rivals. The chapter will then concentrate on a discussion of the track record of this method.

Essentially, until very recently, most surgeons in the West had only rudimentary experience with the liver and were taught the 19th Century technique of Kousnetzoff and Pensky [3] and Auvray [4] which was the blunt technique of passing mattress sutures through the liver to control bleeding but taking no account of the anatomy of the organ during this procedure. Keen [5] at the turn of the Century, did try to develop a pedicle in which the blood vessels could be controlled but Sir Heneage Ogilvie [6] in 1951 described the method of cutting bluntly through the liver tissue with a hemostat which allowed surgeons to more accurately define this pedicle. Finger fracture was then introduced in 1958 by Lin *et al.* [7] and this technique was a rapid method of getting through the hepatic parenchyma down to the major vessels. However, it also had the major disadvantage of tearing many major vessels as well, but if the Pringle maneuver [8], introduced in 1908 was used, where the hilar vessels were compressed, at least inflow bleeding could be kept under some control. Lin recognized this problem and introduced his clamp [9] to also reduce blood loss from the draining veins in 1973. Although this and other variants are used widely in Asia, it has not generally been accepted in the West where the relatively bloody finger fracture technique, or digitoclasia, has continued to be used in association with placement of heavy mattress sutures. Indeed, even when liver clamps are used, control of bleeding is still achieved by the placement of heavy interlocking mattress sutures before the clamp is removed. These techniques do involve a great deal of surgical skill if the patient is not to be lost on the operating room table and as a consequence, very few centers have attempted to perform large numbers of liver resections. Nonetheless, these techniques did allow major advances in liver surgery to occur in the 1970's [10–12]. Such success could not have occurred without the clinical application of hepatic anatomy which particularly took place in Japan, France and America, commencing perhaps first with Honjo and Araki [13] who probably performed their first resection in 1952 but did not publish until 1955. Lortat-Jacob and Robert [14] also carried out preliminary hilar ligation and did a lobectomy based on vascular anatomy in 1952. In America, Pack and Baker [15] used the same technique. Quattlebaum [16] used the back of a knife to carefully break open the parenchyma for his dissections. Early resections by Brunchwig [17] resulted in a mortality of 30%. Lesser mortals were frightened off and only in the 1980's has interest begun to resurface. On the other hand, our Asian colleagues were quietly increasing their experience and soon developed the largest worldwide series [9, 18–21].

In terms of technique, Starzl has contributed much; first by defining the right trisegmentectomy in 1975 with only a minimal morbidity, and then in 1982 he defined the left trisegmentectomy [22, 23]. However, this work would not have been possible without Couinaud's demonstration in 1950 of the eight hepatic segments [24]. Bismuth [25] has been to the fore in applying this knowledge clinically.

Those experienced surgeons who are comfortable with their own methods for hepatic tumor resection, do not need a new approach. They are too few in number to perform the thousands of operations required every year if all resectable cases of hepatic cancer, primary or secondary, were referred. Therefore, we have arrived at the situation where hepatic anatomy has been defined, but the majority of surgeons in practice today have not had the tools to apply this knowledge.

The first surgical tool which allowed the surgeon to find hepatic vessels before they were lacerated was the ultrasonic dissector. This instrument skeletonizes hepatic vessels by removing mesenchymal tissue from them in a controlled manner and the surgeon is able to see and feel the difference. The dissector has a free-standing control and power console and has a separate gas sterilizable lightweight handpiece. The power console simply uses regular operating room electricity and is self-contained (Fig. 1). A 15 foot disposable cable is attached to the handpiece which is designed like a pencil grip (Fig. 2). This contains a magneto-strictive transducer placed in an electric coil. Therefore, when an alternating current is passed through this coil, the transducer oscillates longitudinally at 23 kHz. These oscillations then pass through the connecting body to a hollow conical titanium tip which acts as an amplifier. At a

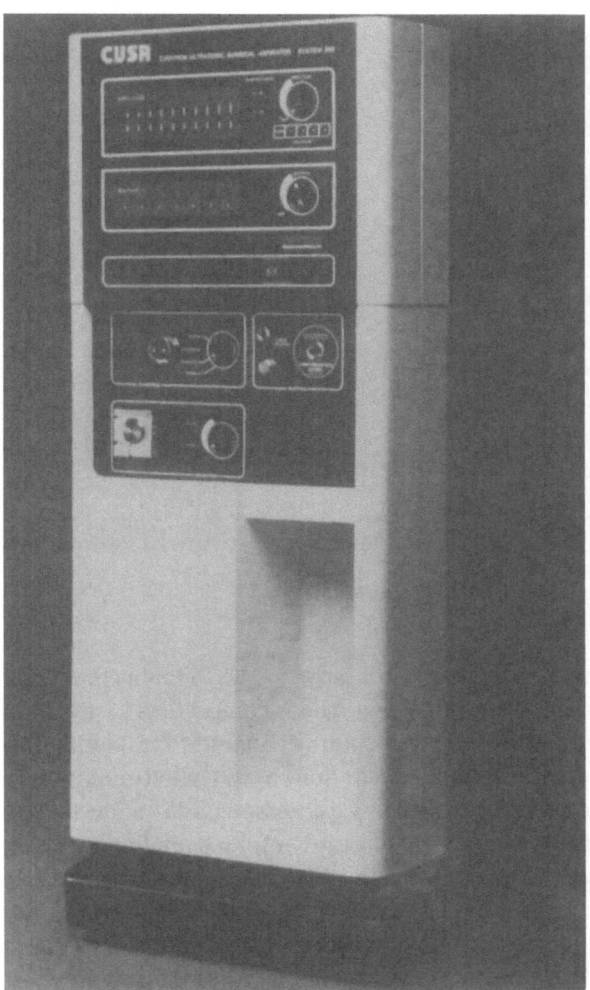

Fig. 1. Ultrasonic dissector.

maximum power of about 100 watts, the excursion of the tip is up to 300 microns. Heat is developed by this process within the handpiece and therefore cooling water must be run around the magneto-strictive transducer through a stainless steel jacket. There is a separate stream of saline solution irrigation which runs under a plastic flue surrounding the tip except at its very end and this helps to remove the fragmented tissue from the operative site. The plastic flue also protects the tissues from undue contact with the handpiece.

The mechanism of action is that when the exposed tip contacts target tissue, cavitation occurs with the resultant implosion and fragmentation. Cavitation

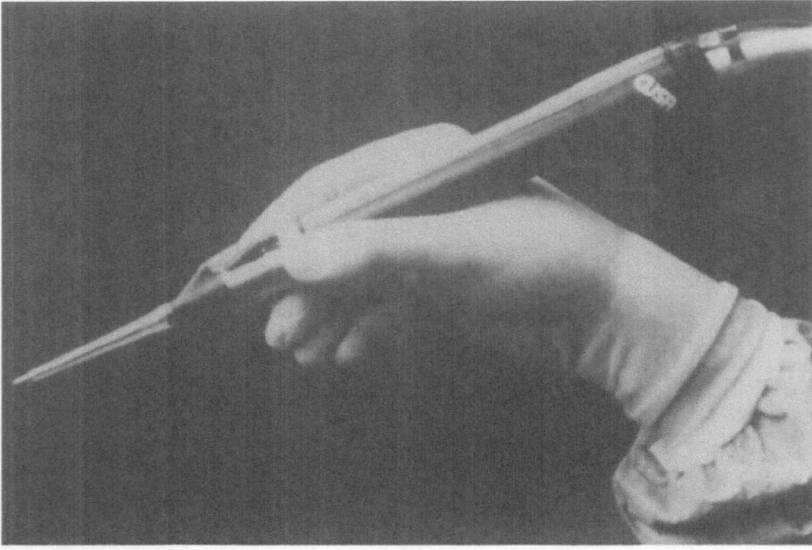

Fig. 2. Handpiece from the ultrasonic dissector.

may be explained as an inability of target tissue to follow the oscillation of the ultrasonic tip. This is because the tissue is compressed by the outward move-ment of the tip but is, due to its inertia, unable to follow the backward os-cillation. An 'empty' volume (cavitation cavity) with (initially) very low pres-sure is thus created, which allows gas dissolved in tissue to diffuse from a dissolved to a gaseous state. During the continued oscillation, all gas in the gas-eous state cannot return to gas in the dissolved state. This means that there is a net transport of gas to the gaseous state. This is likely to occur also intra-cellularly near the tip and to contribute to tissue disruption by the formation of gaseous bubble ruptures. Whatever the mechanism of action, blood vessels and bile ducts can be dissected out because fragmentation is proportional to the water content of the tissue in that the greater the water content, the easier it is for fragmentation to occur. Tissue with a high collagen and elastin content appear to be more resistant to fragmentation and it may be that they yield somewhat to the vibrations.

When the power is reduced, the total stroke of the tip is also reduced and therefore less tissue is fragmented and so the instrument can be used in various situations and organs which require different power ranges. After the tissue has been fragmented, the irrigating saline suspends the fragments which are then aspirated from the operative field leaving a clear view. Because blood vessels have a high collagen and elastic tissue content, it is relatively easy to spare them and the surgeon can run the tip of the dissector alongside many of these vessels and feel them during the course of dissection and avoid direct injury to them.

Histological studies indicate that the depth of cell damage used in the ultrasonic dissector is in the same range as that caused using an ordinary steel scalpel [26, 27]. Damage is therefore far less than that caused by the cautery or laser. The final appearance of the cut liver is of a smooth almost glossy surface and histologically red cells appear to adhere as a coating to the surface [26, 27].

In a recent study on liver resection in dogs, an ultrasonic dissector (CUSA system) was compared with the Nd-YAG laser and the standard blunt dissection technique. The caudal halves of the two left lobes of the liver were resected with each technique in eight dogs. The CUSA and the YAG laser reduced the operation time, with the laser being the faster of the two. Blood loss was not significantly reduced, but there was a clear tendency towards a decrease in bleeding with increasing familiarity with the two new modalities. The ultrasonic dissector caused significantly less tissue damage on light and electromicroscopic examination than the other two methods, and this finding agreed well with the incidence of bacterial infection. Although not quantifiable, a real advantage with the ultrasonic dissector was a clear visualization of vessels and bile ducts, which gave a better control and safer resection and no unforeseen major hemorrhage [28]. Other investigators have reported the same experience [29, 30].

The Nd-YAG laser has a considerable ability to cut and coagulate tissues simultaneously but its use has so far been limited because it causes more tissue damage than other methods and because it is expensive. The recent development of the contact YAG laser scalpel, using sapphire rods, may change the situation because contact method apparently causes little, and controlled, tissue necrosis with preserved cutting and coagulating properties [31]. However, it is very difficult to translate the results of surgery in the rat to the patient.

Another alternative, which has not yet been compared directly, is the microwave tissue coagulator which appears to reduce bleeding and may be especially helpful in the cirrhotic liver [32]. Cryoresection [33] has also been tried but does not appear to have been generally accepted.

At present there are three ultrasonic dissectors on the market: The Cavitron Ultrasonic Surgical Aspirator (CUSA System, Cooper Medical Corp., Moutainview California), Sonotec (Sumitomo Bakelite Co., Tokyo) and Sonocut (Comair Co., Stockholm). Ultrasonic vibration is generated in a magnetostrictive transducer in the CUSA system. The other two machines utilize electro-strictive transducers (piezoceramics), which means that the degree of efficiency is higher. In Sweden, Tranberg tested all three brands and found their performance and ease of handling to be essentially identical. The irrigation fluid is led through a separate cannula in the Sonotec and Sonocut and through a plastic mantle covering the tip in the CUSA system. The latter arrangement is somewhat more convenient because it avoids the 'foaming' that otherwise appears at high irrigation rates. However, foaming is not a problem with any brand of ultrasonic dissector in liver resection. The major advantages with the Sonocut are that its cost is less than half that of the other two machines (it is also available in a 'stripped' version, with a simpler irrigation system and no in-built suction, thus reducing costs by a further 40%) and the other improvement is that the handpiece can be sterilized in an ordinary autoclave at 120 degrees C. Nonetheless, the CUSA system has been in use for the longest period of time and has been demonstrated to be reliable and almost indestructable. The cheaper units may not have this advantage. Further, the CUSA system is also available in a stripped, cheaper, tabletop version.

The ultrasonic dissector is a totally different instrument to anything else previously used by surgeons and this must be recognized. It cannot be simply picked up and used and the method employed by neurosurgeons is not the technique which must be used by general surgeons. Mastery of the technique is rapid for most surgeons provided a laboratory session is first attended or a surgeon already using the technique can be watched in the operating room.

Surgical technique

Hodgson uses the ultrasonic dissector after first of all mobilizing the liver and visualizing the inferior vena cava, much after the method of Schwartz [34]. For right-sided tumors, hepatocaval veins are serially clamped, divided and tied from below upwards and large veins are left intact. Sometimes the dorsal hepatic vein can be as large as a centimeter in size and it is preferable in these cases to oversew the vein rather than to tie it off. Therefore it is easier to leave it until later in the procedure. The same thing applies to the right hepatic vein or even the left hepatic vein. Since only about 40% of these veins are extrahepatic [35], it has not been Hodgson's practice to clamp them prior to division of the liver. However, they are visualized beforehand whenever possible.

The next step is to carry out a dissection of the porta hepatis and to isolate and ligate the appropriate hepatic arterial branch. This is usually done by blunt dissection with a right angle clamp and peanut but occasionally the ultrasonic dissector has been used to carry out this portion of the dissection according to the technique described by Putnam [30]. The gallbladder is normally taken at this stage of the procedure as it is a useful way of tracing the cystic duct down to the common duct and also providing traction during exposure of the portal vein. After the appropriate portal vein branch has been isolated, heavy ties are applied and then the vein is clamped, divided and tied again and also suture ligated. Finally, the appropriate hepatic duct is clamped, divided and tied.

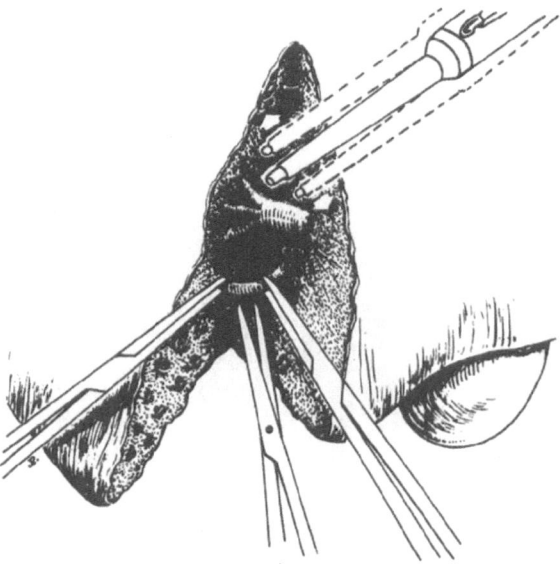

Fig. 3. Use of ultrasonic dissector during deep dissection of the liver showing lateral sweeping motion clearing mesenchymal tissue from blood vessels which can then be clamped, cut and sutured (Reprinted from Surgery 1984; 95: 230 with permission).

At this point the Bovie is used to score the surface of the liver from front to back to indicate the plane of dissection. The Bovie can also be used to divide the first centimeter of liver without fear of significant bleeding although sometimes it is quite useful to use the ultrasonic tip to dissect out the vessels first using a side to side motion so that these vessels can then be cauterized (Fig. 3). It is best to use clips in the slightly larger vessels for speed but anything over 2 mm in size should really be tied off. #3–0 silk is a safe way of doing this. Essentially, the surgeon who is using the ultrasonic dissector stands on the side of the patient from which the lobe of the liver is to be removed. The surgeon then takes the lobe in the left hand and exerts an upward and outward pressure which puts the anterior surface of the liver slightly on the stretch. This then allows mesenchymal tissue to be easily removed and using a combination of vision and tactile sensation, veins can be dissected out and cleared of mesenchymal tissue (Fig. 4) before being isolated, clamped, divided and tied. The operation is tedious, but safe and occasional uncontrolled bleeding points can be dealt with with a #3–0 silk figure of eight suture but a #0 vicryl suture is also used from time to time where necessary. Using this technique, there should be no blood loss at all unless a vein is violated. Even then, it is sometimes possible to quickly dissect alongside the vein with the ultrasonic dissector in order to find where the hole is in the vein and then to repair this hole. The last portion of the procedure is to complete the removal of the mesenchymal

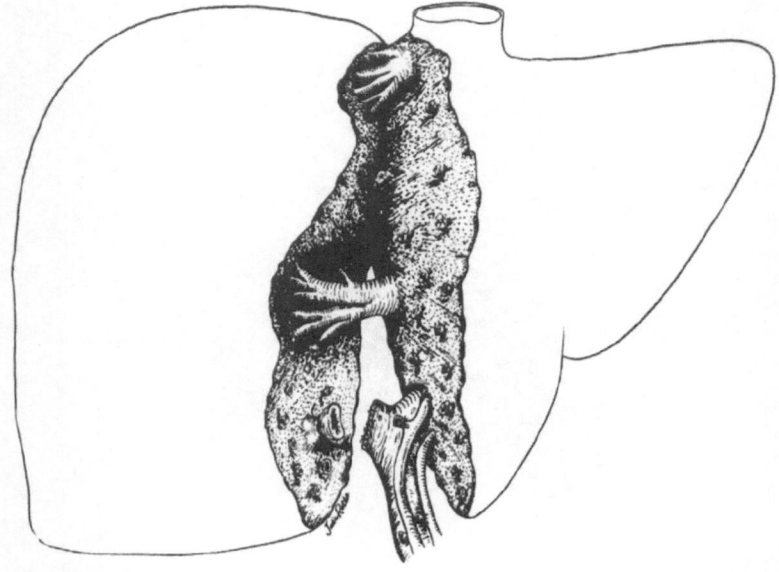

Fig. 4. Illustration of the ability of the ultrasonic scalpel to dissect out the branches of major hepatic vascular structures before clamping, which allows a highly controlled division of these vessels to take place without the chance of a caval or portal tear (Reprinted from Surgery 1984; 95: 230 with permission).

tissue from the large veins running directly to the cava.

On the other hand Tranberg indicates that in Sweden the direct parenchymal approach is preferred and in this method, the vessels are controlled inside the liver. They ligate the hepatic veins at the end of the parenchymal transection, i.e. inside the liver, and not before transecting the parenchyma. Positive pressure ventilation is used throughout the transection in order to avoid the danger of air embolism. If major bleeding occurs during liver transection, they try temporary occlusion of the porta hepatis during which bleeding from individual, intra-parenchymal structures is controlled. There is no difficulty with this since it has been recently reported that the human liver tolerates warm ischemia for an hour without demonstrable ill-effects [36].

Intraoperative ultrasonography helps in diagnosing liver tumors and in making liver resections safe. Its ability to delineate the tumors and to establish the relationship between tumor and vascular structures aids in avoiding damage to major vessels and in making limited, but still sufficient, resections of neoplastic tissue, for instance in patients with multiple tumors or in patients with liver cirrhosis [37].

Kemeny makes the point that with the ultrasonic dissector it is quite possible to perform a metastasectomy, i.e. removal of the metastases with a rim of nor-

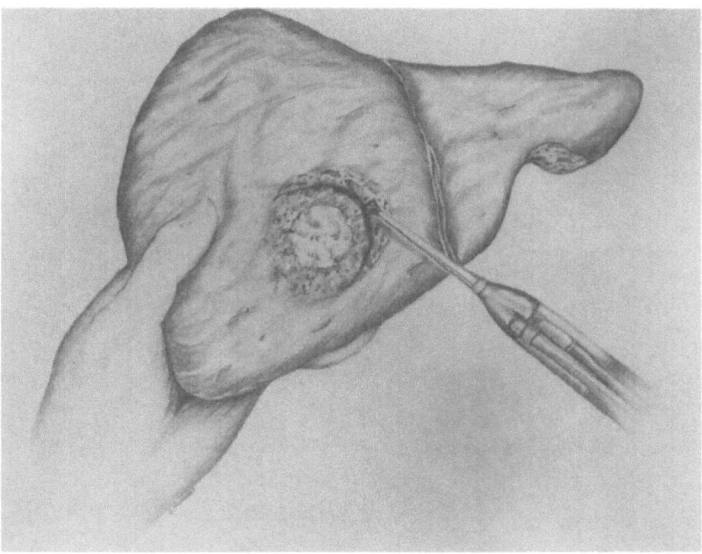

Fig. 5. Illustration of the use of the ultrasonic dissector during the performance of a metastasectomy.

mal liver around each (Fig. 5). Her average blood loss at the City of Hope Hospital in Durante, California and average hospital stay and postoperative complication rate was lower for metastasectomy than with anatomic lobectomy [38].

As Hodgson and DelGuercio [29] demonstrated, the technique for this procedure is to mobilize the liver so that the hand can be placed underneath the lobe for control. Then, exerting a little traction, a dissection of the hepatic parenchyma can take place with the ultrasonic dissector in a parellel direction to the edge of the metastasis. As the smaller vessels are identified, they are cauterized and then slightly larger vessels are clipped. As these vessels are exposed and divided, the trench which appears is gradually extended around the metastasis and under the metastasis and larger vessels are recognized and clamped, divided and tied. Usually, these more superficial tumors extend into the liver for about 2–3cms. and the largest vessels which are encountered are of the order of 8mm in size. Gradually, the dissection then extends under the tumor which is slowly lifted up by pressure upon the liver from below and eventually, the dissection reaches the other side of the metastasis and extends back towards the liver surface at which point it can be removed under complete control. As previously published [29], blood loss with this type of procedure was in the order of 611ml.

In Erlangen, in the Federal Republic of Germany, Scheele has indicated

152

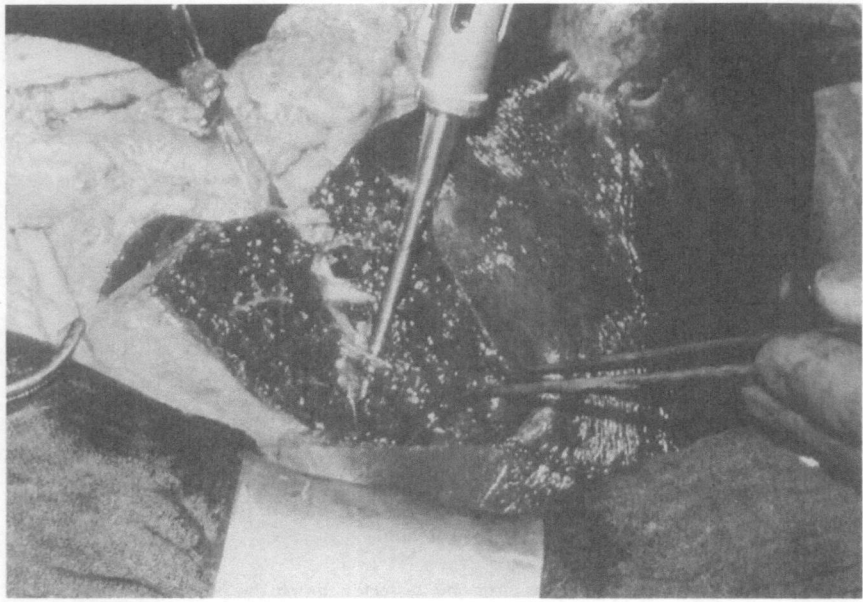

Fig. 6. Isolated resection of segment IVb for a follicular nodular hyperplasia, compressing the junction of the bile duct; use of the ultrasonic dissector results in an even and dry cut surface along the falciform ligament and enables preparation of portal structures radiating into segment IV.

that the University Hospital has demonstrated an intense interest in preservation of normal hepatic tissue during tumor resections. And they have been using the ultrasonic dissector since 1982, noting that it permits a precise fragmentation of liver tissue and that small vessels and bile ducts running within the resection plane remained intact so that they can be dealt with individually (Fig. 6). This resulted in a very accurate preparation of important hepatic structures (Fig. 7) and resulted in smooth, unusually dry wound surfaces. Infrared coagulation or a fibrinogen sealant was used to manage any residual bleeding (Fig. 8).

Although the ultrasonic dissector has proven advantageous in their experience for liver resection in general, it was of particular value if an exact segmentectomy was intended. Once the intersegmental plane was reached, dissection proceeded unusually easily and quickly, since no crossing vessels or bile ducts remained, and the two parts of the liver separated apart as if spontaneously. This method has been used since 1984 and involved primary transection of the hepatic tissue along anatomical planes, but without previous ligation of hilar structures. It was based on the subdivision of the liver into Couinaud's eight independently resectable units (Fig. 9) [24]. This intersegmental anatomy demonstrated that in the longitudinal axis, the borders of these segments

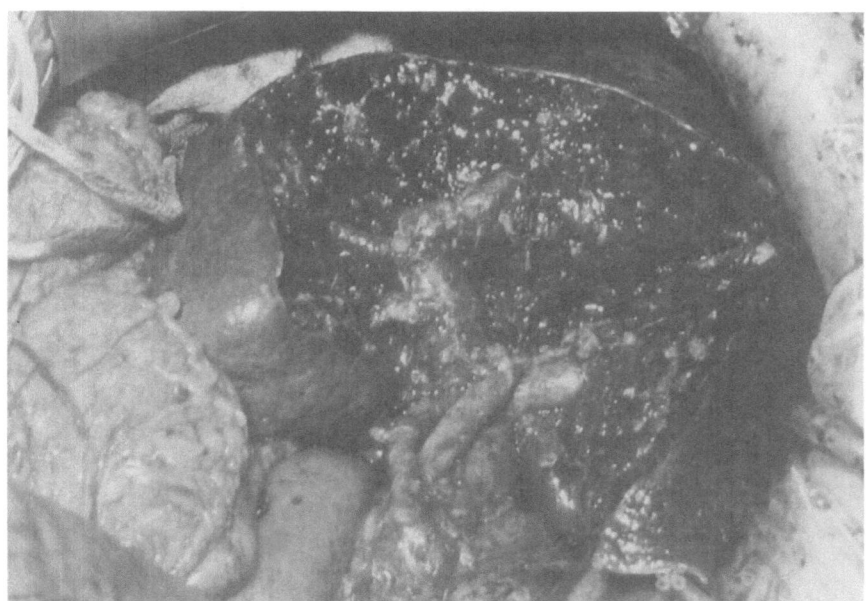

Fig. 7. Resection of a cholangiocarcinoma by resection of segment III, IV and V. The portal structures and their intrahepatic branching are clearly visible.

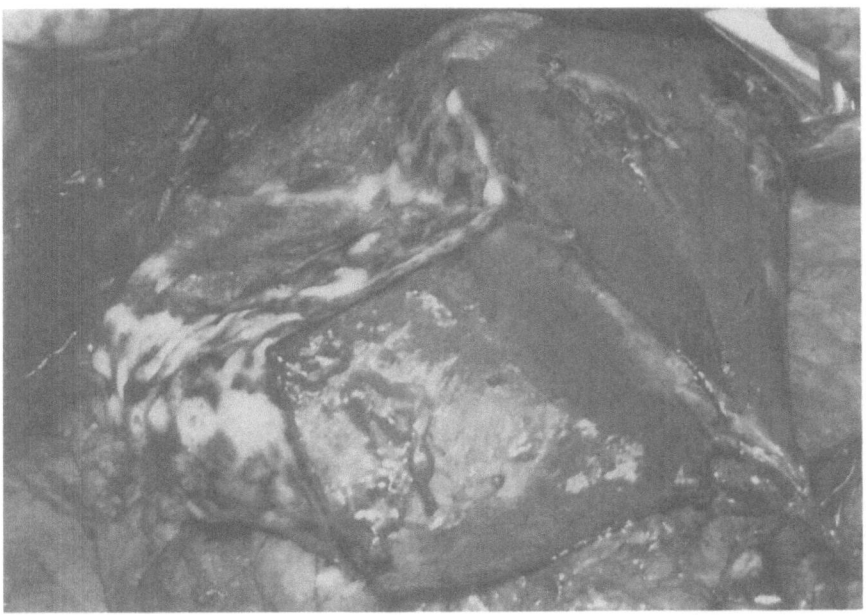

Fig. 8. Raw surface of the liver, following a pleurisegmentectomy IVa + (V–VIII), covered by fibrin tissue adhesive; in the vicinity of the hepatic veins a combination of collagen fleece, and in the other regions a spray technique was used.

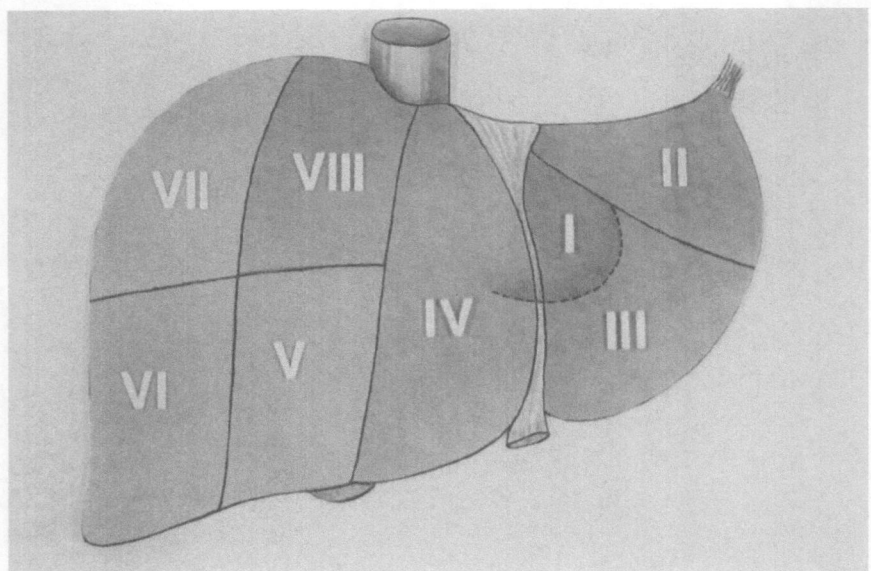

Fig. 9. Liver segments according to Couinaud.

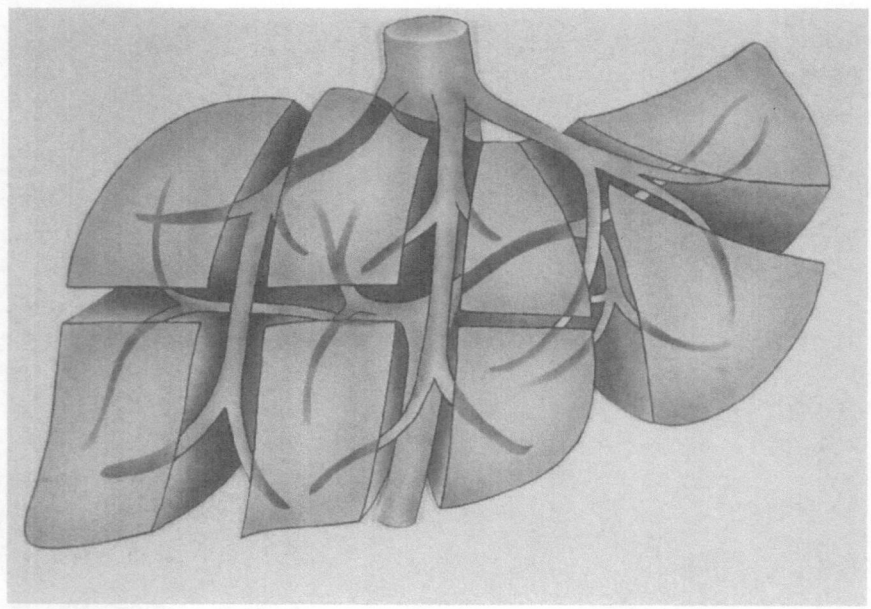

Fig. 10. Segmental borders of the liver; segment IV can also be subdivided into a cranial part (IVa) and a caudal part (IVb).

155

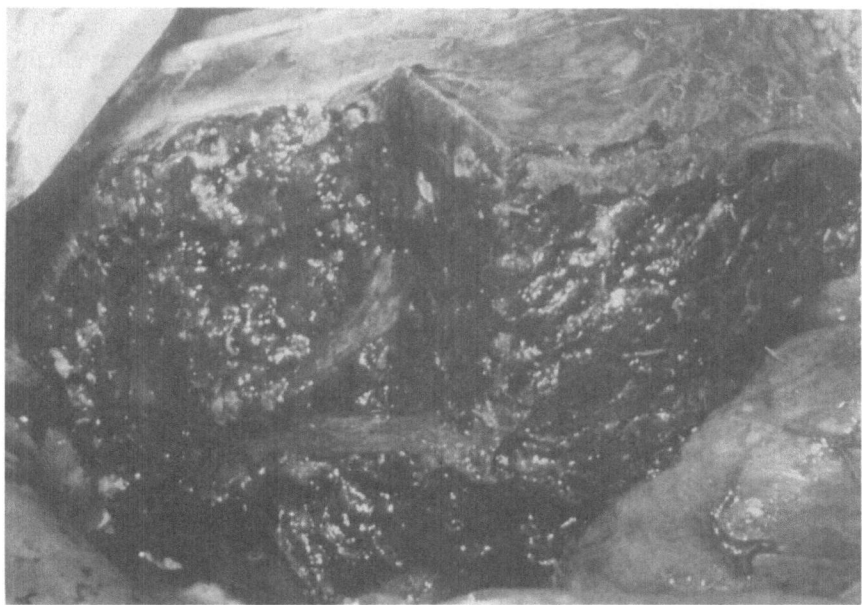

Fig. 11. Pleurisegmentectomy IVa + (V–VIII); if compared to a right lobectomy, the noninvolved segment IVb is preserved. The middle hepatic vein and a branch of the left hepatic vein are visible.

are characterized by the course of efferent hepatic veins, and in the transverse direction by the intrahepatic branching of the portal structures (Fig. 10).

These intersegmental planes, it was noted by Gall and Scheele [39] were almost never transgressed even by very large tumors. For this reason, a segment oriented resection technique appeared to offer, for smaller nodules, the advantage of safe radical surgery. In cases of more pronounced tumors, it could, compared with common hepatectomies, keep additional parenchymal regions intact (Fig. 11) thus resulting in a greater postoperative functional reserve.

For the exact determination of the intersegmental borders, they found intraoperative ultrasound very helpful. By exact determination of the intrahepatic extent of the tumor and of the distance between the tumor and the intended resection line, it facilitated an individual decision concerning the type and extent of resection. Supplementary to the preoperative diagnostic workup, it furthermore permitted a re-examination of the liver by direct view and simultaneous palpation. This resulted in superior accuracy regarding the detection of small, previously undiscovered metastases and enabled suspicious intrahepatic nodules to be diagnosed by a well directed biopsy.

At the Westchester Medical Center, intraoperative ultrasound has been found useful in trying to define tumors which did not appear as expected. This may have been because such abnormalities have been overread during CT scanning as tumors and in fact turned out to be due to hemangiomata or cirrhotic nodules. However, because at the Westchester Medical Center in Valhalla we have been using the technique of CT arterial portography (CTAP) routinely, the infusion of dye through the superior mesenteric artery has resulted in a high detection rate of tumors as small as $\frac{1}{2}$ cm in size when the CT scanning is done during the portal phase.

Results

Worldwide experience with the Cavitron ultrasonic dissector now involves some hundreds of resections. Experience with the Sonotec and Sonocut is still limited. Generally, most centers using the ultrasonic dissector still have limited numbers and unfortunately some have given up the technique after initial disasters. This problem has been defined as inadequate training and there is no doubt that the technique is totally different from any previously employed in the liver.

The authors of this chapter have a combined experience of hepatic resections in over 230 patients.

Hodgson [2] demonstrated in a small group of patients in 1979 that, using the ultrasonic dissector, it was quite possible to resect hepatic tumors without having to perform lobectomy. In addition to performing these wedge excisions, in contradistinction to wedge biopsies, it was also shown that formal lobectomy appeared to be simplified [40]. Indeed, in a subsequent paper, Hodgson demonstrated that the wedge resection could be huge, as in resection of a 12 cm. hemangioma and safe with the ultrasonic dissector [41]. Furthermore, normal liver was preserved without performing right lobectomy.

Subsequently, Hodgson and DelGuercio [29] published their paper in 1984 which demonstrated that the average blood loss per wedge resection was 611 cc and for left lateral segmental resection it was 644 cc. For formal lobectomy it was 1580 cc. This was a major improvement on other techniques previously employed. They also indicated in this paper that it was possible to excise multiple tumors individually from the same patient, even if bilateral, having first done this in 1981.

Kemeny [38] took this concept a stage further and, at the City of Hope, performed a randomized study comparing patients with resection using the liver-conserving technique of the ultrasonic dissector and patients who also had continuous hepatic artery infusion (CHAI) of FUDR as well. She found the best survival in patients with solitary metastases with eight of eleven patients still alive 9–54 months post-resection with an average survival of 24 months. For the eleven patients who had CHAI of FUDR five were alive 15–51 months post-resection with an average survival of 25 months. Five of these patients had four or more metastases and eight had bilobar disease. On the other hand, in the group of patients with similar disease loads receiving only CHAI, six of the 15 were alive at 14–22 months with an average survival of 20 months. There is no statistically significant difference between the two groups but a trend towards resection is indicated.

Hodgson *et al.* [42] noted that there was a clear difference, but reserved CHAI and FUDR treatment for patients with advanced disease and in this group the median survival was only six months. In the group who had resection and CHAI, the median survival could not be calculated as the overall survival was prolonged. Further, in Hodgson's patients with bilateral disease, the longest survivor after resection lived 51 months, and the shortest 21 months. There did not appear to be any difference in survival between patients with unilateral and bilateral disease resected where the volume of metastatic colon carcinoma of the liver was similar.

As previously indicated, Scheele has really expanded segmentectomy, which was introduced in Erlangen in October 1984. Using the ultrasonic dissector, in 18 months they did 110 liver resections and in 78 patients both lobes of the liver were affected. 63 of these patients had malignant tumors, nine had a benign tumor and six had other indications. A total of 30 tumors (26 malignant, 4 benign), and two other lesions were removed by segmentectomy.

In this group, Scheele performed 13 monosegmentectomies for limited tumors, and all were histologically complete. However, when using wedge resection only, three of 19 excisions demonstrated tumor infiltration of the resection margin histologically. Of 17 bi and poly-segmentectomies, only one was incomplete. This was about the same as in his 23 right hepatic lobectomies, where two showed tumor at the resection margin.

Scheele's segmentectomy patients only had two minor complications, but liver failure occurred in 22% of his lobectomy patients which resulted in three out of his four deaths. Similarly, Kemeny and Hodgson noted minimal complications from local resection and Hodgson had one intraoperative death in a right lobectomy, due to tumor invasion of the inferior vena cava and one late death in a trisegmentectomy due to liver failure.

Discussion

During the last ten years, liver resection has become a routinely performed surgical procedure. Operative risk has become remarkably reduced and it seems that there is a case for its oncological effectiveness.

For example, at the Mayo Clinic, which probably has as much experience in the management of colorectal liver metastases as anywhere in the world, the five year survival of a group of patients with single colorectal metastases to the liver, after resection of these metastases, was 25% but that without resection was 2% [43]. It was also noted at the Mayo Clinic that patients who had two or three metastases in one lobe had a similar five year survival after resection as those with single metastases [43]. At the Memorial Hospital in New York City a report on a group of patients with unilateral or bilateral disease resected appeared to show no difference in survival [44].

In another report from the National Cancer Institute on 33 patients with multiple metastases there was no survival difference in the patients with unilobar disease versus bilobar disease and between patients with solitary metastases or those with two or three lesions [45]. However, patients with four metastases did significantly poorer.

The scope of the problem of malignant liver disease can be appreciated by examining metastatic colorectal carcinoma which is the second most common noncutaneous malignancy in the United States with approximately 44,000 new cases anually [46]. In about 12,000 cases metastatic disease affects only the liver [47, 48]. Very few of these cases are actually resected.

Perhaps the lack of a generally accepted reproducible safe technique is the problem.

In this article, the authors demonstrate an increasingly accepted technique, the ultrasonic dissector, which, when combined with increasing anatomical knowledge, appears to reduce intraoperative blood loss. Further, the usual postoperative complications of biliary leakage and abscess formation also appear to be diminished by this technique. In addition, the understanding of hepatic physiology and regeneration is important. For example, when most of a lobe is replaced by a large tumor mass (Fig. 12) the other lobe frequently compensates by hypertrophy. In such a case postoperative functional capacity is not a problem. However, when an extended resection becomes necessary because of multiple or awkwardly placed small tumors, and there is no such compensatory hypertrophy, then the risk of postoperative acute liver failure increases considerably. It is in this group in particular that wedge excision, or subsegmentectomy or segmentectomy should be considered. Andrus and Kaminski [49] have independently come to the same conclusion, using the liver-sparing techniques of segmental hepatic resection. They feel that utilization of the ultrasonic dissector to perform such resections may increase our versatility in the management of various hepatic and biliary tract diseases. On the other hand, Makuuchi et al. [50] have shown it is possible to perform such procedures using intraoperative ultrasound scanning, but without the ultrasonic dissector.

Experienced surgeons comfortable with their own techniques will not find much improvement with the ultrasonic dissector. Indeed, they could find the dissection tedious with this method and this could increase their unease. The

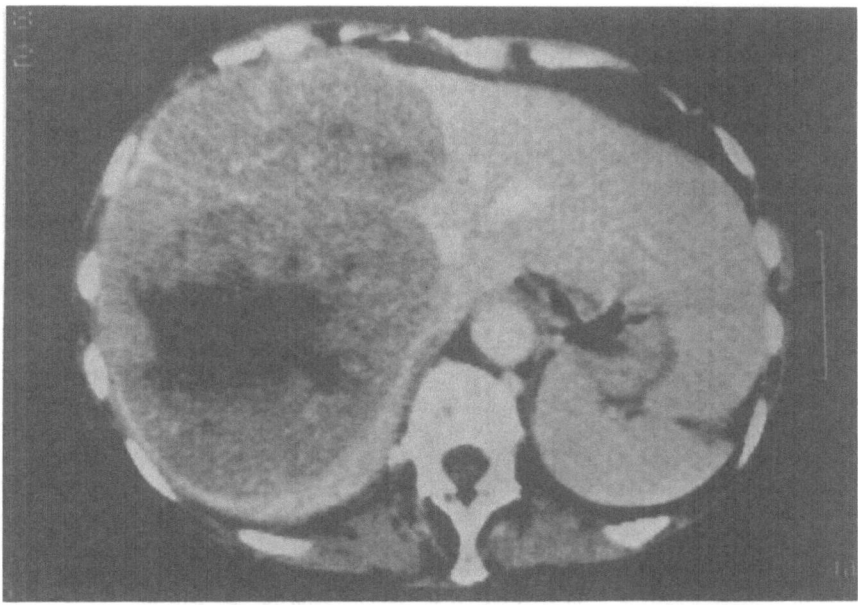

Fig. 12. Metachronous liver metastases of a small bowel sarcoma, located in segment VII and VIII; compensatory hypertrophy of the left liver lobe (segments II and III) extending into the splenic hilum.

authors strongly feel that the technique must be properly taught, and when mastered it may allow some surgeons to perform local resections. This is a relatively simple ability with the ultrasonic scalpel, but in most hands is difficult without it. Also, such localized resections appear to reduce the risk of liver failure, and long-term survival after local resection of tumors appears possible.

Conclusion

Does the ultrasonic dissector improve the quality of HPB surgery? To the experienced surgeon – probably not. However, it is conceded that there are occasions when it could be useful in particularly difficult hepatic resections.

For the problems of hepatic surgery are still formidable, and the results of disastrous bleeding intraoperatively, and postoperative bile leaks, abscesses and liver failure are well known. However, the experience presented here seems to indicate that disastrous intraoperative bleeding is rare using the ultrasonic dissector, so that operative mortality is no longer significant. Also, postoperative complications seem minimal. The problem of post-resectional liver failure with massive resection remains, but local resection is simplified with the

160

ultrasonic dissector and very accurate segmentectomy is possible. Tumor resection appears adequate with this method and survival seems compatible to that obtained by hepatic lobectomy for a similar tumor volume.

In summary therefore, the authors believe that the answer to the question may be positive, in that when the technique is properly taught, it does seem to be a useful, reproducible and safe technique.

References

1. Hodgson WJB, Poddar PK, Mencer EJ, *et al.*: Evaluation of ultrasonically powered instruments in the laboratory and in the clinical setting. Am J Gastroenterol. 72: 133, 1979
2. Hodgson WJB, Aufses Jr AH: Surgical ultrasonic dissection of the liver. Surgical Rounds Aug: 1968, 1979
3. Kousnetzoff M, Pensky J: Études cliniques et experimentales sur la chirurgie du foie sur la résection partielle du foie. Rev Chir 16: 954, 1896
4. Auvray M: Études experimentales sur la résection du foie chez l'homme et chez les animaux. Rev Clin 17: 318, 1897
5. Keen WW: Report of a case of resection of the liver for the removal of a neoplasm with a table of 76 cases of resection of the liver for hepatic tumors. Ann Surg 30: 267, 1899
6. Ogilvie H: Partial hepatectomy. Brit Med J 2: 1136, 1953
7. Lin TY, Tsu KY, Mien C, Chen CS: Study on lobectomy of the liver: A new surgical suggestion on hemihepatectomy of the liver. J Forum Med Ass 11: 742, 1958
8. Pringle JH: Notes on the arrest of hepatic hemorrhage due to trauma. Ann Surg 48: 541, 1908
9. Lin TY: Results in 107 hepatic lobectomies with a preliminary report on the use of a clamp to reduce blood loss. Ann Surg 177: 413, 1973
10. Foster JH, Berman MM: Solid liver tumors. Maj Prob Clin Surg 23, W.B. Saunders, Phila, 1977
11. Fortner JG, Maclean VJ, Kim DK, *et al.*: The 70's evolution in liver surgery for cancer. Cancer 47: 2162, 1981
12. Adson MA, van Heerden JA: Major hepatic resections for metastatic colorectal cancer. Ann Surg 191: 576, 1980
13. Honjo I, Araki C: Total resection of the right lobe of the liver. J Int Col Surg 23: 23, 1955
14. Lortat-Jacob JL, Robert HG: Hépatectomie droit réglée. Princ Med 60: 549, 1952
15. Pack GT, Baker HW: Total right hepatic lobectomy. Report of a case. Ann Surg 138: 253, 1953
16. Quattlebaum JK: Massive resection of the liver. Ann Surg 137: 787, 1953
17. Brunchwig A: The surgery of hepatic neoplasms with special reference to secondary malignant neoplasms. Cancer 6: 725, 1953
18. Ong GB, Chan PKW: Primary carcinoma of the liver. Surg Gynecol Obstet 143: 31, 1976
19. Tung, TT: Chirurgie d'exérèe du foie. Hanoi, 1962
20. Honjo I, Mizumoto R: Primary carcinoma of the liver. Amer J Surg 128: 31, 1974
21. Balasegaram M: Hepatic resection for malignant tumor. Surgical Rounds September: 14, 1979
22. Starzl TE, Bell RH, Beart RW, Putnam CW: Hepatic trisegmentectomy and other liver resections. Surg Gynecol Obstet 141: 429, 1975
23. Starzl TE, Iwatsuki S, Shaw BW, *et al.*: Left hepatic trisegmentectomy. Surg Gynecol Obstet 155: 21, 1982

24. Couinaud C, Le foie: Études anatomiques et chirurgicales. 9–12 Masson et Cie. Paris, 1957
25. Bismuth H: Surgical anatomy and anatomical surgery of the liver. World J Surg 6: 3, 1982
26. Williams JW, Hodgson WJB: Histologic evaluation of tissues sectioned by ultrasonically powered instruments. (A preliminary report) Mt Sinai J Med 46: 105, 1979
27. Chopp RT, Shah BB, Addonizio JC: Use of the ultrasonic surgical aspirator in renal surgery. Urology 22: 115, 1983
28. Tranberg KG, Rigotti P, Bracket KA, et al.: Liver resection: A comparison using the Nd-YAG laser, an ultrasonic surgical aspirator, or blunt dissection. Am J Surg 151: 368, 1986
29. Hodgson WJB, DelGuercio LRM: Preliminary experience in liver surgery using the ultrasonic scalpel. Surgery 95: 230, 1984
30. Putnam CW: Techniques of ultrasonic dissection in resection of the liver. Surg Gynecol Obstet 157: 475, 1983
31. Joffe SN, Bracket KA, Sankar MY, Daykuzono N: Resection of the liver with the Nd-YAG laser. Surg Gynecol Obstet 163: 437, 1986
32. Tabuse K, Katsumi M, Kobayashi Y, et al.: Microwave surgery: Hepatectomy using a microwave tissue coagulator. World J Surg 9: 136, 1985
33. Kotsko NI, Sandomirskii BP, Kostia PI: Cryoresection of the liver in metastatic lesions. Klin Chir 5: 53, 1982
34. Schwartz SI: Right hepatic lobectomy. Amer J Surg 148: 668, 1984
35. Nakamura S, Tsuzuki T: Surgical anatomy of the hepatic veins and the inferior vena cava. Surg Gynecol Obstet 152: 43, 1981
36. Huguet C, Nordlinger B, Bloch P, Conard J: Tolerance of the human liver to prolonged normothermic ischemia. Arch Surg 113: 1448, 1978
37. Gozetti G, Mazziotti A, Bolondi L, et al.: Intraoperative ultrasonography in surgery for liver tumors. Surgery 99: 523, 1986
38. Kemeny MM, Goldberg D, et al.: Results of a prospective randomized trial of continuous regional chemotherapy and hepatic resection as treatment of hepatic metastases from colorectal primaries. Cancer 57: 492, 1986
39. Gall FP, Scheele J: Die operative Therapie von Lebermetastasen. In: TW Schildberg (ed) Chirurgische Therapie von Tumormetastasen. Bibliomed, Melsungen (in press)
40. Hodgson WJB: Ultrasonic surgery. Ann Roy Coll Surg Engl 62: 459, 1980
41. Hodgson WJB: The technique of ultrasonic dissection in cavernous hemangiomas of the liver. Surgical Rounds, March: 30, 1984
42. Hodgson WJB, Friedland M, Ahmed T, et al.: Treatment of colorectal hepatic metastases by intrahepatic chemotherapy alone or as an adjunct to complete or partial removal of metastatic disease. Ann Surg 203: 430, 1986
43. Adson MA, Van Heerden JA, Adson MH, et al.: Resection of hepatic metastases from colorectal cancer. Arch Surg 119: 647, 1984
44. Butler J, Attiyeh FF, Daly JM: Hepatic resection for metastases of the colon and rectum. Surg Gynecol Obstet 162: 109, 1986
45. August DA, Sugarbaker PH, Ottow RT, et al.: Hepatic resection of colorectal metastases. Ann Surg 201: 210, 1985
46. Silverberg E, Lubera J: Cancer Statistics 1986. Ca-a Cancer Journal for physicians 36: 9, 1986
47. Welch JP, Donaldson GA: Clinical correlation of an autopsy study of recurrent colorectal cancer. Ann Surg 189: 496, 1979
48. Kemeny N, Yagoda A, Braun D, et al.: Therapy for metastatic colorectal carcinoma with a combination of methyl-CCNU, 5-Flurouracil, Vincristine and Streptozoticin (MOF-Strep). Cancer 45: 876, 1980
49. Andrus CH, Kaminski JL: Segmental hepatic resection utilizing the ultrasonic dissector. Arch Surg 121: 515, 1986

50. Makuuchi M, Hasegawa H, Yamazaki S, Takayasu K: Four new hepatectomy procedures for resection of the right hepatic vein and preservation of the inferior right hepatic vein. Surg Gynecol Obstet 164: 69, 1987

9. Hepatic arterial infusion chemotherapy: rationale, results, credits and debits

C.J.H. VAN DE VELDE, L.M. DE BRAUW, P.H. SUGARBAKER and K.G. TRANBERG

Introduction

The chemotherapy of primary and secondary neoplasms of the liver has evoked over the past decades passing through phases of single agent systemic treatment, regional infusion chemotherapy, combination chemotherapy and finally continuous regional drug delivering. This latter development has been made possible through the development of a very sophisticated biomedical device: the totally implantable pump. Since it's introduction for continuous hepatic arterial chemotherapy in 1980 it is estimated that over 5000 implantations have been performed of the Infusaid® pump, suggesting a therapeutic fad in the treatment of liver metastases. Although the Infusaid pump represents a substantial technological advance, it is important to distinguish the device itself, it's reliability and the role it plays in regional chemotherapy, from the efficacy of the regional approach to metastatic colorectal cancer in the liver. This chapter will mainly focus on this latter complex problem in which the pump is merely a device for the delivery of agents which, like the method itself, will be subject to a critical review of credits and debits.

Rationale

Although resection is the only therapeutic option with a chance of cure, the majority of patients present at the time of diagnosis with irresectable hepatic metastases [1]. Systemic treatment of colorectal hepatic metastasis with 5-Fluorouracil (5-FU) until now the most effective agent, results in a transient partial response without survival benefit in 20% of the patients.

In an effort to improve the results of chemotherapy, local approaches have been devised. The rationale behind hepatic artery infusion of cytotoxic drugs is based on:
1. the concept of exploiting the dose-response relationship by generating high

local drug concentrations, while maintaining low systemic drug levels, and
2. the premise that effective local (hepatic) tumor control will result in increased therapeutic effect or cure.

High local drug exposure

For over 60 years the blood supply of established hepatic metastases was thought to be entirely of (hepatic) arterial origin. Only (clinically occult) tumors weighing less than 30 mg were reported to be dependent on the portal blood flow as well [2]. This view was challenged by more recent studies using human autopsy livers [3] and rat livers [4]. Also large hepatic metastases exhibited frequently portal blood supply, especially the periphery of the metastases containing the highest proliferation zone. Furthermore, recent studies showed that arteriovenous communications exist between hepatic artery and portal vein [5], and that these arterioportal connections may open up when arterial occlusion is implemented [6]. The frequent portal blood supply could explain some of the therapeutic failures after local infusional chemotherapy via the hepatic artery.

Low systemic drug levels

Based on a pharmacological model it was assumed that 5-FU, among a few other drugs, would show a significant increase in therapeutic benefit when infused intra-arterially as compared to the results obtained with systemic administration of the drug [7]. Hepatic extraction of 5-FU would result in higher drug concentrations in the liver combined with low systemic drug levels [8]. The benefit of regional infusion of 5-FU and FUDR was based on measurements of the unchanged drug in the afferent and efferent blood flow of the liver. FUDR has been assumed to have therapeutical advantage over 5-FU because of the greater first pass uptake of the drug (95% versus 20–50% for 5-FU) [8]. However, these studies lack determination of the drug in tumor tissue, and measurements of rapidly formed non-cytotoxic catabolic products of 5-FU, which can be released immediately during administration [9, 10]. Therefore, higher hepatic extraction ratios do not necessarily implicate increased tumor cell uptake of 5-FU. Furthermore, a high hepatic extraction ratio is associated with low systemic drug levels after arterial infusion of fluorinated pyrimidines, so that microscopic extra-hepatic tumor may reside as an important unexposed site of recurrence [11].

Dose-response relationship

Although the exact parameters of 5-FU action may be unknown, two essential criteria must be met for any anticancer drug to exert its optimal activity, that is:
1. attainment of adequate high concentration of the drug in tumor tissue, and
2. sufficient duration of drug exposure in the tumor. Important pharmaco-kinetic data for pharmacological evaluation of various administration methods of chemotherapy could be obtained when efforts are devoted to measure drug (and metabolites) concentrations within the tumor.

The question whether increased 5-FU levels locally will result in a substantial increase in tumor cell kill should be answered with care. The parent drug itself is not cytotoxic: 5-FU has to be anabolized into the presumed active metabolites 5-fluorouridine triphosphate (FUTP) and 5-fluoro-2'-deoxyuridine monophosphate (FdUMP) schematically represented in Fig. 1. Although FUTP appeared to contribute significantly to the cytotoxic action of 5-FU [12], most investigators believe that the primary chemotherapeutic effect of the drug results from inhibition of thymidylate synthetase by FdUMP, preventing DNA-synthesis [13]. Numerous investigations to elucidate the biochemical determinants of 5-FU action revealed no clear relationship between tumor effect and tumor cell concentration of 5-FU or its metabolites [14].

Benefit of local tumor control

Whether any local therapy of hepatic metastasis will have a major impact on survival depends not only on the effectivity of local treatment, but also on the presentation of the disease. In an autopsy study it was found that the liver is the sole site of initial tumor recurrence in upto 30% of patients with metastatic colorectal disease [15]. Several studies reported 5-year survival rates of 25–35% after resection of liver metastases of colorectal origin [16]. The absence of 5-years survival rates after resection of hepatic metastases of other than colorectal origin (pancreas, biliary tract, stomach, melanoma, breast and other) points at a different tumor biology and limits the ratio for a liver-only directed treatment. Colorectal hepatic metastases are currently considered resectable-for-cure when their number is limited to three or less, in the absence of extra-hepatic tumor deposits. The failure pattern after resection of more than three hepatic metastases indicates the presence of systemic metastatic disease. The question whether irresectable hepatic metastases are always an expression of widespread incurable disease is not answered yet, and will be discussed later. Although a majority of patients will die from their disease after aggressive local therapy directed at liver-only tumor growth, it seems worthwile for a significant number of patients in terms of local tumor control. Furthermore, it

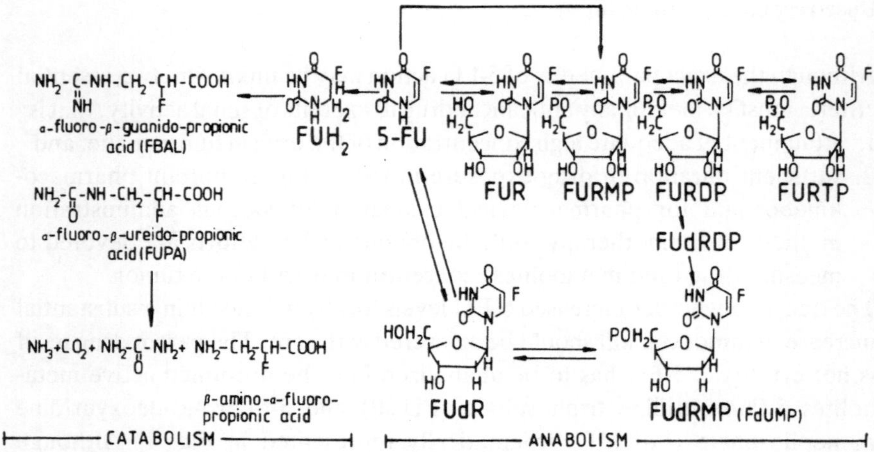

Fig. 1. Schematic diagram of the metabolic pathways of 5-FU and FUDR.

has been shown that hepatic metastases exert a dominant influence upon survival of the patient, despite the presence of concurrent extra-hepatic tumor recurrences [17]. Thus, aggressive (chemotherapeutic) treatment directed at irresectable hepatic metastases appears to have a rational basis.

Hepatic artery infusional chemotherapy

Despite theoretical and pharmacological advantages of hepatic artery infusion (HAI) with fluoropyrimidines, there is no sound proof of its clinical superiority. Randomized studies evaluating HAI versus a no-treatment control group are non-existent. In uncontrolled studies with HAI a disparity was apparent for reported responses, ranging from 35–80%, and median survival times. These non-randomized studies with HAI suggested increased response rates as compared to the results obtained with systemic administration of 5-FU. However, the most definitive randomized trial comparing short term HAI and systemic administration of 5-FU in 61 evaluable colorectal cancer patients with hepatic metastases failed to show significant differences in response rate and mean survival time [18]. Response rates were 34% and 24% for the HAI and systemic treated groups respectively. This study has been criticized on grounds of short duration of HAI, the limited number of evaluable patients, the percutaneous placement of the intrahepatic catheters and ineffective evaluation of perfusion [11, 19].

Controlled trials can be performed more easily in the experimental situation. Rats (n = 25) with hepatic tumors were randomly assigned to three treatment modalities including hepatic artery infusion, jugular vein infusion (both continuously during 7 days) and oral administration (7 days) of 5-FU. Tumor volumes were evaluated at day 11 after inoculation of the syngeneic hepatic Walker carcinoma. Tumor volumes were significantly smaller in the hepatic artery infusional group as compared to the results obtained with systemic administration or no treatment (and the other groups). Survival times were similar in all groups [20].

Dissatisfaction with the therapeutic results from short-term hepatic artery infusion, and operative- and treatment related complications resulted in fading enthousiasm for this approach, but a recent burgeoning of interest followed the advent of the totally implantable pump for continuous infusion of chemotherapy [21].

Protracted infusional therapy

Technical advances made continuous delivery of chemotherapy possible, but is there evidence that prolonged administration might be more effective than intermittent chemotherapy? Theoretical principles that may favor continuous administration include:
1. continuous exposure would offer a greater opportunity for destroying more tumor cells, since most chemotherapeutic agents display greater activity against the relatively small fraction of proliferating cells in solid tumors, and
2. destruction of proliferating cells would induce an increased number of cells coming into cycle, which again would make them more sensitive to treatment [22].

With respect to clinical data, only one randomized study is available in the literature, which evaluated the effectiveness of protracted infusion of 5-FU [23]. Seventy patients with advanced colorectal cancer were randomly assigned to rapid bolus injection (5 days each month) or continuous infusion (for 5 days, each month) administering intravenously equitoxic doses of 5-FU. A higher response rate was observed among the continuously infused patients (15 of 34 patients versus 8 of 36 in the rapid injection group). Also median survival times showed benefit for the protracted infusion group (8 months versus 2 months for the bolus injection group). However, definitive conclusions from this trial are precluded by the different distribution of measurable lesions and uneven patient distribution among the groups. In view of this inclusive evidence, there is, in fact, no current data that clearly support the superiority of continuous infusion over intermittent administration of chemotherapy.

Table 1. Uncontrolled studies evaluating the pump: number of patients, % of patients with extrahepatic metastases; % of responses as assessed by imaging technique, CEA; median survival in months from pump implantation and from time of diagnosis of liver metastases; and toxicity including chemical hepatitis gastro-intestinal toxicity and biliary complications.

	No. of pts	extra-hep. mets. (% of pts.)	Responses (%)		Med. survival (mo)		Toxicity (%)			Reference
			Imag.	CEA	From pump	From diagnosis	Chem. hep.	G.I.	Biliary	
Balch 1983	81	15[b]	.	88	.	26	90	17	0	27
Weiss 1983	17	–	29	65	13	17	53	38	15	28
Cohen 1983	17	12	59	.	.	.	24	18	0	30
Niederhuber 1984	93	46	76	91	18[c]	25[c]	32	56	24	31
Kemeny 1984	41	–	44	42	.	.	71	46	5	34
Johnson 1985	40	20[b]	47	.	±13	.	50	10	5	32
Schwartz 1985	25	–	15	74	(>10)	(>15)	.	10	20	29
Shepard 1985	62	15	32	.	17[c]	.	49	18	.	40
Summarized: (n =)	376	(x =)	43	72	15	23	53	27	10	

[a] biliary complications including (clinically evident) jaundice, biliary sclerosis and/or strictures.
[b] extrahepatic metastases were resected in these patients.
[c] median survival of patients without extrahepatic metastases.

Summary of trials employing continuous arterial chemotherapy

The advent of a light-weight, totally implantable infusion pump [24] provided a practible and reliable means to deliver chemotherapy continuously [25].

Table 1 summarizes the results of uncontrolled studies evaluating continuous intrahepatic chemotherapy delivered by the implantable pump in patients with metastatic colorectal carcinoma. This table contains only larger series, considerably fewer than have been treated with the pump. Comprising approximately 577 cases reported in the literature (Tables 1 and 2), only an estimated 11% of all pump-treated patients is properly evaluated and reported on, suggesting that clinicians are already convinced of the therapeutical benefit of the pump. Initial feasibility studies gave encouraging results, suggesting substantial therapeutical advantage over previous intrahepatic infusion chemotherapy. Ensminger and collaborators have reported a 83% response rate, with a median survival time exceeding 21 months [26]. These findings were corroborated by Balch and co-workers, who reported a 88% response rate, with an associated median survival time of 26 months [27]. However, other investigators employing similar techniques and patient selection did not come up to these promising results [28, 29].

It must be recognized that the pump-treated patients are a highly selected group. Eligibility criteria included a life expectancy of more than 2–4 months, a good performance score (Karnofsky >60), and absence of signs of liver failure (serum bilirubin level <2–4 mg/dl). The reported series are heterogeneic with respect to eligibility of patients with concurrent extrahepatic metastases. Five studies included these patients [27, 30, 32, 40] of which in two, the extrahepatic tumors were resected prior to pump implantation [27, 30]. It should be realized that these eligibility criteria may create a selection bias, since these patient characteristics are well known and important prognostic factors [33]. In all series patients were included who received prior chemotherapy, most often systemic 5-FU.

Treatment schedules were comparable, employing continuous infusion rates of initially 0.3 mg FUDR/kg/day for 14 consecutive days, alternated with a period of 2 weeks of saline and heparin. In most series, mitomycin-C was added via the side port if there was evidence of lack of response of the hepatic lesions, or of progression of intrahepatic or extrahepatic tumors. Occasionally, BCNU or cisplatinum were used in addition. FUDR was used exclusively in only one study [28].

The reported responses varied from 15–88% (Table 1) and the variability appears at least in part to be due to the response parameters used. The highest response rate of 88% was reported by Balch *et al.* [27], using a CEA-reduction of 30% as indicative of response. In other studies, response rates were recorded as assessed by imaging techniques as well as by CEA reduction. Re-

Table 2. Randomized studies.

	Arm	No. pts.	Crossing over	Resp. %	Med. surv.	2 years surv.	Extrahep. failures	Reference
Kemeny '86	ia	45	+	46*	15	–	43%	37
	iv	49		22,5	15	–	15%	
Sugarbaker '87	ia	32	–	67*	±17	40%	24%	38
	iv	32		17	±10	18%	4%	
Niederhuber '85	ia	12	–	58	.	–	.	39
	iv	13		38	.	–	.	
	both	18		56	.	–	.	

* ia and iv group: difference considered significant (p<0.05).

sponse rates were 65% versus 29% [28] and 74% versus 15% [29] as indicated by CEA and imaging technique respectively. Obviously the results of the two methods did not correlate well. These findings were in contradistinction to the results of Lokich et al., who reported that CEA was a sensitive and reliable indicator of tumor response in patients with colorectal carcinoma [35]. Also, Kemeny et al. reported similar response rates as assessed by the methods [34]. On average, response rates were 27% higher when CEA reduction was used (Table 1). Not discussed here is the related problem of the variable criteria for response and duration of response. There is an obvious need for a uniformous system of response assessment, which was recognized during a workshop on the methodology in the clinical study of hepatic metastases. As a result an international staging system for hepatic metastases and reporting of response criteria was designed [36].

A similar disparity was evident of reported median survival times, ranging from 13–26 months. The longest median survival time of 26 months was noted by Balch, but this figure was based on the period from diagnosis of liver metastases to death [27]. The average median survival time as measured from time of pump implantation appeared to be 8 months shorter (Table 1).

Toxicity occurred in up to 100% of patients receiving continuously FUDR, requiring dose reductions, or even cessation of therapy. The most common finding was chemical hepatitis (20–90% of all patients) with significant elevation of alkaline phosphatase, SGOT and serum bilirubin levels. Most reports did not clearly distinguish chemical hepatitis and the more severe biliary complications due to development of biliary sclerosis, with marked elevation of bilirubin or clinically evident jaundice, and a persistent elevation of alkaline phosphatase. The latter finding was absent in the series of Balch et al. [27], but occurred in 24% of the patients in another study [31]. Also gastrointestinal toxicity with severe gastritis, or duodenitis with or without ulceration was frequently found, although not all reported cases were documented endoscopically. Overall the pump appears to be a reliable and accurate device acceptable to patients with a failure rate of below 1%. Morbidity of therapy with FUDR however was considerable.

Data from (ongoing) randomized trials

The considerable variability of reported response rates and median survival times and possible introduction of a selection bias preclude meaningful comparisons of the results of pump-treatment and conventional infusional chemotherapy. The difficulty to reach any conclusion from looking at these results demonstrates the need for randomized trials, which might shed light on the issue of selecting the best treatment. Yet, data from randomized trials is only

172

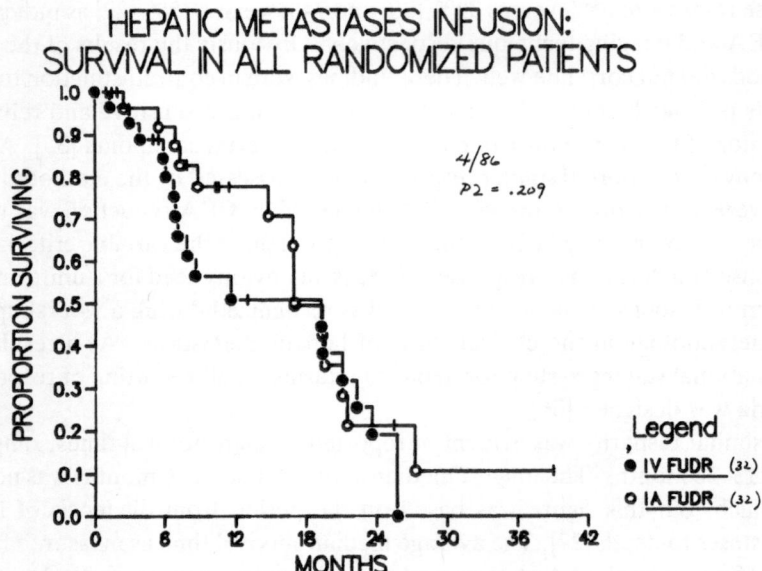

Fig. 2. Overall survival (months).

available in abstract form (Table 2). Two ongoing studies [37, 38] and one completed study [39] compared continuous infusion of FUDR systemically and intra-arterially [37, 38], and both [39]. Although the results are preliminary, several conclusions are tempting. The two largest series provided evidence for a significantly increased response rate in the intra-arterially infused group [37, 38]. The results from the third study showed a similarly trend, with comparable response rates in the regional and combined regional and systemic treatment arms [39]. This increased reponse rate was associated with a (not significantly) prolonged median survival time in one study [38] (Fig. 2). The other study reported similar survival rates, but is not appropriate to address the important issue of survival benefit, since it allows failures in the systemic arm to receive the alternate treatment [37]. Moreover there is no current data available, that supports the premise of a correlation of response and survival. A subset of patients without nodal involvement (n = 26) significantly showed a prolonged survival time for the regional treatment arm, providing the first indication of possible survival benefit for these patients [38] (Fig. 3).

Interestingly, the initial advantage of a higher tolerable dose with regional infusion as compared to systemic administration diminished due to toxicity requiring dose reductions in the regional treatment arm. After 7–8 chemotherapy cycles the dosages were similar in both arms [38] (Fig. 4).

A major flaw in the intra-arterially treated groups was the appearance, in all reported series, of extrahepatic metastatic disease, even when the hepatic met-

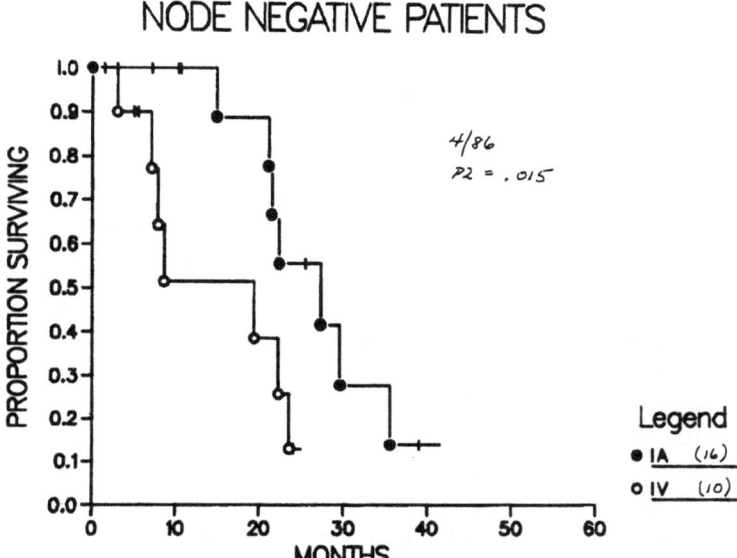

Fig. 3. Survival (months) in node negative patients.

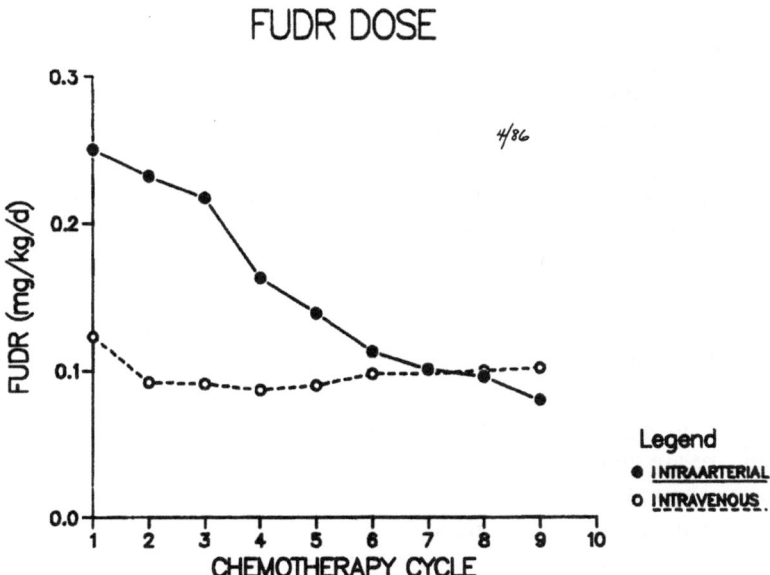

Fig. 4. Mean FUDR doses administered during the treatment course.

Table 3.

	Toxicity				
	Arm	Chem. hep.	Peptic ulcer	Diarrhea	Bil. sclerosis
Sugarbaker [38]	ia	79%	39%	13%	13%
	iv	7%	7%	59%	0%

astases were controlled. Often survival was determined by the progression of extrahepatic metastatic disease, pointing at the possible underlying weakness of the strictly regional therapeutic approach. The preliminary data from the randomized trials indicate an increased rate of extrahepatic failures in the regional treatment arm as compared to the systemic arm (Table 3). Theoretically, this change in natural history of the disease prompts the addition of systemic treatment to the regional approach, but no data is yet available to support this hypothesis.

Conclusions

In evaluating if regional chemotherapy plays a definitive role in the treatment of patients with hepatic metastases one should realize that on the basis of tumor biology and metastatic patterns this treatment option is only justified in patients with colorectal primaries. In this selected patient group the rationale for a regional therapeutic approach was substantiated by anatomic, pharmacological, experimental and clinical data. This review specifically focused on the use of the implanted pump for continuous drug delivery which results in a high total dose of the administered drug with a relatively low fractional cell kill. On the basis of present clinical and pharmacological data the fluorinated pyrimidines are the only established therapeutic option for use in this technically very reliable device.

After having defined our armamentarium and target one should look at the goals we are aiming at in cancer treatment. A first goal is improving overall survival and attaining cure of patients with colorectal malignant disease. This latter goal has not been attained. A second (best) goal is the prolongation of life. The uncontrolled studies reported here pointed at survival benefit, but these data could support a selection bias favouring pump treated patients with a greater likelihood of prolonged survival. No clear-cut survival advantage was demonstrated by the data from the ongoing randomized trials. A related problem is that all comparisons of treatment results to date have been more or less in vain because the investigators have never referred to standardized criteria for patient selection, magnitude of the metastatic spread or definition of response to the treatment. In fact, the lack of a worldwide accepted classification of liver metastases is responsible for the present difficulty of assessing any treatment in relation to untreated controls. So far no randomized trial including a no-treatment control arm has been performed. The reported response rates varied widely among the uncontrolled series. Preliminary data from the three randomized trials provided evidence for increased response rates in the intra-arterially treated groups. A third goal is the maintenance or restoration of quality of life. One should realize that liver disease is often asymptomatic until very close to the end, and among the routes of exodus for the cancer patient, liver failure is not the worst. At this moment it remains unclear what the outcome of the cost/benefit ratio is of making symptomatic patients asymptomatic and vice versa. The lack of uniformity of reporting treatment responses is even more true for the interpretation and quantitation of the quality of life data of this until now palliative treatment method. Quality of life data would be especially relevant if there were similar survival statistics provided in two different treatment plans within a clinical trial. Then, the treatment that had the lowest morbidity and allowed for the best quality of life would be recommended for broad application. Patients treated with continuous hepatic chemotherapy all experience to some extent toxicity, most commonly chemical hepatitis. A more serious complication is sclerosing cholangitis (biliary sclerosis) which may be fatal. Acute cholecystitis has commonly been reported and most investigators will routinely remove the gallbladder at the time of catheter placement. At present there is no conclusive answer to the questions related to quality of life.

A final goal of cancer treatment is to gain information on tumor biology, and the influence of the therapeutic option to alter the metastastic pattern. Despite the shortcomings of many studies, a number of studies have addressed important issues in regional cancer treatment. The answer to the question, if by effective regional therapy the natural history of the disease can be altered, seems to be affirmative. A definitive shift towards extrahepatic treatment failures is noticed indicating a intervening effect on tumor at the (clinically) dominant site: the liver.

Current trials must be completed. Yet, even at this point, available data point to the continued need for innovation in the treatment of hepatic metastatic colorectal cancer. The delivery of FUDR by the infusion pump has improved our understanding of the therapeutic problems of such an approach. The need to test hypotheses under the restrictions of a clinical trial-setting is evident with standardization of our definitions of response criteria. Only in this setting the use of the implantable pump is justified so that through a cooperative approach answers can be given to a few of the myriad of questions to be addressed. Also the 'combined modality treatments' concerning the combination of resection therapy with (adjuvant) continuous regional chemotherapy should be fui ther explored [41, 42]. Not enough data are presently available to make definitive statements concerning utility, applicability and indications of regional, continuous cytotoxic drug delivery. However, the need for exploration of alternative approaches is already evident.

Acknowledgements

The authors gratefully acknowledge the participation of W. John B. Hodgson, J. Pettavel, Seymour I. Schwartz, Peter Schlag and Margaret Kemeny for their assistance and contributions to the session.

References

1. De Brauw LM, Van de Velde CJH, Bouwhuis-Hoogerwerf ML, Zwaveling A: Diagnostic evaluation and survival analysis of colorectal cancer patients with liver metastasis. J Surg Oncol 34: 81–86, 1987
2. Ackerman NB, Lien WM, Kondi ES, Silverman NA: The blood supply of experimental metastasis: I. The distribution of hepatic artery and portal vein blood to 'small' and 'large' tumors. Surgery 66: 1067–1072, 1969
3. Strohmeier T, Haugeberg G, Lierse W: Vaskularisation von Lebermetastasen: eine korrosionsanatomische Studie. Acta Anat 12: 172–176, 1986
4. Ackerman NB: Experimental studies on the role of the portal circulation in hepatic tumor vascularity. Cancer 58: 1653–1657, 1986
5. Cho KJ, Lunderquist A: Experimental hepatic artery embolization with Gelfoam powder: Microfil perfusion study of the rabbit liver. Invest Radiol 17: 523–527, 1982
6. Lin G, Lunderquist A, Hägerstrand I, Boijsen E: Postmortem examination of the blood supply and vascular pattern of small liver metastases in man. Surgery 96: 517–526, 1984
7. Chen HSG, Gross JF: Intra-arterial infusion of anticancer drugs: theoretic aspects of drug delivery and review of responses. Cancer Treatm Rep 64: 31–40, 1980
8. Ensminger WD, Rosowsky A, Raso V, et al.: A clinical-pharmacological evaluation of hepatic arterial infusions of 5-fluoro-2'-deoxyuridine and 5-fluorouracil. Cancer Res 38: 3784–3792, 1982
9. McDermott BJ, Van den Berg HW, Murphy RF: Non-linear pharmacokinetics for the elimination of 5-fluorouracil after intravenous administration in cancer patients. Cancer Chemother Pharmacol 9: 173–178, 1982
10. De Bruijn EA, Remeijer L, Tjaden UR, et al.: Non-linear pharmacokinetics of 5-fluorouracil as described by in-vivo behaviour of 5,6 dihydro-5-fluorouracil. Biochem Pharmacol 35: 2461–2465, 1986
11. Schein PS: Management of hepatic metastases: A general overview. In: Van de Velde CJH, Sugarbaker PH (eds) Liver Metastasis, Basic aspects, Detection and Management. Martinus Nijhoff Publ, Boston/Dordrecht/Lancaster, 1984, pp 169–177
12. Mandel HG: The target cell determination of the antitumor actions of 5-FU: Does 5-FU incorporation into RNA play a role? Cancer Treatm Rep 65: 63–71, 1981

13. Heidelberger C: Pyrimidine and pyrimidine nucleoside antimetabolites. In: Holland JF, Frei E (eds) Cancer Medicine. Philadelphia, Pens., Lea and Febiger, 1973, pp 768–791
14. Washtien WL, Santi DV: Assay of intracellular free and macromolecular bound metabolites of 5-fluorodeoxyuridine and 5-fluorouracil. Cancer Res 38: 3397–3404, 1979
15. Welch JP, Donaldson GA: Detection and treatment of recurrent cancer of the colon and rectum. Am J Surg 135: 505–511, 1978
16. Hughes KS, Simon R, Songhorabodi S, et al.: Resection of the liver for colorectal carcinoma metastases: A multi-institutional study of patterns of recurrence. Surgery 100: 278–284, 1986
17. Jaffe BM, Donegan WL, Watson F, et al.: Factors influencing survival in patients with untreated hepatic metastases. Surg Gynecol Obstet 127: 1–11, 1968
18. Grage TB, Vassilopoulos PP, Shingleton WW, et al.: Results of a prospective randomized study of hepatic artery infusion with 5-fluorouracil vs intravenous 5-fluorouracil in patients with hepatic metastases from colorectal cancer: a Central Oncology Group study. Surgery 86: 550–555, 1979
19. Opfell RW, Bowen J: Regional chemotherapy of liver cancer. In: Bottino JC, Opfell RW, Muggia FM (eds) Liver Cancer. Martinus Nijhoff, Boston, 1985, pp 247–263
20. Cotino H, Zwaveling A: Treatment of experimental liver tumors by continuous intra-arterial chemotherapy. Eur J Cancer 12: 177–180, 1976
21. Blackshear PJ: Implantable drug-delivery systems. Scientific American 241: 66–73, 1979
22. Frei E, Garnick MB, Ensminger WD, et al.: Biochemical pharmacology in medical oncology. Cancer Treatm Rep 65, Suppl. 3: 21–26, 1981
23. Seifert P, Baker LH, Reed ML, et al.: Comparison of continuously infused 5-fluorouracil with bolus injection in treatment of patients with colorectal adenocarcinoma. Cancer 36: 123–128, 1975
24. Blackshear PJ, Dorman FD, Blackshear PL, et al.: The design and initial testing of an implantable infusion pump. Surg Gynecol Obstet 143: 54–56, 1972
25. Buchwald H, Grage TB, Vassilopoulos PP, et al.: Intra-arterial infusion chemotherapy for hepatic carcinoma using a totally implantable infusion pump. Cancer 45: 866–869, 1980
26. Ensminger W, Niederhuber J, Gyves J, et al.: Effective control of liver metastases from colon cancer with an implanted system for hepatic arterial chemotherapy. Proc Am Soc Clin Oncol (Abstr) 1: 82, 1982
27. Balch DM, Urist MM, Soong SJ, McGregor M: A prospective phase II clinical trial of continuous FUDR regional chemotherapy for colorectal metastases to the liver using a totally implantable drug infusion pump. Ann Surg 198: 567–573, 1983
28. Weiss GR, Garnick MB, Osteen RT, et al.: Long-term hepatic arterial infusion of 5-fluorodeoxyuridine for liver metastases using an implantable infusion pump. J Clin Oncol 1: 337–344, 1983
29. Schwartz SI, Jones LS, McCune GS: Assessment of treatment of intrahepatic malignancies using chemotherapy via an implantable pump. Ann Surg 201: 560–565, 1985
30. Cohen AM, Greenfield A, Wood WC, et al.: Treatment of hepatic metastases by transaxillary hepatic artery chemotherapy using an implanted drug pump. Cancer 51: 2013–2019, 1983
31. Niederhuber E, Ensminger WD, Gyves J, et al.: Regional chemotherapy of colorectal cancer metastatic to the liver. Cancer 53: 1336–1343, 1984
32. Johnson LP, Wasserman PB, Rivkin SE: The implanted pump in metastatic colorectal cancer of the liver. Am J Surg 149: 595–598, 1985
33. Lahr CJ, Soong SJ, Cloud G, et al.: A multifactorial analysis of prognostic factors in patients with liver metastases from colorectal carcinoma. J Clin Oncol 1: 720–726, 1983
34. Kemeny M, Daly J, Oderman P, et al.: Hepatic artery pump infusion: toxicity and results in patients with metastatic colorectal carcinoma. J Clin Oncol 2: 595–600, 1984
35. Lokich JJ, Kinsella T, Perri J, et al.: Concomitant hepatic radiation and intra-arterial fluo-

rinated pyrimidine therapy: Correlation of liver scan, liver function tests, and plasma CEA and tumor response. Cancer 48: 2569–2574, 1981

36. Van de Velde CJH, Veenhof CHN, Sugarbaker PH: Methodology in the clinical study of heaptic metastases. In: Van de Velde CJH, Sugarbaker PH (eds) Liver Metastasis, Basic aspects, detection and management. Martinus Nijhoff Publ Boston/Dordrecht/Lancaster, 1984, pp 358–375

37. Kemeny M, Reichman D, Oderman P, et al.: Update of randomized study of intrahepatic vs systemic infusion of fluorodeoxyuridine in patients with liver metastases from colorectal carcinoma. Proc Am Soc Clin Oncol (Abstr) 5: 349, 1986

38. Sugarbaker PH: Unpublished results, 1987

39. Niederhuber JE: Arterial chemotherapy for metastatic colorectal cancer in the liver: hepatic tumor study group. In: Abstract-book II Int Conf Adv Reg Cancer Ther, Giessen, W-Germany, 1985, p 23

40. Shepard KV, Levin B, Karl RC: Therapy for metastatic colorectal cancer with hepatic artery infusion chemotherapy using a subcutaneous implanted pump. J Clin Oncol 3: 161–169, 1985

41. Kemeny MM, Goldberg D, Beatty, et al.: Results of a prospective randomized trial of continuous regional chemotherapy and hepatic resection as treatment of hepatic metastases from colorectal primaries. Cancer 57: 492–498, 1986

42. Hodgson WJB, Friedland M, Mittelman A, et al.: Treatment of colorectal hepatic metastases by intrahepatic chemotherapy alone or as an adjuvant to complete or partial removal of metastatic disease. Ann Surg 203: 420–425, 1986

10. Primary cancer of the liver: considerations about resection

M.A. ADSON

Cancer may arise from any of the great variety of cells that comprise the liver, and each type of cell may be incited to malignant change in a variety of ways [1]. Therefore, the spectrum of primary hepatic malignancies that may or may not be resectable is so broad as to preclude generalizations about therapy.

The uncommon primary malignancies

Primary hepatic sarcomas, cystadenocarcinomas, mesenchymal malignancies and localized lymphomas are so uncommon that resectability rates and results of resective treatment cannot be studied well. However, enough is known about such lesions [2] that most often rational judgments about treatment can be made. Surgical decisions have to do with: the tumors location in relation to portions of the liver that must be saved; the nature of the tumor's periphery (whether it is inclined to push or to invade); and to tendencies to multicentric growth or hematogenous or lymphogenous spread. There is some evidence to show, and good reason to believe on empiric grounds, that these less common primary liver cancers may be treated by resection more often and more successfully than are the more common malignant lesions that arise from intrahepatic biliary ducts or from hepatocytes. This has to do with the fact that some of these uncommon tumors are less invasive of resective margins, lymphatics and blood vessels, and because some may respond to adjuvant biological manipulations by use of radiation, immunotherapy or chemotherapy.

Hepatic cholangiocarcinomas

The next more common tumor is cancer that arises in the intrahepatic biliary ducts. Histopathologically, all cholangiocarcinomas are seen to be much the same. There are variations in the degree of cellular undifferentiation that affect the incidence of distant spread and the chance for invasion beyond resectable margins. But, the site of origin of such tumors and their extent of growth when found are the major determinants of prognosis.

There are some problems in the anatomical classification of 'hepatic' versus 'ductal' cholangiocarciomas when the same cells line the biliary tree from its periphery through the hilar ductal conguries to the major ducts that drain the liver into the gut. It is possible to make an arbitrary distinction between cholangiocarcinomas that arise in intrahepatic ducts and present as 'hepatic' tumors rather than major ductal lesions that start to grow outside the liver. Nevertheless, studies of 'hepatic' cholangiocarcinomas are faulted by the anatomic contiguity of intra and extrahepatic biliary ducts, by intraductal or parenchymal extensions of some one sided tumors to the other side, and by some tendency to multicentric growth.

David Nagorney [3] has studied 32 patients seen in our Clinic between 1965 and 1980 who had histologically proven *cholangiocarcinomas* that appeared to have arisen from intrahepatic ducts and presented as 'hepatic' rather than major ductal tumors. More than three-fourths of the tumors were *not* removed because of co-existent cirrhosis [7], sclerosing cholangitis [2], or because lesions were either bilobar or so centrally sited that no functioning portion of the liver could have been preserved had the tumors been removed. Only seven of the 32 tumors (22 percent) were resected – six with intent of cure and one for palliation. The mean survival of patients who had tumors removed was three years, and one patient was still living without recurrence 4.6 years after the tumor was taken out. These results of resective treatment can be compared with a mean 3.6 month survival of patients who had tumors that were not removed. However, the influence of natural history is seen in two untreated patients: one is alive 4.5 years after diagnosis of an unresectable tumor, and another patient died three years after having only a palliative resection. Slow growth related to histopathologic differentiation likely accounts for such longevity. Nevertheless, resection of resectable tumors seems to have value even though the major determinants of survival too often are related to proximity of 'hepatic' cholangiocarcinomas to major biliary ducts, coexistent cirrhosis, intrahepatic ductal extensions of tumor, and multicentric growth. Thus, primary hepatic cancers that arise in the minor biliary ducts are less amenable to resective treatment than are malignant tumors that arise from hepatocytes.

Primary hepatocelluar malignancy

Hepatocytic cancer (hepatocellular carcinoma) the most common primary hepatic malignancy occurs worldwide in a variety of forms determined by regional epidemiologic factors. Thus, the tumor must be considered hemispherically [4–6].

Hepatocellular cancer in the western hemisphere

Resectability. In the *Western world,* co-existent cirrhosis (present about half the time) most often is considered to be a deterrent to resective surgery. However, malignancy that develops in otherwise normal livers often can be resected with acceptable risk and enhanced survival. Despite general agreement about the value of resection of such lesions, a clear view of the true incidence and resectability rates of such tumors after resection is not evident in the existing literature. The tumor is as common as is Hodgkin's disease in North America [7]; but hepatocytic cancer is surgically obscure when its true *incidence* is hidden by co-existent cirrhosis, and overlooked in studies of advanced disease reported prior to common use of good techniques for hepatic imaging. Also, mass 'medical' surveys [8, 9] of treated populations reflect low *resectability rates* (less than 10 percent) without stating how often proper surgical consultation had been obtained. Moreover, such low estimates of resectability are hard to reconcile with exaggerated 'surgical' views reported when the resectability rates are calculated with reference to a partial sample of patients who came to surgical evaluation.

Confusion stems from indiscrimate use of the words *operability* and *resectability* and from the fact that few surgeons are able to account for those patients (who have obviously unresectable tumors) that they have not been asked to see. Surgeons in the West report resectability rates which range from 21 to 44 percent [1, 2, 4–6, 10–20]. However, most often these figures have been exaggerated by selective bias or by patterns of referral. In such calculations, the numerator (the patients who have had their tumors resected) is easily identified: but the denominator (comprised of an undefined partial sample of unseen total population) remains obscure. As a consequence, a broad view of the true value of resective surgery done for hepatocytic cancer is difficult to obtain.

Our institutional study of *resectability* [21] likely is faulted by patterns of referral, but offers a realistic and somewhat hopeful view. Of 123 patients who had histologically proven hepatocytic cancers seen at the Mayo Clinic between 1972 and 1982, 60 had co-existent cirrhosis. None of them was treated surgically. But, for 34 (54 percent) of the 63 patients who had cancers that grew in normal livers, all gross evidence of tumor could be removed. Only one early operative death followed these 'curative' resections, and 25 percent lived five years or more. Obviously, the frequent presence of cirrhosis contaminates the scene: overall resectability rate was 28 percent; but 54 percent of patients who had cancer which grew in non-cirrhotic livers had tumors which could be removed.

Operative mortality. The risk of hepatic resection relates to problems with hemostasis, to injury of blood vessels or biliary ducts that serve portions of the

Table 1. Resective treatment – Western experience. Most reported analysis involve *all* primary hepatic malignancies. Only in the reports of Huguet and Adson could other lesions be excluded for separate analysis of experiences with hepatocellular cancers.

	El-Dameiri (1971)	Foster Berman (1977)	Flatmark (1977)	Smith (1979)	Sorenson (1979)	Hanks (1980)	Fortner (1981)	Bengmark (1982)	Starzl Iwatsuki (1983)	Thompson (1983)	Lim/Bongard (1984)	Adson (1985)	Huguet/Mouiel (1983)	Huguet/Mouiel (1983)
Tumors resected[a]	26	134	16	48	31	10	42	21	43	35	22	47	134	75
With cirrhosis – %	?	20%	0	?	16%	10%	?	0	12%	20%	43	4%	0%	100%
Hepatocellular carcinoma[a]	19	109	16	22	25	7	30	15	29	26		47	134	75
Other primary malignancies	7	25	0	23	6	3	10	4	10	9		0		
Hospital mortality, %	42%[b]	21%	6%	7%	26%	20%	17%	14%	9%	20%	37%	5%	22%	33%
Long-term survival, % at														
1yr		80%					85%		78%				72	58
2yr		68%	73%	28%	62%			38%	60%				50	35
3yr		53%			42%		50%		56%		Median,	54%	36	19
4yr		37%						20%					27	12
5yr	16%	30%		11%	16%		37%		46%	31%	16 months	35%	23	4
10yr												20%		
Hospital mortality														
Included	X			X					X	X	X	X		
Excluded		X	X	X	X	X	X	X					X	X

[a] Observations that could not be tabulated conveniently are: 1) exclusion from El-Dameiri's report of wedge resections of histologically unclassified lesions, 2) Smith's failure to distinguish between intraoperative and hospital mortality in his reference to patients 'who survived operation', and the disparity between his tabulated classification of 48 primary hepatic malignancies and his reference in his text to '60 patients undergoing lobectomy', the 3) the fact that many of Fortner and coauthors' patients had palliative resections, and 9 of Bengmark and associates' 21 patients had either tumor at the margin of resection or lymph node metastases.

[b] Wedge resections excluded because types of tumors not reported.

liver to be saved, and to hepatic functional reserve. The risk of standardized anatomical major resections done by experienced surgeons for patients who have no co-existent hepatic disease is less than five percent (Table 1). Higher reported rates of operative and early postoperative mortality reflect operative inexperience evident in broad surveys [1, 20] or early publications [10]; the presence of co-existent cirrhosis of the liver [19, 20] or anatomical problems associated with very large or centrally sited tumors.

Each of these determinants of increased risk is easy to explain: experience with parenchymal hemostasis is not easy to acquire; cirrhosis may beget technical difficulties with hemostasis and may compromise convalescence when hepatic functional reserve is low; and the proximity of tumors to the vena cava, major hepatic veins or the hepatic hilus is an obvious cause of surgical misadventure.

Operative risk can be reduced by better understanding of surgical anatomy and by surgical experience as well as by avoidance of or very selective surgical management of cirrhotic patients. However, the only other way to reduce operative mortality involves surgical judgments that are hard to objectify and to justify – the denial of resection for patients who have tumors so large or so sited as to be surgically available only at increased risk.

Specific analyses of the risk involved in what may at times be seen as undue surgical aggressiveness cannot be found in our literature. However, the influence of this factor in the reported operative risks of resection of primary hepatic malignancies can be seen clearly between the lines. The reported operative risk involved in the resection of primary hepatic malignancies is much greater than the risk involved in removing either benign or metastatic liver lesions [4, 5]. This has to do with the increased incidence of cirrhosis that co-exists with hepatocytic cancer; but also, it has to do with the fact that primary hepatic malignancies are so often symptomatic and with the fact that so often the hepatic growth of such lesions appears to be the major determinants of prognosis. The increased risk involved in resection of large asymptomatic *benign* liver lesions that are surgically uninviting is easy to avoid. Also, reluctance to take great risk for resection of unfavorably sited *metastatic lesions* is easily rationalized (and most often can be rationally justified) either by absence of symptoms or by the frequent presence of other major determinants of prognosis (other metastases that are present but cannot be seen).

Therefore, there is good evidence of show that increased risk associated with resection of primary hepatic malignances has to do with the presence of concomitant cirrhosis, and also with the fact that increased surgical aggressiveness is fostered by the presence of symptoms, the lack of therapeutic alternatives, and by the appearance of the hepatic lesion as a major determinant of prognosis.

Longterm survival. Length of survival of patients who have primary liver cancer is determined mostly by the natural history of this disease. Unfavorable determinants include: 1) the tumor's frequent association with cirrhosis of the liver, 2) the usual appearance of symptoms only after extended growth, 3) predisposition to hematogenous metastases, and 4) some tendency to multicentric growth.

Nevertheless, a significant number of patients in whom such lesions grow may be cured or palliated by resection of their tumors. About one-half of patients have cirrhosis which increases operative risk and limits longterm survival; and about one-half of tumors that grow in non-cirrhotic livers are found only after having extended beyond the limits of resection. However, for the rest, resection offers five-year survival to about one-third of treated patients. Results of resective treatment reported by surgeons in the Western World, are summarized on Table 1. Although longterm survival is determined in part by operative mortality, the table shows that some authors have *not* included this factor in their calculations.

The influence of cirrhosis upon operative mortality and upon longterm survival is evident in careful comparative analysis and can be seen in the table in two reports. Lim and Bongard's [19] experience was greatly influenced by patients derived from shifting Asian populations to the western coast of North America; and Huguet and Moniels' [20] broad survey of the experience of 100 members of the French Surgical Society shows most clearly the unfavorable influence of co-existent cirrhosis by specific comparative analysis.

Whether or not the extent of resection affects longterm survival is difficult to determine from available reports. There is no doubt that limited tumor-free resective margins are a source of residual or recurrent growth. However, good correlations between width of unaffected margins and incidence of local recurrence have not been made. Also, specific studies that relates tumor size and site (in relation to major veins or hilar structures) have not been done.

Smalley's [22] study of patterns of recurrence following resective surgery done in our Clinic showed loco-regional (liver only) recurrence to have developed in 50 percent of our resected patients. However, because good correlations between width of resective margins and hepatic recurrence could not be made, we could not determine whether recurrence came from marginal residua or from multicentric growth. Having personal experience with most of the patients studied, I do know that many of the tumors were very large and unfavorably sited and that (at least for me) the widest available resective margins had been obtained.

Starzl's remarkable experience [17] suggests that extent of resection may influence survival. His group has performed hepatic trisegmentectomy and lobectomy with an operative mortality no greater than that of lesser resections, and their rates of survival after resection are better than those of others (Table

1). Whether this survival is related to the extent of resection, to patient selection, or to the method of analyzing longterm survival rates is unclear.

Fibrolamellar hepatoma, a more or less distinct variant which occurs more often in somewhat younger patients (median age 26 years) has been shown to have a more favorable prognosis than other hepatocytic cancers [23–25]. However, our institutional study of this lesion [26] showed that one-fourth of such tumors contain foci of non-fibrolamellar hepatocytic cancer. Also, survival *after* resection was similar to survival after removal of type ordinaire hepatocytic cancers. Thus, the more favorable *overall* prognosis was determined by higher resectability rate of the fibrolamellar variant (75 percent versus 50 percent of nonfibrolamellar tumors seen).

The risks, limitations and benefits of resection or primary hepatic malignancies have been reasonably well defined. It is likely that only small gains will come with technological advances in diagnostic imaging or in surgical technique. The need for biological manipulations for use as primary or adjuvant therapy is all too clear.

Hepatocellular cancer in the east – A western view

Most Western surgeons are reluctant to treat hepatocytic cancer associated with cirrhosis when operative mortality is seen to exceed five-year survival rates by far. However, in the East, surgeons have made thoughtful efforts to prevail [27–35]. The screening of patients with viral hepatitis or cirrhosis has identified patients with small 'early' hepatic cancers which are resectable. Also, early detection has been combined with careful measurement of hepatic functional reserve and use of limited sublobar resections. Reported results reflect impressively low operative mortality, and reports of postoperative survival are encouraging so far as they have gone. However, few Eastern surgeons have considered the importance of the natural history of disease in a convincing way. Calculated survival rates do not take into account the time that smaller lesions might have taken to become symptomatic or clinically evident (or to kill), and postoperative studies give evidence of rising levels of alpha-feto-protein which must signify development of multicentric neoplasia. Even if Eastern surgeons are seen to be effective, efforts to duplicate their experience in the West must be studied separately – because both hepatocytic cancer *and* cirrhosis may differ markedly from East to West [36].

References

1. Popper H: Hepatic cancers in man: quantitative perspectives. Environmental Research 19: 482, 1979

2. Foster JH, Berman MM: Solid liver tumors. In: Major Problems in Clinical Surgery. WBSaunders, Philadelphia, 22: 1, 1977
3. Schlinkert RT, Nagorney DM, van Heerden JA, Adson MA: Intrahepatic cholangiocarcinoma. (Submitted for publication)
4. Adson MA: Liver resection in primary and secondary liver cancer. In: S Bengmark and LH Blumgart (eds) Liver Surgery. Churchill Livingstone, Edinburgh, 1986, pp 63–80
5. Adson MA: Primary hepatocellular cancers – Western experience. (in press)
6. Nagorney DM, Adson MA: Major hepatic resections for hepatoma in the West. In: HJ Wanebo (ed) Hepatic and Biliary Cancer. Marcel Dekker, Inc, New York, 1987, pp 167–185
7. Cancer Statistics: CA 1980, pp 30: 23
8. Axtell LM, Asire AJ, Meyers MH: Cancer patient survival report number 5. In: Asire and Meyers (eds) DHEW publication No. NHI 77–992, Axtell. Government Printing Office, Washington, D.C., 1976, pp 60, 124
9. Smart CR: Progress in cancer patient management in community hospitals. American College of Surgeons Bulletin 5–13, (sept) 1981
10. El-Domeiri AA, Huvos AG, Goldsmith HS, Foote Jr FW: Primary malignant tumours of the liver. Cancer 27: 7, 1971
11. Flatmark A, Frethem B, Knutrud O, Lande G: Surgical treatment of primary liver carcinoma. Scand J Gastroent 12: 571, 1977
12. Smith R: Bradshaw Lecture 1977: tumors of the liver. Ann Royal Coll Surg Eng 61: 87, 1979
13. Sorenson TIA, Aronsen KF, Aune S, et al.: Results of hepatic lobectomy for primary epithelial cancer in 31 adults. Am J Surg 138: 407, 1979
14. Hanks JB, Meyers WC, Filston HC, Killenberg PG, Jones RS: Surgical resection for benign and malignant liver disease. Ann Surg 191: 584, 1980
15. Fortner JG, Maclean BJ, Kim DK, Howland WS, Turnbull D, Goldiner P, et al.: The seventies evolution in liver surgery for cancer 47: 2162, 1981
16. Bengmark S, Hafstrom L, Jeppsson B, Sundqvist K: Primary carcinoma of the liver: Improvement in sight? W J Surg 6: 65, 1982
17. Iwatsuki S, Shaw Jr BW, Starzl TE: Experience with 150 liver resections. Ann Surg 197: 247, 1983
18. Thompson HH, Tompkins RK, Longmire Jr WP: Major hepatic resection. A 25-year experience. Ann Surg 197: 375, 1983
19. Lim Jr RC, Bongard FS: Hepatocellular carcinoma. Changing concepts in diagnosis and management. Arch Surg 119: 637, 1984
20. Huguet CI, Mouiel J: Les tumeurs primitives du foie chez l'adulte. Masson, Paris, 1983
21. Smalley SR, Moertel CG, Adson MA, Creagan ET, Fleming T, Hilton J, Nagorney DM: Treatment of hepatocellular carcinoma in the noncirrhotic liver. Proc Am Soc Clin Oncol 3: 148, 1984
22. Smalley SR, Gunderson LL, Schray MF, Adson MA, Moertel CG, Weiland LH: Patterns of failure following complete resection of hepatomas (in press)
23. Craig JR, Peters RL, Edmondson HA, Omata M: Fibrolamellar carcinoma of the liver. A tumor of adolescents and young adults with distinctive clinico-pathologic features. Cancer 46: 372, 1980
24. Berman MM, Libbey NP, Foster JH: Hepatocellular carcinoma: Polygonal cell type with fibrous stroma – an atypical variant with a favorable prognosis. Cancer 46: 1448, 1980
25. Collier NA, Weinbren K, Bloom SR, Lee YC, Hodgson HJF, Blumgart LH: Neurotensin secretion by fibrolamellar carcinoma of the liver. Lancet 1: 538, 1984
26. Nagorney DM, Adson MA, Weiland LH, Knight CD, Smalley SR, Zinsmeister AR: Fibrolamellar hepatoma. Am J Surg 149: 113, 1985
27. Okuda K, Musha H, Nakajima Y, Kubo Y, Shimokawa Y, Nagasaki Y, Sawa Y, et al.: Clin-

icopathologic features of encapsulated hepatocellular carcinoma. A study of 26 cases. Cancer 40: 1240, 1977

28. Okuda K and the Liver Cancer Study Group of Japan: Primary liver cancers in Japan. Cancer 45: 2663, 1980
29. Tobe T: Current status of surgical therapy for primary liver cancer in Japan. Jpn J Surg 13: 86, 1983
30. Tobe T: Hepatectomy in patients with cirrhotic livers: Clinical and basic observations. Surg Annu. 16: 177, 1984
31. Tang A, Yu Y, Lin Z, Zhou X, Yang B, Cao Y, Lu J, Tang C: Small hepatocellular carcinoma. Clinical analysis of 30 cases. Chin Med J (Engl) 92: 455, 1979
32. Wu M, Chen H, Zhan X, Yao X, Yang J: Primary hepatic carcinoma resection over 18 years. Chin Med J (Engl) 93: 723, 1980
33. Shinagawa T, Ohto M, Kimura K, Tsunetomi S, Morita M, Saisho H, Tsuchiya T, Saotome N, Karasawa E, Miki M, Ueno T, Okuda K: Diagnosis and clinical features of small hepatocellular carcinoma with emphasis on the utility of real-time ultrasonography. A study of 51 patients. Gastroent 86: 495, 1984
34. Okuda K, Munemasa R, Takayoshi T: Surgical Management of Hepatoma. The Japanese Experience. In: JH Wanebo (ed) Hepatic and Biliary Cancer. Marcel Dekker, Inc, New York, 1987, pp 219–238
35. Okuda K, Ohtsuki T, Obata H, Masahiko T, Ozazaki N, Hasegawa H, Nakajima Y, Ohnishi K: Natural history of hepatocellular carcinoma and prognosis in relation to treatment. Study of 850 patients. Cancer 56 (4): 918–28, 1985
36. Bismuth H, Houssin D, Ornowski J, Meriggi F: Liver resections in cirrhotic patients: A Western experience. W J Surg 10: 311–317, 1986

11. Liver resection for colorectal metastases: who, when, and to what extent?

M.J. KORETZ, K.S. HUGHES and P.H. SUGARBAKER

Progress in the understanding of the natural history of liver metastases from colorectal cancer as well as improvements in the techniques and technology have permitted the development of curative hepatic surgery over the past two decades. With the accumulation of a large amount of retrospective data from numerous institutions, the time has now come when critical questions must be investigated such as: 1) who are candidates for liver resection, 2) when should resection be performed after the diagnosis of liver metastasis, 3) what is the extent of liver resection necessary for optimal survival rates, and 4) what criteria preclude hepatic resection? These questions will best be answered prospectively, but by analysis of personal experience and review of the available data we hope to provide an initial framework with which to begin to analyze the problems.

Natural history

In the United States, approximately 130,000 cases of colorectal cancer were expected in 1986 and 60,000 deaths due to disease. Liver metastases are an important factor as a cause of mortality, being the cause of death in at least 30% of cases and occurring at some point in 70% of patients who eventually die of colorectal cancer [1]. Long-term survival of patients with liver metastases as measured at five years is quite rare. Analysis of retrospective series reveals that even though short-term survival of two and three years may be common with early stage disease, survival at five years is extremely rare [2, 3]. These dismal survival figures stimulated investigation into the surgical treatment of liver metastases.

   In order to gain a perspective on the impact of surgery for colorectal liver metastases, it is imperative to calculate the number of patients who might be eligible for surgical resection. Between 10 and 20 percent who undergo initial surgery for colorectal cancer will be found to have metastasis only to the liver, and one quarter of those will be resectable. Of those patients resected for cure, another 25 percent will develop metachronous liver metastases, of whom perhaps 25% will be resectable. Therefore roughly about 10% of patients with colorectal cancer will at some point be candidates for curative hepatic resection, or approximately 13,000 cases. It is thought that less than a 10th of this number underwent liver resection in 1986, probably to some extent due to fatalistic opinion by physician.

Diagnosis of liver metastasis

We advise careful, frequent follow up of the colorectal cancer patient to detect signs of postoperative recurrence. A large number of so-called liver function tests have been utilized to screen for liver metastases; unfortunately, their sensitivity is not acceptable to detect disease until an advanced stage (Fig. 1). The discovery of CEA (carcinoembryonic antigen) over twenty years ago has dramatically aided the early diagnosis of colorectal cancer recurrence, especially in the liver. The CEA level is elevated in over 90% of patients with liver metastases and currently remains the most accurate test, followed by physical examination. Once a patient is found to have signs or symptoms suggestive of liver metastases, a thorough workup should be undertaken. Although there are no long term prospective studies proving the efficacy of CEA monitoring in improving the outlook for colorectal cancer, the experience to date suggests that a certain percentage of patients may expect long term benefit by surgical resection of recurrent disease, especially in the liver. Once the CEA level is elevated suggesting disease recurrence, the test should be repeated at least once, since laboratory variations as well as benign inflammatory conditions may cause a false-positive result. If consecutive CEA tests are elevated and the physical examination is not helpful, further workup is indicated. Endoscopy of the colonic suture line is mandatory to rule out anastomotic recurrence. Imaging studies of the abdomen are usually the next tests ordered. The development of radiological imaging techniques over the past ten years has revolutionized the approach to diagnosing recurrent cancer. Computerized tomography of the liver is the most common study for detection of liver tumors in the U.S., especially since it images other areas at risk for recurrence within the peritoneal cavity. In addition, the anatomy and function of the urinary tract can be delineated when water-soluble intravenous contrast is administered. Hepatic vascular structures can also be differentiated from biliary radicles with contrast imaging. Contrast-enhanced CT scans reliably detect lesions as small as 2 cm.

A number of techniques are being utilized in order to increase the accuracy of CT scanning. It has been suggested that the rapid examination of the liver

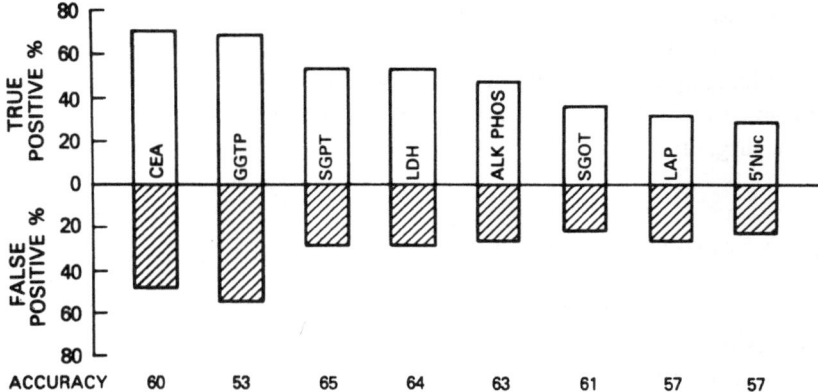

Fig. 1. Accuracy of CEA and liver function tests in predicting liver metastases.

during bolus administration of intravenous contrast can improve the detection rate. To be useful, the entire liver must be imaged within two minutes of the end of the infusion, prior to the equilibrium phase. In addition, the infusion of a large volume of water-soluble intravenous contrast with delayed scanning has been used to improve opacification of the liver and thereby detect very small lesions. Such scanning is done approximately four hours after the initial scan and is therefore too cumbersome for routine use. Another technique to improve liver opacification is that of CT angiography, when the liver is imaged following administration of contrast into the superior mesenteric circulation. Such techniques as described have been reported to accurately diagnose lesions as small as 1 cm, but their clinical utility awaits further trials.

In selected series, ultrasound of the liver has been demonstrated to be as accurate as CT scan in imaging liver metastases [4]. Ultrasound examinations are widely used, especially in Europe, to diagnose and serially follow hepatic tumors. Ultrasound is quite 'observer-dependent' however, and results may differ between institutions. Four sonographic patterns of hepatic metastases are typically seen: foci of increased or decreased echogenicity, cystic appearing or diffuse parenchymal abnormalities without a discrete identifiable focus. One of the advantages of ultrasound is its capability to differentiate cysts from solid tumors. In addition, it displays the anatomic relationship of metastases to hepatic vasculature and the inferior vena cava.

Magnetic resource imaging (MRI) of the liver offers great promise for further improved imaging and treatment planning in patients with liver metastases. MRI uses difference in tissue proton density, spin-lattice relaxation time (T1) and spin-spin relaxation (T2) to produce images of the liver. The metastasis will appear either hypo- or hyperdense compared to the normal liver parenchyma, depending on the technique utilized. MRI is a technique currently undergoing continuous change due to manipulation of image recovery techniques, but we believe it will eventually become the procedure of choice in imaging the liver. In particular, MRI exhibits the precise anatomic relationship of liver lesions to major vascular structures, which is a great benefit to the surgeon.

Diagnosis by percutaneous biopsy

If a patient with a history of colon cancer develops a liver lesion suspicious for metastases on imaging studies, it is usually unnecessary to do a needle aspiration of the liver prior to surgical exploration. When the diagnosis is in doubt, or when there are multiple liver lesions, demonstrations of a benign process by needle biopsy may radically alter the treatment plan. Fine needle aspiration can be performed commonly under CT or ultrasound guidance as an outpatient technique utilizing an 18 to 22 gauge needle. The lesion is initially localized and the skin marked. The needle is then inserted to the previously measured depth and the scan is repeated to confirm proper needle placement.

Investigative techniques

The development of monoclonal antibody technology during the past decade has permitted the production of a 'pure' antibody to cancer antigens such as CEA. When antibodies are tagged with radioactive isotopes, foci of metastases may be imaged utilizing conventional scintiscanning. Due to current limitations including lack of antibody specificity and uptake by the reticuloendothelial system and blood pool, lesions smaller than two centimeters are not reliably imaged. There is little doubt that as the technology improves, monoclonal antibodies will become more useful in the diagnosis of cancer.

Preoperative workup and preparation

Prior to surgical exploration, full workup to exclude distant metastases is mandatory. Computerized tomography of the lung will detect evidence of lung metastases in approximately 15% of patients initially thought to have only liver involvement. Many surgeons obtain a bone scan to rule out bony metastases, but positive results are quite uncommon in the setting of normal laboratory values and lack of symptoms.

Selective hepatic angiography is usually performed prior to surgery to define the hepatic arterial anatomy, which will assist the surgeon in operative dissection of the portal structures. Knowledge of hepatic arterial anomalies such as the right hepatic artery originating from the superior mesenteric artery may simplify the operative dissection.

Prior to liver resection, standard mechanical and antibiotic bowel preparation should be given, in the event that bowel resection becomes necessary. Of course, major concurrent medical problems should be investigated preoperatively including cardiac and pulmonary disease. Severely compromised pulmonary function can cause major postoperative morbidity since thoracoabdominal incisions are often necessary in patients with large tumors.

Surgical considerations

The centennial marking the first reported elective liver resection will occur in 1988. Many of the early advances in liver surgery were reported from Europe including the technical details (Table 1). The publication by Foster and Berman in 1977 of their Liver Tumor Survey [5] served as a milestone in the development and acceptance of hepatic surgery for cancer.

The actual technique for transecting liver parenchyma has been a focus of lively debate among liver surgeons. In 1958, Lin and others described the finger fracture technique, by which the hepatic parenchyma is digitally fractured, preserving the larger bile ducts and vessels. Foster pioneered the technique of utilizing a suction cannula for parenchymal dissection. Technologically advanced instruments such as the laser, ultrasonic dissector and microwave tissue coagulation have been proposed as aids for surgical dissection. The Nd-YAG laser aids liver resection primarily by vaporizing and coagulation actions. In comparison with ultrasound dissection however, the laser appears to cause more local tissue necrosis and bleeding which may lead to complications such as abscesses and biliary leaks due to sloughing of the liver surface. Results from at least two randomized controlled studies comparing ultrasonic dissection, laser transection, and conventional techniques agree that ultrasonic dissection is associated with the least amount of blood loss and the least trauma to hepatic parenchyma [6, 7]. As we have gained further experience with the ultrasonic dissection, we have come to recommend it as the technique of choice. The ultrasound scalpel (or CUSA as it is popularly known) contains a transducer that converts electrical energy into 23 kHZ longitudinal vibrations of a titanium tip. The hepatic parenchymal tissue is fragmented and sucked out of the operative field. Blood vessels and bile ducts can easily be dissected free because fragmentation is proportional to tissue water content and because collagen and elastic yield to the ultrasonic vibrations. This allows careful dissection and ligation of major vessels and directs in a precise unhurried manner while minimizing tissue necrosis and bleeding (Fig. 2). We believe this will di-

Table 1.

Suggested data base record for patients undergoing hepatic resection

Resection of colorectal hepatic metastases clinical record

Patient name: _____ Hospital: _____

Hospital number: _____ Surgeon: _____

Birthdate: _____

(A) Primary colon or rectal tumor

1. Date of resection: ___/___/___

2. Location:
   Ascending
   Transverse
   Descending
   Sigmoid
   Rectum

3. Duke's stage (Astler-coller)
   A B1 B2 C1 C2

4. Nodes resected:

   _____/_____
   Pos.   Total

5. Contiguous structures invaded:
   Omentum   Small bowel
   Prostate   Abdominal wall
   Bladder   Pelvic side wall
   Ovaries   Other _____
   Uterus   None

6. Histology:
   Adenocarcinoma
   Signet ring adenocarcinoma
   Carcinoma simplex
   Mucinous adenocarcinoma
   Scirrhous

7. Grade:
   Poor
   Moderate
   Well

8. Other treatment prior
   to liver metastases:
   None
   Radiation therapy
   Chemotherapy

(B) Preoperative to hepatic resection

1. Date of diagnosis: ___/___/___

2. Determined By:
   L/S scan   Rising CEA
   CT scan   Ultrasound
   Laparotomy   Other

3. Symptoms:
   Present
   Absent

4. Number of metastases
   suspected _____

5. Bilirubin (mg%):

6. Alkaline phosphatase:

7. Albumin (g%):

(C) Operation for hepatic resection

1. Date: _____/_____/_____

2. Number of metastases found:

3. Percent hepatic

replacement =

   <25
   25–75
   >15

4. Wedges # L _____

5. Wedges # R _____

6. Major resection:
   L lobe
   R lobe
   L lat. seg.
   Triseg

7. Extrahepatic disease:
   None
   Nodes
   Contiguous
   Discontinuous

8. Other organs involved:
   None   Small bowel
   Diaphragm   Abdominal wall
   Adrenal   Omentum
   Kidney   Other _____

9. Made NED:
   Yes
   No

Table 1. Continued.

(D) Postoperative

1. CEA (Nadir):   2. Complications: 3. Chemotherapy and route:

_____ Date: _____

None	None	IV (periph)
Bleeding	5-FU	Intra-peritoneal
Infection-intraabdominal	FUDR	Intra-arterial
Infection-wound	Other	Intra-portal
Other _____		

Resection of colorectal hepatic metastases pathologic record

Patient name: _____ Hospital: _____

Hospital number: _____

(F) GROSS EXAM

1. Total number of nodules on the surface of specimen: _____

2. Total number of nodules seen upon cutting specimen into 1 cm slices: _____

3. Location of individual metastases:

	1.		2.		3.		4.		5.	
Left/Right:	L	R	L	R	L	R	L	R	L	R
Med./Lat.:	M	L	M	L	M	L	M	L	M	L
Ant./Post.:	A	P	A	P	A	P	A	P	A	P

4. Closest margin: 5. Extrahepatic invasion:

Gross inspection: _____   None

Microscopic: _____   Nodes

Contiguous

Discontinuous

(G) Analysis of individual metastases

	#1	#2	#3	#4	#5
1. Size (greatest diameter)					
2. Grade (1 [poor] to 3 [well])					
3. Histologic type					
4. Hepatic venous invasion (Y/N)					
5. Lymphatic invasion (Y/N)					
6. Portal venous invasion (Y/N)					
7. Inflammatory response (Y/N)					
8. Tumor border (1= pushing, 2= infiltrating)					
9. Necrosis (0 [least] to 4 [most])					
10. Daughter metastases (number)					

Key: 2. 1 = Poor   2 = Moderate   3 = Well

3. 1 = Adenocarcinoma   2 = Scirrhous   3 = Mucinous   4 = Signet ring

5 = Carcinoma simplex

(H) Hepatic lymph nodes

1. Number (total) ... _____ 2. Size ... _____ 3. Number positive ... _____

4. Histopathology ....

1 = Sinus histiocytosis   2 = Paracortical activity   3 = Germinal center activity

(I) Mediastinal nodes

1. Number (total) ... _____ 2. Size ... _____ 3. Number positive ... _____

4. Histopathology ....

1 = Sinus histiocytosis   2 = Paracortical activity   3 = Germinal center activity

Comments: _____

_____

_____

_____

_____

_____

196

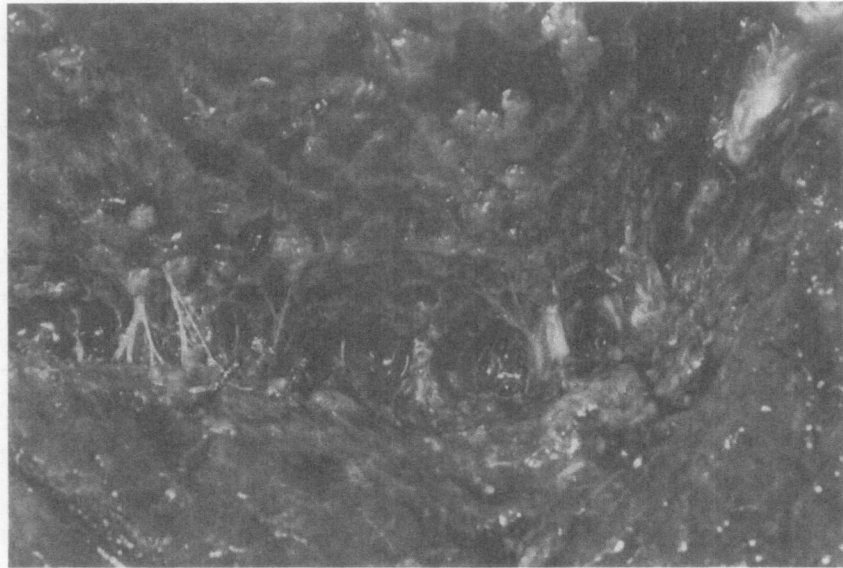

Fig. 2. Exposure of bile ducts and vessels by ultrasonic dissection allowing controlled division.

rectly result in a negligible incidence of bile leaks and infections when performed properly.

A thorough knowledge of vascular and ductal anatomy is necessary for safe hepatic surgery [8]. Liver anatomy allows five major resections (Fig. 3). Small or peripheral tumors can be removed by a wedge resection, although anatomic lobular resections will transverse fewer major blood vessels and ducts than major wedge resections and we believe are often safer to perform. For large metastatic lesions in the right lobe, thoracic extension through the diaphragm allows improved and safer exposure, while the remainder of hepatic resections can usually be performed through the abdominal incision alone.

Prior to the actual performance of liver resection, a thorough exploration at laparotomy is indicated to detect extrahepatic disease. Despite the best efforts in imaging the liver and abdominal cavity, in approximately one third of cases additional disease will be detected, usually extrahepatic, which will lead to abandonment of the liver resection. Therefore thorough exploration remains the 'gold standard' for staging patients with liver metastases [9]. Extrahepatic involvement of either portal or celiac nodes has been conventionally felt to be a contraindication to liver resection. Localized extrahepatic soft tissue recurrence may not represent an absolute contraindication to resection, as will be discussed later. Once examination has confirmed limitation of disease to the liver, a number of preliminary steps are helpful prior to actual liver transection. A large self-retaining retractor should be positioned so that the operative

Date	Author	Country	Comment
1888	Garrè (Bruns)	Germany	Metastatectomy
1899	Keen	USA	Left lateral segmentectomy
1908	Pringle	Great Britain	Temporary occlusion of the portal pedicle
1910	Wendel	Germany	Right lobectomy, partial hilar dissection
1952	Lortat-Jacob and Robert	France	Preliminary hilar ligation for anatomic lobectomy
1958	Lin	Taiwan	Finger fracture technique
1971	Storm and Longmire	USA	Liver clamp
1975	Starzl, et al.	USA	Right trisegmentectomy
1977	Foster and Berman	USA	Liver Tumor Survey, Suction dissection technique
1979	Hodgson and Aufses	USA	Ultrasonic dissector
1981	Fortner, et al.	USA	High voltage cautery
1982	Starzl, et al.	USA	Left trisegmentectomy

Fig. 3. Milestones in hepatic surgery.

field is widely exposed and stabilized (Fig. 4). Dissection is begun by dividing the attachments between the liver and diaphragm, usually identifying the appropriate hepatic veins. For a right hepatic lobectomy, the liver is next mobilized off the inferior vena cava by controlling and dividing the numerous branches draining the caudate lobe (Fig. 5). Following this, the liver may be reflected superiorly, allowing excellent exposure of the portal hepatis during dissection of the vessels and duct to the involved lobe. The hepatic arterial and portal venous branches to the lobe to be resected are then divided, at which point a line of demarcation of the non-viable parenchyma is evident, identifying the border for transection. Following hepatic transection the surface is usually healthy and dry; no approximation of liver capsule or oversewing with omentum is necessary (Fig. 6). Closed suction drains are placed for a short time and can usually be withdrawn within a week when drainage has abated. Postoperatively liver resection is usually well tolerated but septic complications remain the major cause of morbidity. Commonly, alterations in liver enzymes are seen which usually soon resolve, although the alkaline phosphatase is often persistently elevated for a number of weeks postoperatively (Fig. 7).

198

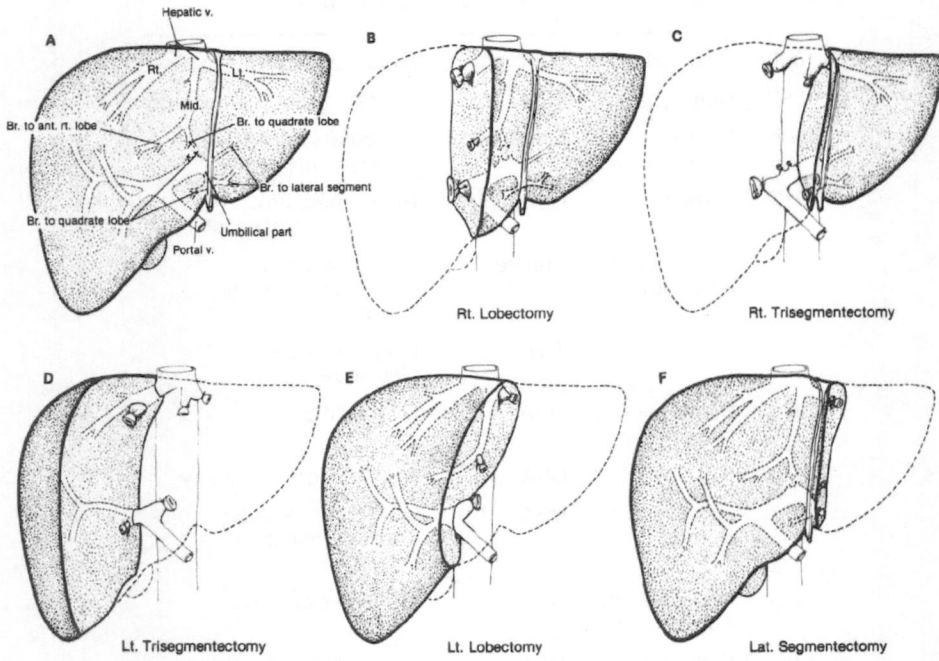

Fig. 4. Conventional anatomic hepatic resections.

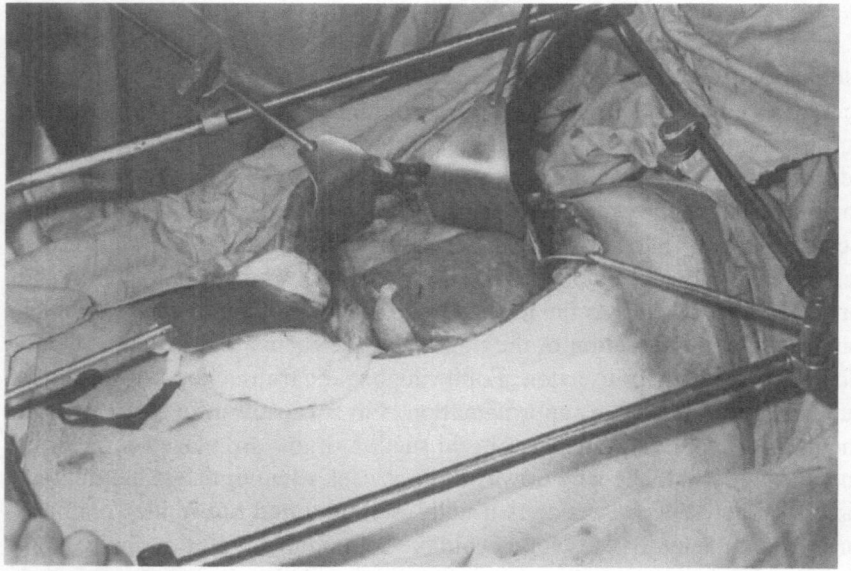

Fig. 5. Excellant exposure achieved with Thompson self-retaining retractor.

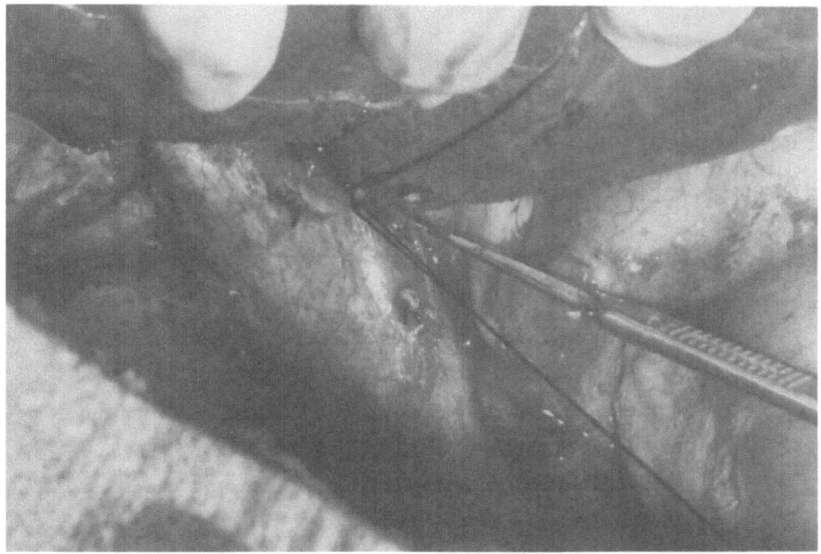

Fig. 6. Control of caudate lobe veins during liver mobilization for right hepatic lobectomy.

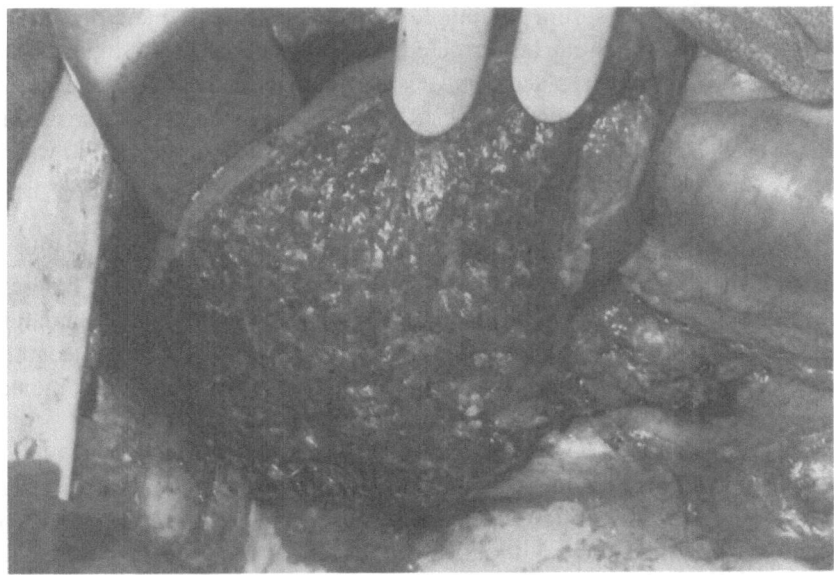

Fig. 7. Healthy viable liver surface following parenchymal transection with ultrasonic dissector.

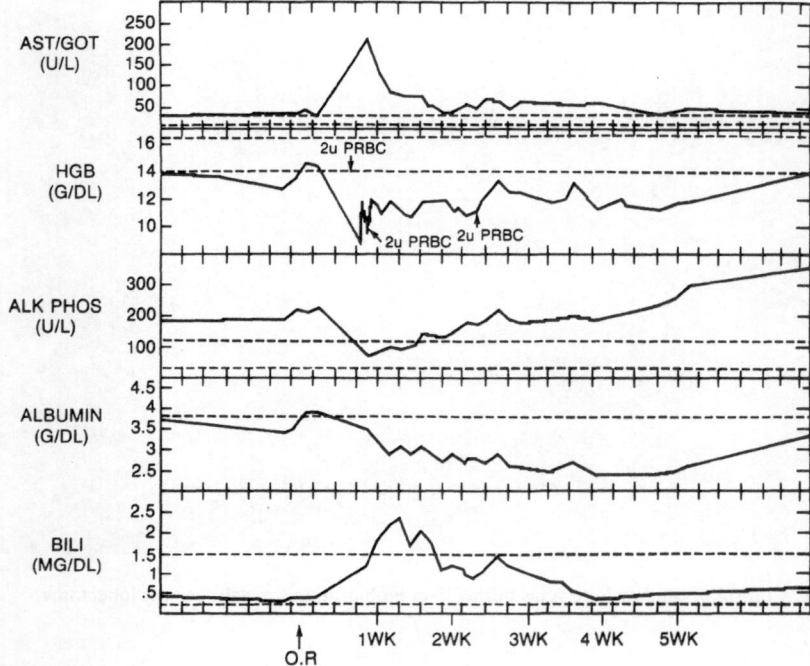

Fig. 8. Representative pattern of metabolic alterations following major hepatic resection.

During the first week serum albumin levels may be decreased and prothrombin time elevated which can be corrected by appropriate albumin, fresh frozen plasma, and vitamin K replacement. Postoperative complications were noted in the NCI series to be directly associated with blood loss and the time of surgery (Fig. 8). Therefore, proper use of techniques such as the CUSA which permits safe relatively bloodless dissection with minimal tissue necrosis will result in low morbidity and mortality.

The overall mortality of liver resections in major centers performing large numbers of cases has been reported to be as low as 0–5%. The field has progressed to the point now when hepatic resection carries with it approximately the same mortality as a primary colon resection. Now that it has been demonstrated in many centers that hepatic surgery can be performed safely, indications for hepatic resection will be further investigated.

In 1986 Hughes at *et al.* reviewed the records of over 850 patients who underwent liver resection for metastatic colorectal cancer in a cooperative effort among numerous institutions to identify indications for liver resection and prognostic variables. The authors collected data in the Hepatic Metastases Registry [10] which serve as the largest numbers of such patients intensively investigated retrospectively.

Liver resection – when?

The belief that metachronous liver metastases represent a select disease with an inherently favorable prognosis still persists currently. Proponents of this theory advocate a period of observation following the diagnosis of liver metastasis and operate when no further distant metastases develop [11]. However, the available data in the literature does not show a significantly increased survival in patients with metachronous lesions over those in whom metastases were resected at the time of or shortly after surgery. Indeed, in Foster's update Liver Tumor Series in 1978, no statistical difference was noted. The five year survival of patients with synchronous metastases was 21% while 23% of patients survived after removal of metachronous deposits. Indeed Foster wrote in 1981 that 'these data pretty much put to rest the older, perhaps reasonable but theoretical concept that the patient with a long interval between the recognition and therapy of the primary tumor and the hepatic metastases will do better [12].' Data from Iwatsuki [13], Wanebo [14], and Adson [15] among others suggest that differences in survival between resection of synchronous and metachronous metastases are insignificant. Cady and McDermott however have been the main proponents of the biological determinant view [11]. According to their theory, host factors prevent growth and spread of already present metastases, thus waiting a period of months to pass following diagnosis with the expectation of discovering further distant metastatic disease will prevent unnecessary liver resections. Since there never has been, nor will there ever probably be, a prospective randomized trial comparing immediate to delayed surgery for newly diagnosed liver metastases, we advocate prompt surgical exploration following diagnosis, considering that patients with synchronous metastases do not appear to be a subset with an inherently unfavorable prognosis. In addition, experimental evidence and clinical observation suggest that metastases themselves may metastasize [16]. Therefore a period of observation may result in development of further distant metastatic disease. Metastatic cells are probably clonal variants which allow their growth in distant sites, and thus allow further spread. Observation of metastases to lymph nodes in the portal, celiac and mediastinal areas (Fig. 9) lends support to the theory of spread from a metastatic focus.

However, as in many other cancers, patients with a longer disease free interval tend to have a longer survival time. Data from the hepatic resection registry showed a trend towards longer survival when the disease free interval was greater than twelve months.

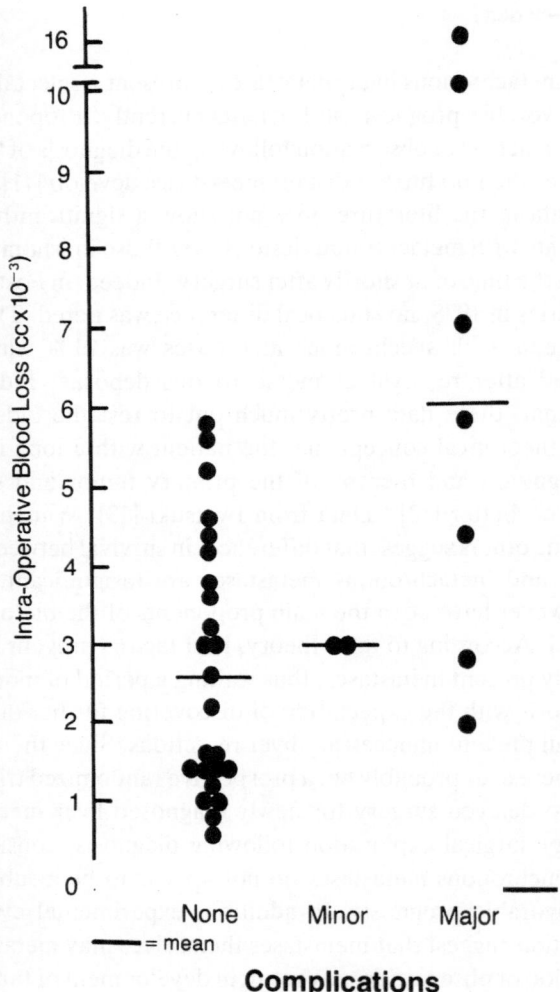

Fig. 9. Complications from hepatic surgery are directly related to magnitude of blood loss.

Liver resection – Who?

Twenty-five years of hepatic surgery have produced gratifying results in patients with resectable colorectal liver metastases. The data from numerous institutions is quite uniform in reporting a five-year survival rate of approximately 30% [11, 13, 17]. Although these represent a highly select group of patients judged to benefit the greatest from surgery, there is no doubt that hepatic resection has salvaged a significant number of patients.

Numerous variables have been investigated in an effort to identify patients with factors prognostic for a poor survival that does not justify hepatic resection. Data from several series have confirmed that Duke's stage of the original primary tumor is associated with an affect on prognosis [13, 15, 17]. Disease-free survival examined in the Registry at five years of patients with Dukes's C lesions (positive mesenteric nodes) following hepatic resection was 18% versus 28% of patients with Duke's B cancers (negative nodes) [10]. Although statistically significant, stage by itself is obviously not an absolute contraindication to liver resection.

The presence of metastases in the portal or celiac lymph nodes appears to be a significant negative determinant survival after liver resection. None of the 24 patients examined in the Hepatic Resection Registry survived five years [10]. Although numbers are small there are no reported 5-year survivors in the literature following resection of liver metastases with nodal spread. There is no question that most hepatic surgeons consider the finding of such metastases as a contraindication to resection, and abandon the procedure.

Not infrequently localized extrahepatic discontiguous disease is encountered at the time of exploration. This may present as local recurrence at the original resection site which is usually unresectable and portends widespread metastatic disease. Occasionally however, localized recurrence in areas such as the abdominal wall or peritoneum may be easily resectable which is tempting to the surgeon in an effort to remove all gross tumor. Results in the small numbers of patients reviewed in the Hepatic Registry in whom all disease was resected and were made clinically disease free showed that although a shorter disease survival was evident, the survival distributions did not appear to differ. Short term follow up did not allow for definitive conclusions. The important question as to whether resection of such extrahepatic disease is justified should be examined prospectively. There is no doubt that historically these patients have not been thought suitable for liver resection and demonstrable benefit may allow application of curative resection to a wider spectrum of patients.

Confusion and controversy exist as to whether patients with multiple liver metastases should be considered for hepatic resection. Adson et al in a large series reported similar survival figures between patients with single and multiple metastases [15]. Iwatsuki et al. [13] in their large series from Pittsburgh and Cady et al. [11] from the Lahey Clinic agreed that survival following liver resection was identical in the patients with one, two or three metastases. The dramatic decrease in survival appeared to occur in patients with four or more metastases. These data are reflected in the Hepatic Registry where the survival dropped from 25% to 7% when three or more metastases were present. Unfortunately there is no widespread agreement among hepatic surgeons as to what constitutes multiple metastases versus a single focus with satellites. There may be in fact a critical difference between patients with a single metastasis and adjacent satellite lesions versus true separate multiple metastases. Many series do not differentiate between these findings but data from Langer *et al.* [18] indicate that resection of the group with satellite nodules associated with a single lesion is indistinguishable from patients with only a solitary metastasis while patients with true multiple metastases fared quite poorly. However, in that series, almost all patients had only one or two satellites and therefore represented a select group. Such criteria should be investigated critically by hepatic resectionists with close cooperation with the pathologist. Inclusion of patients with perhaps one or two satellite nodules into the category of solitary metastases in the future will allow more reproducible and consistent data.

The very high incidence of recurrence in the liver following resection of more than four metastases has been noted by experienced hepatic surgeons. From the available accumulated data there appears to be no significant survival difference between patients with unilobar and bilobar metastases which are totally resected. However recurrence in the liver appears to be more frequent following resection of bilobar metastases.

Liver resection – How much?

Reflecting characteristics of their primary tumor, liver metastases' size does not appear to correlate with survival. This of course may reflect the inherent biologic behavior of a metastatic lesion which allows it to grow to large size without distant metastases. Patients reviewed in the Hepatic Registry appeared to have the same prognosis whether the size of the lesion was less than 2cm, 2–4cm, or 4–8cm [10]. There was a somewhat decreased survival when the metastasis was greater than 8cm. Perhaps a more important question to be answered is how radical one needs to be in resecting liver metastases. Foster's survey [5] suggested a survival rate of 13% in patients who underwent hepatic lobectomy, while 24% of patients who were able to undergo wedge resection survived. However data from larger, more recent series reviewed in the Hepatic Registry did not find any significant differences regardless of the procedure performed. What did become evident was the fact that patients with large (>4cm) metastases did worse following wedge resection compared to formal anatomic lobectomy, suggesting that anatomic resections might be necessary in large lesions to obtain adequate margins. Data on the adequacy of surgical margins is not sufficiently recorded in many retrospective series to permit definitive conclusions and we suggest that this should be definitely stratified in all future prospective studies.

Ekberg *et al.* have reported that no patients who had a positive margin following liver resection survived five years while 30% of patients with greater than one centimeter margin survived. They therefore advocated a minimum of one centimeter tumor free margin if possible. The Roswell Park series found that survival in patients with tumor free margins was 25%, half of that in patients with margins greater than 2 cm. Data accumulated in the Hepatic Registry also suggested that positive margins had a significant impact on survival with only 23% of patients with positive margins alive at five years while 45% of those with greater than 1 cm margins survived. There may be certain situations when the surgeon is forced to accept a thin or positive margin, such as when the tumor abuts hilar structures, hepatic veins, and the inferior vena cava. The ultrasonic detector may be a particular help in these situations, since it allows for safe and precise dissection of major vascular structures and extended dissection into normal hepatic parenchyma adjacent to the tumor. The question as to whether tumors which break through the liver capsule may have an inherent 'positive margin' and therefore signify higher risk for peritoneal surface recurrence has not been addressed.

As mentioned previously, simultaneous resection of localized extrahepatic recurrence has been reported to result in an acceptable overall survival, although disease free survival is quite low. Conceivably, one could advocate such an approach when the extrahepatic recurrence can be safely removed with little added morbidity, such as abdominal wall or small local recurrences. We have quite commonly found adherence of liver metastases to the diaphragm or adrenal gland and have performed standard en bloc resections to encompass all disease. Our impression is that many of these patients have gone on to do quite well, reflecting the importance of adherence to standard surgical oncology principles in hepatic surgery. There is no doubt that oftentimes recurrence at the original resection site will be unresectable. Those patients eligible for simultaneous resection will be ideal candidates for inclusion into adjuvant therapy protocols.

Recurrence following liver resection

Approximately two-thirds to three-quarters of patients will recur and therefore die following 'curative' hepatic resection. Understanding the patterns of recurrence is crucial in selecting appropriate patients eligible for surgery as well as planning for any adjuvant therapies.

The majority of patients who do relapse will do so outside of the liver. The Pittsburgh group reported that only three of twenty-nine patients recurred in the liver alone [13]. Steele *et al.* [20] noted the common finding of recurrence in the lung, which has been confirmed in other large studies. Ekberg *et al.* [19] reported a slightly higher evidence (28%) of liver involvement alone, with intraabdominal relapse being most common.

The Hepatic Registry data has noted the incidence of liver involvement

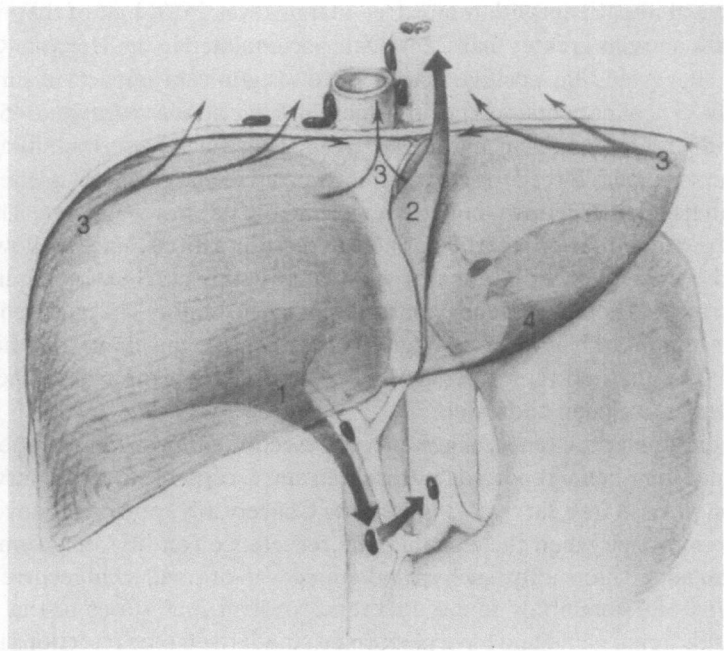

Fig. 10. Possible sites of metastasis from hepatic metastases through lymphatic drainage of the liver.
1. caudad to portal and celiac lymph nodes
2. along the falciform ligament cephalad to mediastinal lymph nodes
3. transdiaphragmatic extension to paracaval and mediastinal lymph nodes and
4. through the gastrohepatic ligament to upper gastric nodes
Adapted from August DA, Sugarbaker PH, *et al.* [16].

alone to be 15% [21], with multiple sites of recurrence, especially on peritoneal surfaces, the most common pattern (Figs. 10, 11). Two variables in particular were predictive of a high incidence of recurrence in the liver. When lesions in both lobes of the liver were resected, the majority of patients did have local recurrence in the liver, although not all were confined to the liver itself (Fig. 12).

The presence of a positive margin following hepatic resection was also predictive of high risk for liver recurrence (Fig. 13).

We have pursued recurrences aggressively and have re-resected metastases in the liver, with gratifying short-term results. Although a majority of patients who recur will be eligible for reoperation, it is possible a significant percentage will expect long-term benefit. Other authors have noted similar success with pulmonary resection for recurrence in the lung. Such positive early results have stimulated us to follow patients closely post-operatively in hopes of detecting resectable disease in those patients who do recur.

SITES OF RECURRENCE AFTER HEPATIC RESECTION

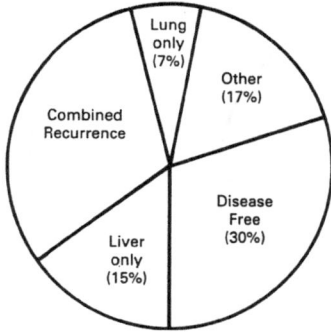

Fig. 11. Patterns of recurrence following curative liver resection.

SITES OF RECURRENCE FOLLOWING HEPATIC RESECTION

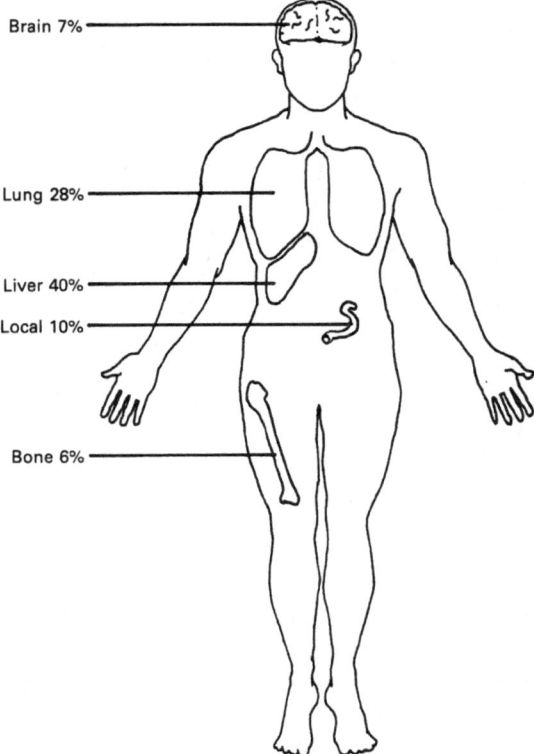

Fig. 12. Site distribution of recurrence.

DISTRIBUTION

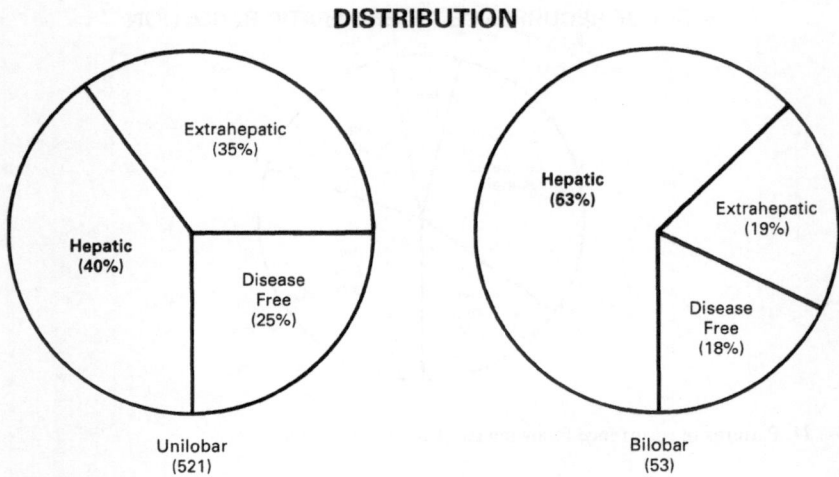

Fig. 13. Effect of bilobar metastases on pattern of recurrence following curative hepatic resection.

PATHOLOGIC MARGIN

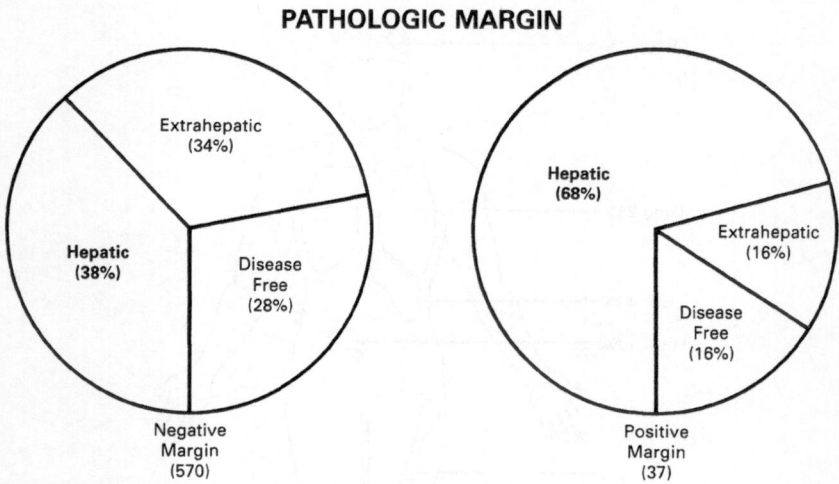

Fig. 14. Notable predominance of recurrence in the liver following resection with positive margins [15].

However, it is evident that the plurality of patients will relapse at multiple sites, most commonly on peritoneal surfaces and in the lungs. It is clear that successful systemic therapy is required to impact significantly on the overall survival following liver resection. Since such therapy is not currently available, thoughtful approaches must be planned to decrease the incidence of recurrence. Patients who have a positive margin or undergo resection of multiple bilobar metastases may be candidates for regional therapy applied to the liver, such as intraarterial chemotherapy. Intraperitoneal chemotherapy may be helpful in limiting recurrences on peritoneal surfaces. Neurochemotherapy or immunotherapy regimens will hopefully soon be utilized to decrease the incidence of systemic spread.

What criteria preclude hepatic resection?

Many of the prognostic variables examined in such retrospective series as the Hepatic Registry have been found to be indicators but not absolute determinants of survival. However, there may be three situations in which hepatic surgeons are in general agreement that patients should not undergo hepatic resection at least outside of a clinic trial:

1. The presence of portal and/or celiac node metastases. These patients do uniformly quite poorly.
2. Patients with more than four liver metastases have a dismal survival expectancy and there are no current data justifying hepatic resection outside of a controlled trial.
3. Institutions or surgeons which have an unacceptably high mortality rate should not carry out major hepatic resections. Today an acceptable mortality rate following liver resections is approximately 5% with 15% of patients developing major complications. There is no place for the occasional hepatic resectionist; institutional support including blood banking and state of the art radiology imaging is mandatory.

While numerous other variables when considered separately or together may predict a decreased survival, such as stage of the original cancer, elevated CEA level, gender, and disease free interval, survival expected from such patients following resection is still far superior to any other current available therapy. It is evident therefore that staging of the recurrence will generally predict outcome. Unfortunately, a widely accepted staging system for liver metastases has not been generally adopted. Acceptance of such a system will permit more reliable analysis of data in the field of liver resection.

Conclusions

The field of curative hepatic surgery has progressed to the point where it is poised to have a major impact on the treatment of colorectal cancer. It is generally agreed that approximately 10–12% of patients with colorectal cancer will at some point present with resectable hepatic metastases [22]. Therefore, the numbers of eligible patients far exceed the total of sarcoma excisions each year and thus assures tremendous importance in surgical oncology today. The fatalistic opinion held by many physicians in the past that liver metastases are inherently not treatable is no longer defensible today. It is clear that in properly selected patients the five-year survival of patients undergoing hepatic resection approximates 30%, far exceeding any non-surgical treatment.

Major advances in surgical techniques and technology have allowed the development of safe hepatic surgery with mortality rates of approximately 5%. There is little doubt that widespread use of CEA monitoring and excellent liver imaging techniques have permitted diagnosis of hepatic metastases at an earlier stage. While numerous retrospective series have attempted to identify variables which might indicate contraindications for resection, it seems most are prognostic indicators, but not determinants of survival. It appears that currently the presence of extrahepatic nodal metastases and numerous, perhaps greater than four metastases are predictive of dismal results and would generally preclude liver resection.

It is a humbling fact to remember that at least two-thirds of patients who undergo hepatic resection will recur. Intra-abdominal recurrence with liver disease is the most common pattern followed by pulmonary metastases. Data suggest that liver recurrence alone happens in approximately 15% of patients who do recur [15]. While there are now encouraging results following resection of hepatic metastases, the overall numbers of survivors will be too small to impact dramatically on survival figures of colorectal cancer. It is evident that patients undergoing liver resection present ideal models for planning adjuvant treatments. While conventional chemotherapy has proved disappointing in preventing recurrences, regional approaches currently being investigated may lead to improvement. Systemic therapy will be necessary to have a major impact on survival figures, since the majority of patients following hepatic resection will fail outside the liver.

The development of biological response modifiers over the past decade will undoubtedly lead to their use in preventing recurrence following liver resection. Numerous lymphokines and cytokines are under intense investigation to discover agents helpful in the treatment of colorectal cancer. Monoclonal antibodies produced against the cancer cells will hopefully assist in the earlier diagnosis of cancer recurrence and may move to be of benefit in treatment when 'tagged' with chemotherapeutic agents or radioisotopes.

Prospective trials will be mandatory in order to answer the crucial questions as to which patients are best served with hepatic resection and what extent of disease can be benefited by surgical extirpation. Only with the close cooperation of many hepatic surgeons in well-planned clinical trials will the field of hepatic surgery for colorectal cancer continue to mature and assume its important role in the treatment of colorectal cancer.

References

1. Pestana C, Reitmeier RM, Moertel CG, *et al.*: The natural history of carcinoma of the colon and rectum. Am J Surg 108: 826–829, 1964
2. Wagner JS, Adson MA, van Heerden JA, Adson MH, *et al.*: The natural history of hepatic metastases from colorectal cancer. Ann Surg 199: 502–508, 1983
3. Bengtsson G, Carlsson G, Hafstrom L, Jonsson P: Natural history of patients with untreated liver metastases from colorectal cancer. Am J Surg 114: 586–589, 1981
4. Ottow RT, August DA, Sugarbaker PH: Surgical therapy of liver cancer. In: Bottino JC, Opfell RW, Muggia FM (eds) Liver Cancer, Boston, Martinus Nijhof Pub., 1985
5. Foster JH, Berman MM: Solid liver tumors. In: Ebert P (ed) Major Problems in Clinical Surgery. Philadelphia: WB Saunders, 1977
6. Tranberg K, Rigotti P, *et al.*: Liver resection: A comparison using the ND-YAG laser, an ultrasonic surgical aspirator, or blunt dissection. Am J Surg 151: 368–373, 1986
7. Ottow RT, Barbaieri SA, Sugarbaker PH, Wesley RA: Liver transection: A controlled study of four different techniques in pigs. Surgery 97 (5): 596–601, 1985
8. Starzl TE, Bell RH, Beart RW, Putnam CW: Hepatic trisegmentectomy and other liver resections. Surg Gynecol Obstet 141: 429–437, 1975
9. Kemey MM, Hogan JM, *et al.*: Preoperative staging with computerized axial tomography and biochemical tests in patients with hepatic metastases. Ann Surg 203: 169–172
10. Hughes KS, Simon R, *et al.*: Resection of the liver for colorectal carcinoma metastases: a multi-institutional study of indications for resection. Surgery (in press)
11. Cady B, McDermott WV: Major hepatic resection for metachronous metastasis from colon cancer. Ann Surg 201: 204–209, 1984
12. Foster JH, Lundy J: Liver metastases. Curr Prob Surg 17 (3): pp 161–202, 1981
13. Iwatsuki S, Esquivel CO, Gordon RD, Starzl TE: Liver resection for metastatic colorectal cancer. Surgery 100: 804–809, 1986
14. Wanebo HJ, Semoglou C, *et al.*: Surgical management of patients with primary operable colorectal cancer and synchronous liver metastases. Am J Surg 135: 81085, 1978
15. Adson MA, van Heerden JA, Adson MH, Wagner JS, *et al.*: Resection of hepatic metastases from colorectal cancer. Arch Surg 119–647–681, 1984
16. August DA, Sugarbaker PH, Schneider PD: Lymphatic dissemination of hepatic metastases. Cancer 55: 1490–1494, 1985
17. Ridge JA, Daly JM: Treatment of colorectal hepatic metastases. Surg Gynecol Obstet 161: 597–607, 1985
18. Coburn CS, Makowka L, Langer B, Taylor BR, *et al.*: Hepatic resection for metastatic disease. (Unpublished data)
19. Ekberg H, Tranberg K, *et al.*: Pattern of recurrence in liver resection for colorectal secondaries. World J Surg 1987 (in press)
20. Steele G, Osteen RT, Wilson RE, Brooks DC: Patterns of failure after surgical cure of large liver tumors. Am J Surg 147: 554–559, 1984
21. Hughes KS, Simon R, *et al.*: Resection of the liver for colorectal carcinoma metastases: Surgery 100 (2): 278–284, 1986
22. Butler J, Attiyeh FF, Daly JM: Hepatic resection for metastasis of the colon and rectum. Surg Gynecol Obstet 162: 109–113, 1986

12. Surgical management in high bile duct tumours

S. BENGMARK and K.G. TRANBERG

Introduction

Despite the fact that cancer of the biliary system is comparatively rare, 4500 new cases are detected each year in the United States – an incidence similar to that of cancer of the tongue. In addition, the number of diagnosed new cases is increasing from year to year. This may, however, not reflect a true increase in incidence but merely improved methods for imaging of the biliary system.

As early as 1922 a review on malignant neoplasms of the extrahepatic bile ducts was published (Renshaw). Renshaw gave credit to Durant-Fardel (1840) for having reported the first case of carcinoma of the common bile duct and Schuppel (1878) for recognizing the first case of carcinoma of the hepatic duct confluence. According to same author, Cotte (1909) seems to have been the first to advise treatment: anastomosing the jejunum to the anterior surface of the left lobe of the liver with the hope that a biliary fistula might develop.

Little attention was given to the tumour until the end of the 1950s and the beginning of the 1960s. Among the rather numerous publications from this time are those of Altemeier et al. (1957, 1966), Alvarez (1958), Ariel and Pack (1962), Benhamou et al. (1959), Braasch et al. (1967), Brown et al. (1961), Caroli (1954, 1956), Champeau and Pineau (1955, 1964), Champeau and Meillere (1965), Champeau and Vialas (1966), Champeau (1967), Couinaud (1967), Dogliotti and Fogliati (1956), Duboucher et al. (1954), Flandreau et al. (1957), Fortner (1958), Gautier et al. (1960), Glenn and Hays (1953, 1954), Goetze (1951), Ham and MacKenzie (1964), Haynes et al. (1964), Hepp et al. (1954), Hepp and Couinaud (1956), Hepp and Mercadier (1956), Klatskin (1965), Kuwayti et al. (1957), Longmire and Sanford (1948), Longmire and Lippman (1956), Quattlebaum and Quattlebaum (1965), Schutt (1964), Smith (1964), Strohl et al. (1963), and Thorbjarnarson (1958, 1959). Longmire and Sanford (1948) described intrahepatic cholangiojejunostomy with partial hepatectomy, a procedure which was used in the early treatment of high bile duct tumours. The first attempt at local resection seems to have been described by

Brown and Myers in 1954. The difficulty of the operation was demonstrated by Longmire *et al.* (1973): surgery was uneventful in only 2 of 13 patients having local or combined local and liver resection for hilar tumour. Most patients developed septic complications: 5 general sepsis, 3 cholangitis and 1 abdominal abscesses. However, one patient subjected to left hepatectomy lived after 4.5 years and another patient was alive, without signs of recurrence, 7 months after an extended right hepatectomy.

Our own attempts started in 1969 and culminated between 1970 and 1975. With regard to complications our early experience was similar to that of Longmire *et al.* (1973) (Evander *et al.* 1980, Bengmark *et al.* 1986). However, there were three 10-year survivors among our first 15 cases (Bengmark *et al.* 1986).

Surgical anatomy

Knowledge of the normal and morbid anatomy of the bile ducts is a prerequisite for understanding carcinomas in this area, their radiologic characteristics and their management. Important contributions to the understanding of the normal anatomy have been given by Hjortsjo (1951), Couinaud (1952, 1957) and Michels (1955). A classical description of the morbid anatomy was given by Edmondson (1967).

The anatomic relationships between bile ducts and blood vessels show great variation. The proximity between the bile duct confluence, the hepatic artery and the portal vein has been considered to render a radical resection at least difficult (Alexander *et al.* 1984, Adson 1981, Waugh 1962). The length of the right hepatic duct averages 0.9 cm and that of the left 1.7 cm. The portion of the left hepatic duct that arises from the lateral segment and which is predominantly extrahepatic averages about 3 cm and recieves branches that drain the medial segment of the left lobe, including the quadrate and caudate lobes of the liver. Sacrifice of these branches thus gives an additional 3 cm, which is of importance in connection with therapeutic considerations. The right duct is almost always short. A large duct draining the anterior segment usually joins the the posterior segment duct at a distance of 0.5–1 cm from the junction. Sometimes the two right hepatic ducts do not join before the confluence with the left hepatic duct. The common hepatic duct has an average length of 4 cm but may vary considerably in length depending upon its point of junction with the cystic duct.

The wall of the extrahepatic bile duct is ordinarily 1 mm or less in thickness. The mucosa consists of a single layer of tall columnar epithelium. The submucosa consists of dense, sparsely cellular, collagenous tissue with a few elastic fibrils. It is especially important to note that blood vessels are few and small within this layer. Further exteriorly there is a loosely arranged layer of coarse collagen bundles with some smooth muscle and a few large elastic fibrils. The muscular layer is not continuous throughout the biliary system, especially not in the upper portions. Most of the muscle tissue is parallel to the long axis of the duct. Many tiny pits – the sacculi of Beale – are present throughout the mucosa. Mucous glands are few and are usually situated around the sacculi of Beale. Some of them are localized within the wall and join the sacculi through short channels.

Successful surgery in this area depends on the avoidance of leakage and stricture. It is important, therefore, to know and understand the arterial supply of the bile ducts. Northover and Terblanche (1979) made an important contribution by describing the so called 3 o'clock and 9 o'clock arteries and the retro-portal artery.

Classification

Bismuth and Corlette (1975) suggested a classification of carcinoma in the liver hilus based on the anatomical location of the tumour:

Type I: unobstructed primary confluence (tumour located in the main hepatic duct)
Type II: obstruction limited to primary confluence (tumour located exactly at the confluence)
Type III: obstruction of the primary confluence with extension to the right or left secondary confluence)

As there are indications that tumours extended to the right or left duct may be treated differently because of the different anatomy, we have suggested (Bengmark *et al.* 1986) that type III is subdivided into two types (Fig. 1):
Type IIIA: extension into the right but not the left duct
Type IIIB: extension into the left but not the right duct

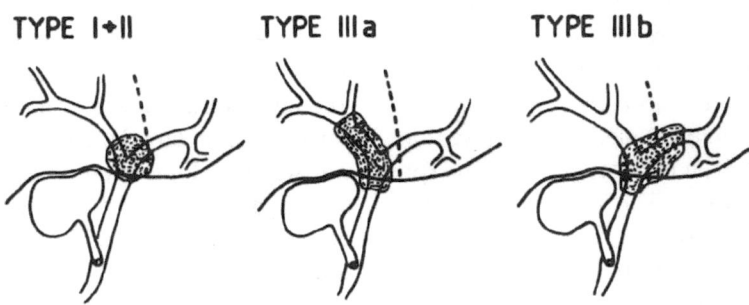

Fig. 1. Modified Bismuth-Corlette classification of high bile duct tumours.

Recently, Weinbren and Mutum (1983) demonstrated that 22/23 malignant neoplasms in the proximal bile duct were of the sclerosing carcinoma type. They also tried to trace the site of origin of the tumour: common hepatic duct (Bismuth Type I) in 16%, confluence (Bismuth Type II) in 53%, right hepatic duct (Type IIIA) in 21% and left hepatic duct (Type IIIB) in 11%.

Biological behaviour of the tumour

As the bile duct has a thin wall, it is natural that the tumour grows into surrounding tissues in most cases. It continues to spread along perineural lymph clefts, periductal lymphatic network and periductal venules and arterioles. It expands through submucosal infiltration and may infiltrate the bile duct wall over a wide distance (Braasch *et al.* 1967, Brown *et al.* 1961, Inouye and Whelan 1978, Thorbjarnarson 1958, Tsuzuki and Uekusa 1978). Orcel (1958) emphasized the importance of regarding this type of carcinoma more as regional than local.

Metastases are rather late. Boerma (1983) reviewed the literature extensively and concluded that regional lymphatic metastases occur in 1/3 of cases with primary bile duct tumours and that the tumour is restricted to the hepatic duct confluence in 1/5 of the cases. He also concluded that metastases to coeliac, mesenteric or other regional lymph nodes occurred in about 15% of the cases. Although the frequency of hepatic metastases varies widely in the literature (0–50%), the impression of most writers is that they are seen in slightly more than 30% of the cases. It is our impression, from the literature as well as from our own experience, that hepatic and/or regional metastases can be expected in every second case at the time of treatment. With the exception of the liver, most distant metastases are located in the lesser omentum and only occasionally in the pancreas, ovaries, spleen and stomach. Dissemination outside the abdomen, mainly to the lungs, is rare. The gallbladder is involved in 10–15%, and it is not clear whether this represents multifocal disease, lymphatic dissemination or local spread.

With few exceptions (Braasch *et al.* 1967), the tumour has been considered as slow-growing (Altemeier *et al.* 1957, 1966, Iwasaki *et al.* 1977, Klatskin 1965, Tompkins *et al.* 1981). A tumour in the hilum of the liver is usually described to be a small, well differentiated, scirrhous, annular adenocarcinoma. However, it is large, multiple and spread diffusely for a long distance in about 10% of cases. The nodular (annular) type of tumour is built up of an unusually strong network of fibrotic connective tissue, which sometimes is so abundant that hardly any epithelial tumour cells are found (Ross *et al.* 1973). In a minority of cases (5–10%) a different structure, usually described as papillary or villous, is found. Despite the scirrhous pattern these tumours are almost always classified as adenocarcinoma. Mucin produced by tumour cells becomes blue-stained by alcaline blue in contrast the mucin of benign cells (Weinbren, personal communication to Boerma). Non-epithelial tumours are extremely rare in this location (Edmondson 1967, Gibson and Sobin 1978). The extensive fibrosis is, together with the small size of the tumour, the main reason why a representative biopsy is difficult to obtain, and, if representative, difficult to interpret, especially if frozen sections are used. It happens that periductal, non-malignant fibrosis is interpreted as bile duct cancer. However, it happens more frequently that no cancer cells are seen and that the condition is described as benign fibrosis.

The aetiology of these tumours is unknown. Chronic inflammation and bile stasis should play important roles (Scott *et al.* 1980) since the disease is over-represented in patients with sclerosing cholangitis (Chapman *et al.* 1980, Kune and Sali 1980), in typhoid carriers (Welton *et al.* 1979), in patients with biliary ductal parasites (Belamaric 1973) and in patients with chronic suppurative cholangitis (Smith 1964). The disease is supposed to be overrepresented also in patients with ulcerative colitis and sometimes presents itself some years after proctocolectomy (Ross *et al.* 1973, Roberts-Thomson *et al.* 1973). It has also been said repeatedly that it is more common in association with biliary malformations like the Caroli disease. The fact that stasis and infection seem to be implicated has led researches to believe that bacterial degradation of bile salts plays an important pathogenic role. In addition, it has been observed that a significant proportion of patients with bile duct cancer are labourers in the rubber industry.

Diagnosis

The symptoms and signs have not changed much since they were described in detail by Altemeier and others (1957) thirty years ago. The onset is invariably insidious and characterized by progressive jaundice, mild epigastric discomfort, anorexia, nausea, and vomiting and is followed by marked weight loss. Progression is characterized by pruritus, increased jaundice, fever, chills, inanition and further weight loss. Finally, evidence of liver and renal insufficiency, spontaneous haemorrhage and septicemia develops and the patient dies.

A careful history will reveal prodromal complaints, sometimes for several months. In the pre-icteric stage the patients may present with vague symptoms and an unexplained elevation of serum alkaline phosphatases or gamma-glutamyl transpeptidase. Such an observation requires immediate and full investigation. In the situation where the bile ducts are not yet completely occluded, there may be obstruction to isolated segments of the liver or the lesion may be early and, if diagnosed, more readily amenable to treatment. It should also be remembered that patients with very rapidly rising bilirubin levels are likely to have malignant disease rather than common duct stones.

Not long ago these tumours were usually detected during exploratory laparotomy for unexplained jaundice. The recent development of techniques like ultrasonography, fine needle percutaneous cholangiography, endoscopic retrograde cholangiopancreatography and CT-scanning has given us new and important tools for early, preoperative diagnosis. In most instances, exploratory laparotomy should no longer be necessary and should be avoided.

Arterial angiography and late phase portography are of great importance in determining resectability and identifying lesions that might require hepatic resection for potential cure.

Indications for surgical treatment

Before 1970 and the early work of Longmire and co-workers (1973), tumours discovered at laparotomy were intubated, if possible. Most patients received no treatment and only limited diagnostic work-up. The pessimistic attitude was summarized by Blumgart *et al.* (1984) to be caused by difficulties in 1) preoperative diagnosis, 2) histological confirmation, 3) excisional therapy, and 4) intrahepatic or subhepatic biliary-enteric anastomosis. However, the situation has changed dramatically in recent years with the availability of modern imaging methods. In addition, liver resection, which used to be hazardous, has become a surgical routine.

Iwasaki *et al.* (1977) set up four criteria for local resectability:
1. the main stems of portal vein and hepatic artery are free of tumour
2. the main branches of portal vein and hepatic artery contralateral to the tumour extension in one of the hepatic ducts are free of tumour
3. distal extension of the tumour leaves a long part of the distal common duct free of tumour
4. proximal extension of the tumour respects at least unilaterally the second duct confluences

These criteria are relative and might be challenged. Most surgeons, including ourselves, have regarded invasion by tumour of the main stem of the portal vein or hepatic artery as a contraindication to attempts at radical surgery, but resection of the portal vein has been performed (Blumgart *et al.* 1984). It remains, however, to be established if resection in such advanced cases leads to prolonged survival. Bilateral invasion of the secondary confluences of the hepatic ducts is generally regarded as a contraindication to liver resection (Corlette and Bookwalter 1980, Imrie and Blumgart 1979, Tsuzuki and Uekusa 1978). Liver metastases as well as distant metastases and a poor general condition are generally accepted contraindications (Akwari and Kelly 1979, Corlette and Bookwalter 1980, Evander *et al.* 1980). A possible exception would be ipsilateral or solitary liver metastases (Quattlebaum and Quattlebaum 1965) but experience is limited in this situation.

Although the aim of this chapter is to discuss resection of high bile duct tumours, palliative measures will be briefly mentioned. Percutaneous, endoscopic or surgical intubation is accompanied by a 30-day mortality rate of some 30% and frequently by a poor quality of life (Blumgart *et al.* 1984, Burcharth *et al.* 1981, Cotton 1982, Dooley *et al.* 1981, Hagenmuller and Classen 1982, Langer *et al.* 1985, Lorelius *et al.* 1982, Terblanche 1976, Tytgat and Huibregtse 1983, Voyles *et al.* 1983). Comparison with biliary-enteric bypass, with or without resection, is difficult because of differences in attitude and patient selection, but it is often noted that the quality of survival is good after surgery and appears better than after intubation alone (Bengmark *et al.* 1986, Blumgart *et al.* 1984, Evander *et al.* 1980, Langer *et al.* 1985). The recent introduction of intracavitary iridium 192 irradiation (Fletcher *et al.* 1981, Mornex *et al.* 1984) may effect a change in policy, but its usefulness remains to be established.

Extent of liver resection

It has been repeatedly emphasized that tumour cells often remain after a macroscopically radical resection of the tumour (Kopelson *et al.* 1981, Todosoki *et al.* 1980, van Heerden *et al.* 1967). Retrospective examination of our first 15 liver resections showed that we were able to obtain free margins in only 4 of 15 cases (Evander *et al.* 1980). Beazley *et al.* (1984) were able to get free margins in 7 out of 16 resected cases. All our patients underwent liver resection as did most of the patients from the Hammersmith hospital.

One would expect the risk of residual cancer to be even greater after local resection. This view is substantiated by the report of Mizumoto *et al.* (1986) in which a free margin was achieved in only 1 of 11 locally resected cases. Although resection of the bifurcation alone is technically possible in many cases, it is likely to leave cancer cells at the margin and to add little to the prospect of life. Residual cancer also increases the risk of early complications related to poor healing of the biliodigestive anastomosis: leakage, abscess formation, sepsis.

Several writers, including ourselves, have regarded the combination of quadrate lobe resection and local resection as the ideal operation for high bile duct cancer (Alexandre *et al.* 1975, Berard *et al.* 1978, Launois *et al.* 1979, Lees *et al.* 1980, Nishimura *et al.* 1978, Stephen 1964). Boerma (1983) collected 12 such operations from the literature. Local recurrence of the tumour was, however, still the main cause of death in these patients, and no 5-year survivor was reported. Available evidence thus favours the opinion that hemihepatectomy is required for curative surgery of a high bile duct tumour.

Early reports indicated (Quattlebaum and Quattlebaum 1965, and others) that the tumours are more common in the left, or the left part of the confluence, than in the right duct. There is little support for such an opinion in the study of Weinbren and Mutum (1983), who found tumours on the right side in 21% and on the left side in 11% of their cases. Longmire *et al.* remarked already in 1973 that the opinion of left side predominance probably reflected the fact that right-sided tumours had been regarded as intrahepatic or untreatable in the past. Most early attempts at hemihepatectomy were thus on the left side. However, the possibility to perform a radical resection and get a good hepatojejunostomy is smaller after left hepatectomy. The right hepatic duct has a maximum length of 1 cm, which means that the tumour usually extends beyond the secondary confluence. (This anatomic fact often makes it difficult to drain the whole right liver by one transhepatic catheter.) The comparatively long, and extrahepatic, left duct offers better possibilities for radical resection on the right side and has led to an increased number of right hemihepatectomies. Most of our recent patients have been operated with right or extended right lobectomies. Of the 12 cases of liver resection reported by Blumgart *et al.* (1984), 9 (75%) were operated with extended right lobectomy. The longest survivor in this material had a tumour affecting the right branch of the portal vein and was treated with extended right lobectomy and reconstruction by hepatojejunostomy.

Caudate lobe resection

Although the importance of resecting the caudate lobe has been emphasized in the literature, it is not until recently that this has been clearly documented. Mizumoto *et al.* (1986) studied the duct anatomy in 106 cadaver livers and found that most of the caudate lobe drained into the left main hepatic duct in 97% of the cases. The distribution of the portal branches was different: in almost half of the patients there were two main branches, one from the left and one from the right main portal branch. The arterial supply to the caudate lobe came from the right hepatic arterial system in 25% of the cases. Of the 24 patients undergoing resection of hilar carcinoma, 8 had invasion of the draining bile duct of the caudate lobe whereas 3 had direct invasion of the parenchyma of the caudate lobe.

Reconstruction of bilio-enteric continuity

Bilio-enteric continuity is usually restored by hepatojejunostomy. To avoid superinfection of the biliary tree a 60cm long Roux-loop is probably the best alternative (Launois *et al.* 1979, Quattlebaum and Quattlebaum 1965, Smith 1964, Way and Dunphy 1972, Whelton *et al.* 1969). It is important to use a well vascularised bile duct and to suture without any tension and with a careful technique. Dissection (cleansing) of the duct should be at a minimum in order to prevent impaired blood supply (Hart and White 1980, Karakousis and Douglass Jr 1977). The anastomosis should be as wide as possible. Some French writers suggest that the duct be closed and that the anastomosis be constructed laterally on the bile duct (Hepp and de Staercke 1960, Salembier 1971). Biliary infection and sepsis are – besides remaining cancer – the greatest threat to success in the treatment of patients with high bile duct tumours. Tsuzuki and Uekusa (1978) emphasized the importance of drainage of all parts of the liver to avoid septic problems and liver abscesses. This view has also been strongly emphasized by Bismuth and Corlette (1975) and Ragins *et al.* (1973).

Although no real evidence has been produced supporting the view, it is usually stated that careful apposition of the bile duct mucosa is essential (Blumgart 1978, Cameron *et al.* 1976, Hart and White 1980, Launois *et al.* 1979, Longmire and Lippman 1956, Malt *et al.* 1980, Smith 1964, Way and Dunphy 1972). Most experimental data indicate that the most important factors are the vascularisation and the presence of bile. The noxious effect of bile is probably produced by bile acids and leads to collagen production, fibrosis and stricture. Douglass *et al.* (1950) demonstrated that the marked fibrotic reaction around the bile duct anastomosis in the dog was avoided if the anastomosis was protected by proximal bile diversion. Later Rains (1959) confirmed the propensity for bile to induce fibrosis. Carlsson *et al.* (1977) showed that bile gained access to mural collagen via mucosal defects leading to rapid collagen turnover and thickening of the duct wall. Cameron and Hou (1962) showed that cross clamping of a bile duct in the guinea pig for 1 min was enough to induce stricture. It seems that a careful approximation is less important than to have a well nourished duct, which we try to dip into the intestine with sutures placed half a cm up on the duct. We try to avoid a catheter through the anastomosis since it could massage the bile into the duct wall and induce fibrosis. If a transhepatic drainage is needed, we favour that the tip of the catheter is placed about 1 cm above the anastomosis. Recently we have frequently placed the blind end of the Roux-loop subcutaneously in order to have easy access to the hepatojejunostomy through an endoscope. So far we have not had to make use of it.

Resection experience

In his review of the literature, Boerma (1983) collected 75 cases of local resection from 30 reports. Most reports were based on 1 case and the largest material consisted of 10 patients (Cameron *et al.* 1982). The operative mortality was 11%. Mean survival was 19 months and there was no 5-year survivor. Local recurrence was the usual cause of death.

Boerma also collected 12 patients, published in 7 reports, in whom resection of the quadrate lobe was added to the local resection of the confluence. The operative mortality was 8% and the mean survival 20 months with no 5-year survivor. Local recurrence was the usual cause of death in these patients, too. Local resection and left hemihepatectomy was performed in 41 patients (reported in 22 papers), and right hemihepatectomy was performed in 9 patients (reported in 7 papers). The results of 15 right lobectomies were published in 8 papers, and the largest experience (4 cases) was that of Rohner (1982). Again, experience with liver resection was usually based on 1 patient, tumour recurrence was responsible for death and survival was not appreciably different from that of quadrate lobe resection. In the right lobectomy group, mean operative mortality was 33% and was caused by liver insufficiency in 3 patients, portal venous thrombosis in 1, and uncontrollable bleeding from a stress ulcer in 1. In addition, one survivor had severe liver insufficiency in the postoperative period. In Boerma's review 7 patients had undergone resection of the portal vein or the hepatic artery in addition to the liver resection. Three of these patients died during the first postoperative month. The mean postoperative survival was 15 months, and 3 of the 4 patients surviving the operation were reported to have died from local recurrence.

The first one center material of liver resection for hilus tumours that comprised a minimum of 10 patients came from our group in 1980 (Evander *et al.*). It was soon followed by four other reports in which liver resection was done for high bile duct tumours: Tsuzuki *et al.* (1981), Blumgart *et al.* (1984), Langer *et al.* (1985), and Mizumoto *et al.* (1986). In addition, a material consisting of 10 patients subjected to local resection was published by Cameron *et al.* (1982).

Tsuzuki *et al.* (1981) reported 15 cases with a 50% actuarial survival time of 24 months and a longest survival of 3 years and months. Blumgart's group reported 12 liver resections with a mean survival of 17 months; seven of their patients were alive at the time of the report. Langer and co-workers (1985) in Toronto performed 12 resections of high bile duct tumours, and all or most of them seem to have included liver resection. They reported a mean survival of 28 months and two 5-year survivors that later died of recurrent disease. In the series of Mizumoto *et al.* (1986) 13 patients underwent resection with a mean survival of 12 months; the longest survival was almost 6 years in a patient having undergone right lobectomy. Our own efforts now comprises 22 patients

(Bengmark *et al.* 1986) and has resulted in a median survival of 6 months, a 33% 1-year survival and 3 patients surviving 10 years.

In conclusion, we believe that patients with high bile duct tumours should be carefully assessed with respect to a resection procedure, which in most cases should include liver resection. This attitude is based on 1) the potential for cure and/or long-term palliation with a good quality of survival, 2) the poor survival and quality of life with non-surgical (or surgical) intubational techniques, 3) an acceptable operative mortality rate (around 10%) in centers experienced in liver surgery, and 4) the possibility to cure patients with benign stricture, supposed to be malignant before surgery. In patients fit for surgery but having disease features that contraindicate resection, it is possible that a surgical by-pass procedure offers the best palliation. This point is, however, not well documented and the relative roles of surgery and intubational techniques, with or without external or intracavitary irradiation, remain to be defined.

References

Adson MA, Farnell MB: Hepatobiliary cancer – surgical considerations. Mayo Clin Proc 56: 686–699, 1981

Akwari OE, Kelly KA: Surgical treatment of adenocarcinoma. Location: junction of the right, left and common hepatic biliary ducts. Arch Surg 114: 22–25, 1979

Alexander F, Rossi RL, O'Bryan M, *et al.*: Biliary carcinoma: a review of 109 cases. Am J Surg 147: 503–509, 1984

Alexandre JH, Chambon H, Poilleux F: La résection dans les cancers des canaux biliaires intra-hépatiques intéressant la convergence. Ann Chir 29: 289–294 (and 304–306), 1975

Altemeier WA, Gall EA, Zinninger MM, Hoxworth PI: Sclerosing carcinoma of the major intra-hepatic bile ducts. Arch Surg 75: 450–461, 1957

Altemeier WA, Gall EA, Culbertson WR, Inge WW: Sclerosing carcinoma of the intrahepatic (hilar) bile ducts. Surgery 60: 191–200, 1966

Alvarez AF: Carcinoma of the main hepatic ducts, within the liver. Ann Surg 148: 773–782, 1958

Ariel IM, Pack GT: Palliative treatment of inoperable cancer of the liver, biliary system and pancreas. In: Pack GT, Ariel IM (eds) Tumors of the Gastrointestinal Tract, Pancreas, Biliary System and Liver. Hoeber, New York, 1962, pp 477–490

Belamaric J: Intrahepatic bile duct carcinoma and C. sinensis infection in Hong Kong. Cancer 31: 468–473, 1973

Bengmark S, Ekberg H, Klöfver-Ståhl B, Evander A, Tranberg K-G: Long-term survival after major liver resection for Klatskin tumour. Ann Surg, accepted for publication, 1986

Benhamou JP, Gottfried A, Darnis F, Fauvert R: Le cancer de la voie biliaire principale. Sem Hop (Paris) 35: 89–100, 1959

Bérard P, Forest G, Cret R, *et al.*: La chirurgie d'exérése des adènocarcinomes excréto-biliaires de la convergence. Ann Chir 32: 126–131, 1978

Bismuth H, Corlette MB: Intrahepatic cholangio-enteric anastomosis in carcinoma of the hilus of the liver. Surg Gynec Obstet 140: 170–178, 1975

Blumgart LH: Biliary tract, obstruction: new approaches to old problems. Am J Surg 135: 19–31, 1978

Blumgart LH, Hadjis NS, Benjamin IS, Beazley R: Surgical approaches to cholangiocarcinoma at the confluence of hepatic ducts. Lancet I: 66–70, 1984

Boerma EJ: The surgical treatment of cancer of the hepatic duct confluence. Thesis, University of Nijmegen

Braasch JW, Warren KW, Kune GA: Malignant neoplasms of the bile ducts. Surg Clin N Am 47: 627–628, 1967

Brown G, Myers N: The hepatic ducts. A surgical approach for resection of tumour. Aust NZ J Surg 23: 308–312, 1954

Brown DB, Strang R, Gordon J, Hendry EB: Primary carcinoma of the extrahepatic bile ducts. Br J Surg 49: 22–28, 1961

Bucharth F, Efsen F, Christiansen LA, et al.: Non-surgical internal biliary drainage by endoprosthesis. Surg Gynecol Obstet 153: 857–860, 1981

Cameron JL, Skinner DB, Zuidema GD: Long term transhepatic intubation for hilar hepatic duct strictures. Ann Surg 183: 488–495, 1976

Cameron JL, Broe P, Zuidema GD: Proximal bile duct tumors. Ann Surg 196: 412–419, 1982

Carlsson E, Zukoski CF, Campbell J, et al.: Morphological, biophysical and biochemical consequences of ligation of the common bile duct in the dog. Am J Pathol 86: 301–312, 1977

Caroli J: In: Hepp, et al. (ed) Les cancers des voies biliaires extra-hépatiques. Arch Mal App Digestif 43: 1041–1057, 1954

Caroli J: Klinik der Gallenwegstumoren. In: Kühn HA, Wernze H (eds) Klinische Hepatologie. Georg Thieme Verlag, Stuttgart, 1979, pp 7.75–7.84

Champeau M, Pineau P: A propos de l'abord du confluent biliaire: voie transhépatique. Acad Chir 81: 635–644, 1955

Champeau M, Pineau P: Voie d'abord élargie transhépatique du canal hépatique gauche. Acad Chir 90: 602–613, 1964

Champeau M, Meillére D: Les anastomoses biliodigestives intra-hépatiques. J Chir (Paris) 89: 281–306, 1965

Champeau M, Vialas M: La mobilisation du segment IV, voie d'abord idéale du confluent biliaire et des pédicules principaux intra-hépatiques. Acad Chir 92: 416–422, 1966

Champeau M: La segmentectomie IV dans l'exposition chirurgicale des voies biliaires intra-hépatiques. Acad Chir 93: 164–174, 1967

Chapman RWG, Arborgh BÅM, Rhodes JM, et al.: Primary sclerosing cholangitis: a review of its clinical features, cholangiography, and hepatic histology. Gut 21: 870–877, 1980

Corlette MB, Bookwalter JR: Individualization of treatment for hilar bile duct cancers. Cancer 46: 415–416, 1980

Cotte (1909): In: Renshaw (ed) malignant Neoplasma of the Extrahepatic Biliary Ducts. Ann Surg 76: 205–221, 1922

Cotton PB: Duodenoscopic placement of biliary prostheses to relieve malignant obstructive jaundice. Brit J Surg 69: 501–503, 1982

Couinaud C: Hépatectomies gauches lobaires et segmentaires. J Chir (Paris) 68: 697–715 and 821–839, 1952

Couinaud C: Le foie. Masson & Cie., Paris, 1957

Couinaud C: Cholangio-jéjunostomies intra-hépatiques gauches. Arch Fr Mal App Dig 56: 295–310, 1967

Dogliotti AM, Fogliati E: Resection of the liver with intrahepatoductogastrostomy or intrahepatoductojejunostomy for biliary obstruction. J Int Coll Surgeons 26: 267–274, 1956

Dooley JS, Dick R, Irving D, Olney J, Sherlock S: Relief of bile duct obstruction by the percutaneous transhepatic insertion of an endoprosthesis. Clin Radiol 32: 163–172, 1981

Douglass TC, Lounsbury BF, Cutter WW, et al.: An experimental study of healing of the common duct. Surg Gynecol Obstet 91: 301–305, 1950

225

Duboucher, Seror, Stoppa: Hépatico-jéjunostomie intrahépatique pour sténose cancéreuse des voies biliaires intra-hilaires. Afr Franc Chir 12: 255–257, 1954

Edmondson HA: Tumors of the gallbladder and extrahepatic bile ducts. In: Atlas of tumor pathology 1967, section VII fasc 26, pp 91–120. Armed Forces Institute of Pathology, Washington DC 20305, USA

Evander A, Fredlund P, Hoevels J, Ihse I, Bengmark S: Evaluation of aggressive surgery for carcinoma of the extrahepatic bile ducts. Ann Surg 191: 23–29, 1980

Flandreau RH, Weber JM, Baird WF: Obstructive jaundice, the problem of differential diagnosis in a patient with carcinoma of the major intrahepatic bile ducts. Gastroenterology 33: 978–984, 1957

Fletcher MS, Brinkley D, Dawson JL, Nunnerley H, Wheeler PG, Williams R: Treatment of high bileduct carcinoma by internal radiotherapy with iridium-192 wire. Lancet II: 172–174, 1981

Fortner JG: An appraisal of the pathogenesis of primary carcinoma of the extrahepatic biliary tract. Surgery 43: 563–571, 1958

Gautier R, Bonnet-Eymard J, Couppie G: Néoplasme des voies biliaires hautes. Dérivation bilio-intestinale intra-hépatique. Mém Acad Chir 86: 680–688, 1960

Gibson LH, Sobin LH: Histological typing of tumours of the liver, biliary tract and pancreas. International Histological Classification of Tumours, no. 20. World Health Organization, Geneva, 31–34, 1978

Glenn F, Hays DM: Carcinoma of the extrahepatic biliary tract. Surg Clin N Am 38: 479–493, 1953

Goetze O: Die transhepatische Dauerdrainage bei der hohen Gallengangsstenose. Langenbecks Arch Klin Chir 270: 97–101, 1951

Hagenmuller F, Classen M: Therapeutic endoscopic and percutaneous procedures for biliary disorders. In: Popper H, Schaffner F (eds) Progress in Liver Diseases, Vol. VII. Grune & Stratton, New York, 1982, pp 299–317

Ham JM, Mackenzie DC: Primary carcinoma of the extrahepatic bile ducts. Surg Gynec Obstet 118: 977–983, 1964

Hart MJ, White TT: Central hepatic resection and anastomosis for stricture or carcinoma at the hepatic bifurcation. Ann Surg 192: 299–305, 1980

Haynes GD, Gingrich GW, Thoroughman JC: Carcinoma of the bile duct: diagnosis and treatment. Am Surgeon 30: 578–582, 1964

Hepp J, Mercadier M, Balansa: Les cancers des voies biliaires extra-hépatiques. Arch Mall App Dig 43: 1041–1057, 1954

Hepp J, Couinaud C: L'ahord et l'utilisation du canal hépatique gauche dans les réparations de la voie biliaire principale. Presse Med 64: 947–948, 1956

Hepp J, Mercadier M: Cancers des voies biliaires extra-hépatiques. Ann Chir 3: 85–96, 1956

Hepp J, Staercke P de: A propos de l'utilisation du grèle en chirurgie biliaire. Acta Chir Belg 59: 682–689, 1960

Hjortsjö C-H: The topography of the intrahepatic duct systems. Acta Anat 11: 599–615, 1951

Imrie CW, Blumgart LH: Tumours of the biliary tree and pancreas. In: Wright R, et al. (ed), Liver and biliary disease. Saunders Comp, London/Philadelphia, 1979, pp 1247–1266

Inouye AA, Whelan Jr TJ: Carcinoma of the extrahepatic bile ducts. Am J Surg 136: 90–95, 1978

Iwasaki Y, Ohto M, Todoroki T, et al.: Treatment of carcinoma of the biliary system. Surg Gynec Obstet 144: 219–224, 1977

Karakousis CP, Douglass Jr HO: Hilar hepatojejunostomy in resection of carcinoma of the main hepatic duct junction. Surg Gynec Obstet 145: 245–248, 1977

Klatskin G: Adenocarcinoma of the hepatic duct at its bifurcation within the porta hepatis. Am J Surg 38: 241–256, 1965

Kopelson G, Galdabini J, Warshaw AL, Gunderson LG: Patterns of failure after curative surgery for extrahepatic biliary tract carcinoma: implications for adjuvant therapy. Int J Radiat Oncol Biol Phys 7: 413–417, 1981

226

Kune GA, Sali A: The practice of biliary surgery, 2nd ed Blackwell Scientific Publ., Melbourne, 1980, pp 252–274

Kuwayti K, Baggenstoss AH, Stauffer MH, Priestley JT: Carcinoma of the major intrahepatic and the extrahepatic bile ducts exclusive of the papilla of Vater. Surg Gynec Obstet 104: 357–366, 1957

Langer JC, Langer B, Taylor Br, Zeldin R, Cummings B: Carcinoma of the extrahepatic bile ducts: results of an aggresive surgical approach. Surgery 98: 752–759, 1985

Launois B, Campion J-P, Brisset R, Gosselin M: Carcinoma of the hepatic hilus: surgical treatment and the case for resection. Ann Surg 190: 151–157, 1979

Lees CD, Zapolanski A, Cooperman AM, Hermann RE: Carcinoma of the bile ducts. Surg Gynec Obstet 151: 193–198, 1980

Longmire Jr WP, Sanford MC: Intrahepatic cholangiojejunostomy with partial hepatectomy for biliary obstruction. Surgery 24: 264–276, 1948

Longmire Jr WP, Lippman HN: Intrahepatic cholangiojejunostomy – an operation for biliary obstruction. Surg Clin N Am 36: 849–863, 1956

Longmire Jr WP, McArthur MS, Bastounis EA, Hiatt J: Carcinoma of the extrahepatic biliary tract. Ann Surg 178: 333–345, 1973

Lorelius LE, Jacobson G, Sawada S: Endoprosthesis as an internal biliary drainage in inoperable patients with biliary obstruction. Acta Chir Scand 148: 613–616, 1982

Malt RA, Warshaw AL, Jamieson CG, Hawk III JC: Left intrahepatic cholangiojejunostomy for proximal obstruction of the biliary tract. Surg Gynec Obstet 150: 193–197, 1980

Meyerowitz BR, Aird I: Carcinoma of the hepatic ducts within the liver. Br J Surg 50: 178–184, 1962

Michels NA: Blood supply and anatomy of the upper abdominal organs. JB Lippincott Co., Philadelphia, 1955

Mizumoto R, Kawarada Y, Suzuki H: Surgical treatment of hilar carcinoma of the bile duct. Surg Gyneol Obstet 162: 153–158, 1986

Mornex F, Ardiet JM, Bret P, Gerard JP: Radiotherapy of high bile duct carcinoma using intra-catheter iridium 192 wire. Cancer 54: 2069–2073, 1984

Nishimura A, Nakano M, Maruyana K, et al.: Successfully resected carcinoma of the bifurcation of the main hepatic ducts. Jap J Surg 8: 123–137, 1978

Northover JMA, Terblanche J: A new look at the arterial supply of the bile duct in man and its surgical implications. Br J Surg 66: 379–384, 1979

Orcel L: Les cancers des voies biliaires. In: DeLarue J, Frühling L (eds) Cancer primitif du foie et des voies biliaires. Masson & Cie, Paris, 1958, pp 111–160

Quattlebaum JK, Quattlebaum Jr JK: Malignant obstruction of the marjor hepatic ducts. Ann Surg 161: 876–889, 1965

Ragins H, Diamond A, Chieng-Hsing Meng: Intrahepatic cholangiojejunostomy in the management of malignant biliary obstruction. Surg Gynec Obstet 136: 27–32, 1973

Rains AJH: Biliary obstruction in the region of the porta hepatis. Ann R Coll Surg Engl 24: 69–100, 1959

Renshaw K: Malignant neoplasms of the extrahepatic biliary ducts. Ann Surg 76: 205–221, 1922

Roberts-Thomson IC, Strickland RG, Mackay IR: Bile duct carcinoma in chronic ulcerative colitis. Aust NZ J Med 3: 264–267, 1973

Rohner A: Analyse d'une série de 85 hépatectomies. Chirurgie 108: 137–143, 1982

Ross AP, Braasch JW, Warren KW: Carcinoma of the proximal bile ducts. Surg Gynec Obstet 136: 923–928, 1983

Salembier Y: Quelques procédés pratiques rares ou originaux en chirurgie biliaire et pancreatique. Masson & Cie., Paris, 1971, pp 63–71

Schutt RP: Bilateral intrahepatic cholangiojejunostomy. Am J Surg 107: 777–780, 1964

Scott J, Shousha S, Thomas HC, Sherlock S: Bile duct carcinoma: a late complication of congenital hepatic fibrosis. Am J Gastroenterol 73: 113–119, 1980

Smith R: Surgery of the gallbladder and bile ducts. Butterworths, London, 1964

Smith R: Hepaticojejunostomy with transhepatic intubation. Br J Surg 51: 186–194, 1964

Stephen JL: Quadrate lobectomy. Proc Royal Soc Med 57: 551, 1964

Strohl EL, Reed WH, Diffenbauch WG, Anderson RE: Carcinoma of the bile ducts. Arch Surg 87: 567–577, 1963

Thorbjarnarson B: Carcinoma of the intrahepatic bile ducts. Arch Surg 77: 908–917, 1958

Thorbjarnarson B: Carcinoma of the bile ducts. Cancer 12: 708, 1959

Todoroki T, Iwasaki Y, Okamura T, et al.: Intraoperative raditherapy for advanced carcinoma of the biliary system. Cancer 46: 2179–2184, 1980

Tompkins RK, Thomas D, Wile A, Longmire Jr WP: Prognostic factors in bile duct carcinoma. Ann Surg 194: 447–456, 1981

Tsuzuki T, Uekusa M: Carcinoma of the proximal bile ducts. Surg Gynec Obstet 146: 933–943, 1978

Tsuzuki T, Ogata Y, Hosoda Y, et al.: Hepatic resection upon patients with jaundice. Surg Gynec Obstet 153: 387–391, 1981

Van Heerden JA, Judd ES, Dockerty MB: Carcinoma of the extrahepatic bile ducts. Am J Surg 113: 49–56, 1967

Voyles CR, Bowley NJ, Allison DJ, Benjamin IS, Blumgart LH: Carcinoma of the proximal extrahepatic biliary tree: radiologic assessment and therapeutic alternatives. Ann Surg 197: 188–194, 1983

Waugh JM: Carcinoma of the extrahepatic bile ducts. In: Pack GT, Ariel IM (eds) Tumors of the Gastrointestinal Tract, Pancreas, Biliary System and Liver. Hoeber, New York, 1962, pp 364–387

Way LW, Dunphy JE: Biliary stricture. Am J Surg 124: 287–295, 1972

Weinbren K, Mutum SS: Pathological aspects of cholangiocarcinoma. Pathology 139: 217–238, 1983

Welton JC, Marr JS, Friedman SM: Association between hepatobiliary cancer and typhoid carrier state. Lancet I: 791–794, 1979

Whelton MJ, Petrelli M, George P, et al.: Carcinoma at the junction of the main hepatic ducts. Quart J med 38: 211–230, 1969

13. Continuing problems in management of benign bile duct stricture

Å. ANDRÈN-SANDBERG and S. BENGMARK

During the last decade a relative decrease in incidence of iatrogenic bile duct strictures following cholecystectomy [1] seem to have occurred. This may be due to several factors: A greater awareness of the problem among surgeons, the more liberal use of pre- or preoperative cholangiography at cholecystectomy, and safer techniques of dissection during biliary surgery. We have recently in more detail characterized some of these avoidable factors [2]. It is extremely important to be aware of the risks as iatrogenic biliary strictures unfortunately most commonly seem to affect otherwise healthy persons in the productive years of their life and may lead to chronic disease which affects their daily life and even eventually shortens it.

The iatrogenic strictures are covered in the literature by a vast number of papers and reviews. Numerous variations of operative and postoperative management have been suggested. So far the ideal management still remains to be developed. After repair of benign biliary strictures, recurrence of symptoms occur in up to 30% of the patients [3] and – in selected materials – even higher frequences [4]. As most reports are based on relatively few patients and the personal experience of each surgeon or team of surgeons with few exceptions is very limited the factors behind recurrence and their prevention are still rather unknown. Due to lack of good experimental models the biliary stricturation process and its regulation has been little studied under experimental conditions. No prospectively randomized studies of treatment have yet been performed and published in the clinical literature.

Quality of the surgery

It has repeatedly been shown [5–9] that the number of further operations for recurrent biliary strictures after the initial cholecystectomy negatively influence the short as well as the long-term outcome. This could be due to a selection of more difficult cases requiring more operations, but it is more likely to indicate the importance of the first repair. Much supports the view that the excellence of the first repair regulates the prognosis. Therefore, pleas for centralizing these uncommon cases to the hands of a few experts and for an early referral of these patients to selected surgeons are not rare in the literature. However, the most important repair is that which is done immediately after the cholecystectomy procedure. If the injury is detected during this operation the most experienced biliary surgeon available should be invited to participate in the repair.

The results of common duct repair have improved for each of the recent decades [6]. In their review Way et al. [10] report good results in 56%, in 1941–50, 77% in 1951–60 AND 91% IN 1961–80. This can partly be explained as due to shorter follow-up, but more probably reflects improved operative skill and a general greater experience.

It is, however, difficult to define and describe the variations in operative details and their importance for the outcome. It is much easier to discuss the use of PTCs, stents, Roux-loops etc, which can be described in more measurable terms, than to describe how an experienced and successful surgeon does during his dissection and anastomosis. It is probable that the most critical objective is to peform a precise, but limited dissection enough to prepare unscarred duct above the stricture – if a delayed repair – and to perform a precise tension-free anastomosis. If these general objectives can be met, the odds for a good result is high, regardless of most other aspects of management. The ability to perform a successful repair is probably related to the surgeons general operative experience, but more important and more specific – to his expertice in this particular anatomical region and with bilienteric anastomoses – often also based on a great experience with cancer operations in the hepato-pancreato-biliary region. The ability to achieve a precise, tension-free anastomosis by the surgeon is, however, also determined by his knowledge in anatomy and pathophysiology, and about factors and conditions to facilitate a per prima healing. This gives the surgeon the ability to chose the best reconstruction for that particular patient and that particular condition.

Anatomical background

The vascular supply to the duct is of utmost importance for success. Northover and Terblanche [11] were able to describe the blood supply to the common duct, based on a series of injection studies. They demonstrated that there are two important arteries that run along the common duct – one on the medial and one on the lateral surface of the duct which they called 3 o'clock and 9 o'clock arteries. In 32% of cases a retroportal artery also contributed to the blood supply. In more than half of the studied cases the vessels got their main blood supply from below, from the superior mesenteric artery. Therefore, to a common duct which has been completely transected, there will often be too little blood supply to the upper part. This could explain the poor healing after common duct injuries. It is also a good argument 1) in hepatoenteric anastomosis to produce a high anastomosis and 2) not to 'cleance' the ends of the duct, especially not on the lateral sides. The more carefully it is cleansed, the more likely it will be stripped of its already tenous blood supply [11–13].

The occurrence of bile duct strictures can fully be explained on the basis of common duct ischemia and subsequent poor healing. Northover and Terblanche [11] further propose that bile duct strictures arise because of ischemia – caused directly by accidental duct clamping or indirectly by trauma – to the bile duct blood supply during operation. Other factors like infection and bile contents – particularily bile acids – are also likely to play a role. Bile acids are known to be fibrogenic. The ischemia might damage ductal mucosa sufficiently to render it permeable to bile, which would then act on the ischaemic tissue within the wall and induce further inflammation and fibrosis. The oedema accompanying such a reaction might occlude adjacent parts of minute vessels in the choledochal arterial plexus. This would produce further ischemia and lead to a spreading cycle of collagen breakdown, followed by fibrosis until a large part of the duct has been destroyed and replaced by condensed fibrous tissue.

It should also be kept in mind that ductal damage not seldom occur during attempts to control bleeding during cholecystectomy. In a series where angiography was performed after the injury more than half of the patients (57%) had had an injury to hepatic artery as well [5].

The biliary system including the gallbladder has no portal blood supply and is hereby in contrast to the liver tissue more vulnerable to hepatic arterial occlusion. To avoid further injuries at reoperations to the branches of the hepatic artery or newly formed collaterals it has been recommended that only the anterior side of the duct should be dissected. This is often sufficient to allow a 3–4 cm long hepaticojejunal anastomos Roux-en-Y [14]. That excessive mobilization of the duct often is unnecessary for repair, has been extensively shown by Smith and associates [15, 16], and is based on their experience from the worlds largest material. On the other hand an experienced HPB surgeon is most often able to get cranial of the stricture and anastomose to a well nourished hepatic duct with good results.

Stenting

The use of stents is very controversial; claimed to be essential [10] or to make more harm than good [17]; necessary to be kept in place for at least six months

[18, 19], or even longer than 12 months [6, 20, 21]. The reason for the variety of diverse views is the lack of experimental as well as randomized clinical studies. Block and Rosemurgy [12] tried to formulate criterias for the ideal stent. It should be nonreactive, not act as a nidus for formation of stones, be pliable and easy to place, change and remove, be radiopaque (or easy in other ways to visualise on X-ray) and have multiple side holes (on the right places). They also tried to give arguments why an indwelling stent should be considered. It should prevent restricture while the fibrotic process continues, and at the same time decompress the ductal system. Further, with a percutaneous stent the biliary tree can be irrigated, cholangiogram can be obtained if necessary and bile can be easily sampled for culture or other investigations. On the other hand, it is easy to find arguments for the opposite view: percutaneous catheters and stents leads to infection, stents leads to mucosal damage and influx of bile into the tissues and thereby further fibrosis.

Three to six months is today often recommended as the optimal period of splintage, with the tube left for 12 months in more difficult cases [5]. In their material of 139 patients with stents Pitt *et al.* [8] found that patients stented for less than one month had the poorest result.

It has been claimed early [22] as well as recently [13] that the longer the stent remains *in situ* the more likely it is to produce good result. For example, better long-term results were obtained in a non-randomized study with anastomosis splinted for longer than 12 months than those splinted for 6 months or less [23]. In their review Warren and Jefferson [6] demonstrate 'excellent or good' results in about 50% of patients treated with stents for 3–6 months, but 90–100% if the stents were left in place for more than 2 years. The theoretical background to this should be that the stents are left in place until maturation of fibrous tissue has occurred [24].

On the other hand, the foreign material in the bile duct in itself predisposes to stasis and infection with resulting calculi and debris occurring in the stent. Therefore, stents are usually not left in place when cholangitis or occlusion, or both, occurs [6]. As no patients have been randomized between short time and long time stenting it could well be that the short stenting is more to be regarded as an indication of complication due to the stenting itself – and the long stenting that no suspected complications occurred. If prolonged stenting is required, the stent may today be exchanged over a guidewire with little difficulty [12]. It is no doubt stents help to increase the accuracy of suture placement especially for the anterior portion of the anastomosis [25]. Most surgeon will probably use stents partly for this purpose. If one do not believe in their value during the healing procedure they can easily be removed immediately or early after the repair. It is important to mention that Bismuth and co-workers rarely use transanastomotic splinting and report excellent results [26]. Also other authors regard transanastomotic splintage is unnecessary [22].

We support that view and have reasons to suspect that stents are to the disadvantage of good healing. It should also be remembered, that most studies compare short and long term stenting but no studies stenting or non-stenting.

Preoperative PTC drainage

Wexler and Smith [16] and Bolton and co-workers [17] advice early hepatic decompression with percutaneous transhepatic drainage of the biliary tree. It is no doubt that PTC is a most useful investigation before reoperation for planning the operation and to map the stricture [9]. The question is more whether a period of drainage between the investigation and the operation helps to improve the results.

Once a PTC-catheter has been positioned and left in place the condition of the patient frequently improves dramatically – especially in the deeply jaundiced and cholangitic patients. Such facts has lead some authors to recommend that the surgical repair is delayed for several months until the inflammation has resolved and the adhesions have matured [27]. On the same basis there has also been proposed a two-stage operation; a hepaticostomy performed initially, and a definitive repair when the physical condition of the patient has improved sufficiently [28].

It should be pointed that in general recent literature does not support routine use of preoperative PTC-drainage. For further information – see chapter 10. Another disadvantage with preoperative PTC-drainage could be that the duct decreases in diameter during the drainage period and hereby the chances for a wide anastomosis. On the other hand the presence of a palpable catheter in the common duct lumen provides a good anatomic landmark in a surgical field which is destroyed by previous operation(s), fibrotic and full of adhesions [25].

Type of anastomosis

In the literature different operations are often described and recommended by different surgeons – unfortunately most often on a very weak scientific basis. We are convinced, however, that there is no oneway approach to the patients with bile duct strictures – all injuries and patients must be treated individually. This does not exclude that in general, some operations are better than others.

End-to-end anastomosis should theoretically be the ideal procedure, as it reestablishes the normal physiologic state. Lord Smith [15] recommend that if it is recognized during the operation that the common bile duct has been damaged, immediate repair should be carried out, employing the smallest number of finest sutures necessary to reconstruct the duct. This is most probably the ideal procedure provided that there is no lack of common duct substance and that the 'Terblanche arteries' are intact. For established strictures and late repair, however, he abandons the end-to-end anastomosis. Bismuth found that following end-to-end ductal repair – even without tension – and usually over T-tube the repair was successful in only about 50% of the cases [26] – despite the fact that most of the injuries were recognized immediately at the operation. In their material of 970 patients – mainly late repair – Warren and Jefferson [6] report satisfactory results in 52% of 493 patients treated with end-to-end anastomosis and 66% of 477 patients operated on which hepatico-jejunostomy.

Also the hepatico-jejunostomy has received some unfavorable reviews with regard to a high incidence of anastomatic stenosis [31, 32]. In spite of that Roux-Y-choledocho- or hepaticojejunostomy is most often recommended [4, 8] either as a hand-sutured Roux-Y-jejunal reconstruction [7, 16, 20, 26, 33–35] or as a sutureless anastomosis Roux-Y [36, 37]. Braasch and co-workers [25] believe that the use of sutures is necessary, but recommend a one-layer suture due to a growing awareness of the possible role of ductal ischemia as a contributing factor to recurrent stricture. A jejunal segment is preferred by some rather than a jejunal loop [38] as the latter often is too bulky to be satisfactorally placed at the hilum of the liver. In addition the food stream is with jejunal segment shunted away from the biliary tree which should decrease the risk of secondary biliary infection. Braasch, however, state that this has no clinical significance [25]. It is likely to be true in the absence of stricture and biliary stasis. In their not randomized study Genest et al. [1] found all operative procedures equally effective in regard to recurrence rate except for direct duct-to-duct anastomosis, which had a higher failure rate. These results are the same as ours [4], and we believe that choledochostomy should very rarely be used.

Distal injuries can be managed by choledochoduodenostomy, especially if the injury is detected during the initial operation and the common bile duct is wide enough. Although this type of repair looks 'more physiological', the practical advantages of hepaticojejunostomy, however, most often make it a far better operation [19, 29, 39]. In a few cases a more special solution of the problem has been recommended. A jejunal interposition between the bile duct and duodenum has been recommended [38, 40]. Also a jejunal patch – in lack of cystic duct remnants – can be used [18]. To us it seems, however, difficult to foresee any situation where these procedures would be superior to more conventional techniques. Intrahepatic biliodigestive anastomoses might be necessary in special cases [42]. The hepatogastrostomy – once a popular procedure – is nowadays virtually abandoned [41].

There is no doubt a proportion of patients, particularly the elderly, in whom an expectant approach may be adopted [5]. Furthermore, there is also place for stricture dilatation in selected cases, carried out surgically or percutanously [43]. Concerning both these procedures we still lack enough knowledge for selection of suitable patients – further studies are needed.

Follow-up

The results of the repair of bile duct injuries are difficult to evaluate. One must take in account morbidity and mortality not associated with operation per se – for example cardiovascular disease – and morbidity and mortality associated with the impaired liver function due to the long term effects of the deranged bile-flow from the liver. As an example of this, Braasch *et al.* [25] describe three cases in which the patients' subsequent clinical course was poor despite the demonstration of an apparently adequate biliary drainage at subsequent re-exploration of the hepaticojejunostomy. In each of these three patients, biliary cirrhosis was present at the time of the first hepaticojejunostomy. Glenn reports [30] nine postoperative deaths among his 100 patients with bile duct strictures; seven were attributed to liver failure secondary to biliary cirrhosis. In addition, the results of simple stricture repair in an uncomplicated case must be separated from the result of those patients with adhesions after bile-peritonitis and fistulas, portal hypertension, lobar liver atrophy etc. Furthermore, there is scant information on relative and absolute morbidity rates related to the level of the stricture. According to Genest and co-workers [1] high-stricture repair have a greater incidence of recurrence – although not significant. From a theoretical point of view one would expect the opposite. In their report Genest *et al.* [1] found that patients who had undergone several previous operations had a higher recurrence rate and greater morbidity and mortality. Warren and Jefferson [6] state that if more than three repairs of a biliary stricture are necessary a satisfactory result is unlikely. Therefore, comparisons between different patient-materials are hazardous.

There has been proposed a well formulated, formal classification of the severity of bile duct strictures by Bismuth [11]. Unfortunately it will only help to some extent as there is no objective definition of satisfactory result. There is a great variation in the way different surgeons accept there results as satisfactory. For example Braasch *et al.* [26] defines as a good result patients without symptoms or with occasional attacks of cholangitis three years after the repair. Others consider the absence of symptoms two years after operation as satisfactory results. Bismuth [12] suggests a follow-up of at least 5 and preferrably 10 years and regards the results as good only if the patients are symptom-free, have normal liver function test and no restenosis.

It should be noted that Pitt and co-workers [8] found that not only the interval from initial surgery till presentation of symptoms increased from 69% at 6

months to 94% at 5 years, but also that the recurrent stricture requiring another reoperation increased from 68% at 3 years to 95% in 12 years, and the
last recognized restricture occurred 19 years after the initial operation. It
seems probable that the operation of a stricture developing many years after
the initial operation has a better over-all prognosis, than those strictures giving
symptoms shortly after the cholecystectomy. Similarly, Walters and Romsdell
[46] had excellent or good results in 73% of their patients followed up 1 to 5
years, but only 61% of their patients followed up 5 to 25 years achieved excellent or good results. Glenn reports a case of recurrent obstruction 11 years after the primary repair [30]. This clearly shows that the true result can not be
evaluated until many years after the re-operation.

Remaining questions

It is not probable that extended clinical studies can give further, conclusive answers to the many questions of management of iatrogenic bile duct strictures.
Instead it is our belief that more laboratory – and laboratorious – work has to
be done.

Firstly, it must be questioned if the fibrotic process is different in the bile
ducts than in other hollow organs. If so, it has to be defined if this is due to a
factor in the tissue itself or in the environment – or both. In particular it is important to know if bile by itself has fibrose-stimulating properties, and if it is
enough to protect the connective tissue with mucosa to inhibite the proposed
fibrosing process. Further, it should be investigated if the process can be inhib-
ited by drugs.

Secondly, the influence of stents have to be further investigated. What happens in a short time perspective if the stent is not entirely surrounded by mucosa – and if the mucosa circumvent the stent, makes it any difference if the stent
is there or not? If there is a lack of mucosa, or if the stent gives a decubital ulcer, will the process of fibrosis be enhanced, or will the stent hinder a stricture
– in a short and in a long time perspective? Not until these questions are answered is it meaningful to discuss type of material in the stent, shape of the
stent, and duration of stenting.

Thirdly, what means infection to the healing process of the common duct? It
is most probable that a stent, from the choledochus to the skin, stomach or the
small bowel – and possibly even when it is only in the common bile duct – will
be infected, and serve as a nidus for the bacteria. Is it then possible to prevent
stricture-formation by a proper antibiotic until the mucosa of the duct has heal-
ed, and in that case: what antibiotic is proper? Should it cover both the aerobic
and anaerobic spectrum and must it be secreted with the bile? Perhaps some
kind of choleretic and viscosity reducing drug increasing the amount of bile

produced and decreasing the viscosity of bile could help to clear the bile ducts from bacterias.

While solving these basic problems, it is probable that the debate will continue among surgeons of the best operative technique. Although one case is never the other quite alike and the management for each has to be individualized some basic principles – and techniques – might be preferable. But instead of each surgeon operating on their own cases we must assume the responsibility and refer those few cases to selected centers where a higher expertice can be reached – and maybe some randomized studies can be done to solve some of the many remaining questions. It should be further emphasized that the results from all studies must be reported in a more uniform way than today – one of the proposed classifications should be generally used – and with a follow-up of at least five years, or, if possible, ten years.

However, one single clinical question can probably be answered less laboratorious – empirically – than the others during the next few years: is there a place for percutaneous dilatation with modern radiologic technique? If a good palliation could be reached for a reasonable length of time, and re-dilatations could be done with an equally low morbidity and mortality, this might be the procedure of choice not only in a few selected cases, but on a wider patient material.

Management of benign bile duct strictures following cholecystectomy remains as a problem, but we are convinced – it is a problem that can be solved!

References

1. Genest JF, Nanos E, Grundfest-Broniatowski S, Vogt D, Hermann R: Benign biliary strictures: An analytic review (1970 to 1984). Surgery 99: 409–13, 1986
2. Andrèn-Sandberg Å, Alinder G, Bengmark S: Accidental lesions of the common bile duct at cholecystectomy. Pre- and peroperative factors of importance. Ann Surg 201: 328–32, 1985
3. Pellegrini CA, Thomas MJ, Way LW: Recurrent biliary stricture. Patterns of recurrence and outcome of surgical therapy. Am J Surg 147: 175–9, 1984
4. Andrèn-Sandberg Å, Johansson S, Bengmark S: Accidental lesions of the common bile duct at cholecystectomy. II. Results of treatment. Ann Surg 201: 452–5, 1985
5. Blumgart LH, Kelley CJ, Benjamin IS: Benign bile duct stricture following cholecystectomy: Critical factors in management. Br J Surg 71: 836–43, 1984
6. Warren KW, Jefferson MF: Prevention and repair of strictures of the extrahepatic bile ducts. Surg Clin North Am 53: 1169–90, 1973
7. Warren KW, Mountain JC, Midell AI: Management of strictures of the biliary tract. Surg Clin North Am 51: 711–31, 1971
8. Pitt HA, Miyamoto T, Parapatis SK, Tompkins RK, Longmire WP: Factors influencing outcome in patients with postoperative biliary strictures. Am J Surg 144: 14–20, 1982
9. Collins PG, Gorey TF: Iatrogenic biliary stricture: Presentation and management. Br J Surg 71: 980–2, 1984
10. Way LW, Bernhoft RA, Thomas MJ: Biliary stricture. Surg Clin North Am 61: 963–72, 1981

238

11. Northover JMA, Terblanche J: A new look at the arterial supply of the bile duct in man and its surgical implications. Br J Surg 66: 379–84, 1979
12. Bismuth H: Postoperative strictures of the biliary tract. In: Blumgart JH (ed) The Biliary Tract. Clinical Surgery International. Vol 5. Edinburgh: Churchill-Livingstone 209–18, 1983
13. Block GE, Rosemurgy AS: A technique for hepaticodochojejunostomy with transhepatic stent. Surg Gynecol Obstet 162: 485–8, 1986
14. Machado MCC, da Cunha JEM, Bacchella T: A modified technique for surgical repair of cicatricial stenosis of the bile duct. Surg Gynecol Obstet 162: 283–4, 1986
15. Smith R: Obstruction of the bile duct. Br J Surg 66: 69–79, 1979
16. Wexler MJ, Smith R: Jejunal mucosal graft. A sutureless technic for repair of high bile duct strictures. Am J Surg 129: 204–11, 1975
17. Bolton JS, Braasch JW, Rossi RL: Management of benign biliary stricture. Surg Clin North Am 60: 313–32, 1980
18. Okamura T, Orii K, Ono A, Ozaki A, Iwasaki Y: Surgical technique for repair of benign stricture of the bile ducts, preserving the papilla of Vater. World J Surg 9: 619–25, 1985
19. Hertzer NR, Gray HW, Hoerr SO, Hermann RE: The use of T-tube splints in bile duct repairs. Surg Gynecol Obstet 137: 413–8, 1973
20. Cameron JL, Gayler BW, Zuidema GD: The use of Silastic transhepatic stents in benign and malignant biliary strictures. Ann Surg 188: 552–9, 1978
21. Warren KW, Braasch JW: Repair of benign strictures of the bile ducts. Surg Clin North Am 45: 617–25, 1965
22. Warren KW, Hardy KJ: The damaged bile duct. Surg Clin North Am 47: 1077–94, 1967
23. Kune GA, Hardy JH, Brown G, McKenzie G: Operative injuries of the common bile duct. Med J Aust 2: 233–6, 1969
24. Moossa AR, Block GE, Skinner DB, Hall AW: Reconstruction of high biliary tract strictures employing transhepatic intubation. Surg Clin North Am 56: 73–81, 1976
25. Braasch JW, Bolton JS, Rossi RL: A technique of biliary tract reconstruction with complete follow-up in 44 consecutive cases. Ann Surg 194: 635–8, 1981
26. Bismuth H, Franco D, Corlette MB, Hepp J: Longterm results of Roux-en-Y hepaticojejunostomy. Surg Gynecol Obstet 146: 161–7, 1978
27. Schwarz W, Rosen RJ, Fitts WT, Mackie JA, Oleaga JA, Freiman DB, McLean GK, Ring EJ: Percutaneous transhepatic drainage preoperatively for benign biliary strictures. Surg Gynecol Obstet 152: 466–8, 1981
28. Cattell RB, Braasch JW: Two stage repairs of benign strictures of the bile duct. Surg Gynecol Obstet 109: 691–6, 1959
29. Saber K, El-Manialawi M: Repair of bile duct injuries. World J Surg 8: 82–9, 1984
30. Glenn F: Iatrogenic injuries to the biliary ductal system. Surg Gynecol Obstet 146: 430–4, 1978
31. Lane CE, Sawyers JL, Riddell DH, Scott HW: Long-term results of Roux-en-Y hepatocholangiojejunostomy. Ann Surg 177: 714–20, 1973
32. Braasch JW, Warren KW, Blevins PK: Progress in biliary stricture repair. Am J Surg 129: 34–9, 1975
33. Longmire WP: Early management of injury to the extrahepatic biliary tract. JAMA 195: 111–3, 1966
34. Lindenauer SM: Surgical treatment of bile duct strictures. Surgery 73: 875–80, 1973
35. Stefanini P, Carboni M, Patrassi N, Basoli A, de Bernardinis G, Negro P: Roux-en-Y hepaticojejunostomy: A reappraisal of its indications and results. Ann Surg 181: 213–9, 1975
36. Smith R: Hepaticojejunostomy with transhepatic intubation. A technique for very high strictures of the hepatic ducts. Br J Surg 51: 186–94, 1964
37. Thorbjarnarson B: Repair of common bil duct injury. Surg Gynecol Obstet 133: 293–6, 1971

38. Wheeler E, Longmire WP: Repair of benign stricture of the common bile duct by jejunal interposition choledochoduodenostomy. Surg Gynecol Obstet 146: 260–2, 1978

39. Hermann RE: Diagnosis and management of bile duct strictures. Am J Surg 130: 519–22, 1975

40. Moreeno-Gonzales E, Sanmartin JH, Azcoita MM, Serna AB: Reconstruction of the biliary tract using biliary-duodenal interposition of a defunctionalized jejunal limb. Surg Gynecol Obstet 150: 678–82, 1980

41. Way LE, Dunphy JE: Biliary stricture. Am J Surg 124: 287–95, 1972

42. Kanematsu T, Sugimachi K, Takenaka K, Inokuchi K: A new secured technique for intrahepatic cholangiojejunostomy and drainage of bile. Surg Gynecol Obstet 159: 85–7, 1984

43. Toufanian A, Carey LC, Martin ET: Transhepatic biliary dilatation: An alternative to surgical reconstruction. Curr Surg 35: 70–3, 1978

46. Walters W, Romsdell JA: Study of three hundred eight operations for stricture of bile ducts: Follow-up periods of one to five or five to twenty-five years. JAMA 171: 872–7, 1959

14. Pancreatic pseudocysts*

M.N. VAN DER HEYDE

Introduction

Before the advent of ultrasonography, computed tomography (CT) and endoscopic retrograde cholangiopancreatography (ERCP), pancreatic pseudocysts were usually not discovered before they became symptomatic: either as a palpable mass in the upper abdomen or as a chance finding in patients with vague upper-abdominal complaints. Barium studies of the stomach, showing the typical compression or displacement (Fig. 1) were the only available information in addition to the patient's history and physical examination.

Nowadays ultrasonography either externally or by way of endoscopy, CT and ERCP offer the opportunity to study prospectively patients at risk of developing pseudocysts (Fig. 2). In addition routine investigation by these methods of patients with unspecific upper abdominal complaints can identify pseudocysts in cases where the relation between complaints and the identified lesion is uncertain. This may lead to the treatment of diagnostic findings. For that reason the time has come to identify those pseudocysts that should be treated and to define the best way of treating them if necessary.

Before the question can be answered why, when and how to treat a pancreatic pseudocyst, information is needed on the nature of these lesions, i.e. how they develop, on the diagnostic criteria and finally on the available treatment modalities.

The development of pancreatic pseudocysts

Pancreatic pseudocysts may develop posttraumatically, as a result of acute pancreatitis or during the course of chronic pancreatitis. It is important to

* In cooperation with: Å. Andrén-Sandberg (Sweden), W.F. Eggink (The Netherlands), H. Obertop (The Netherlands), J.C. Garles (France), A. Schmidt (Denmark), R.C.N. Williamson (United Kingdom).

242

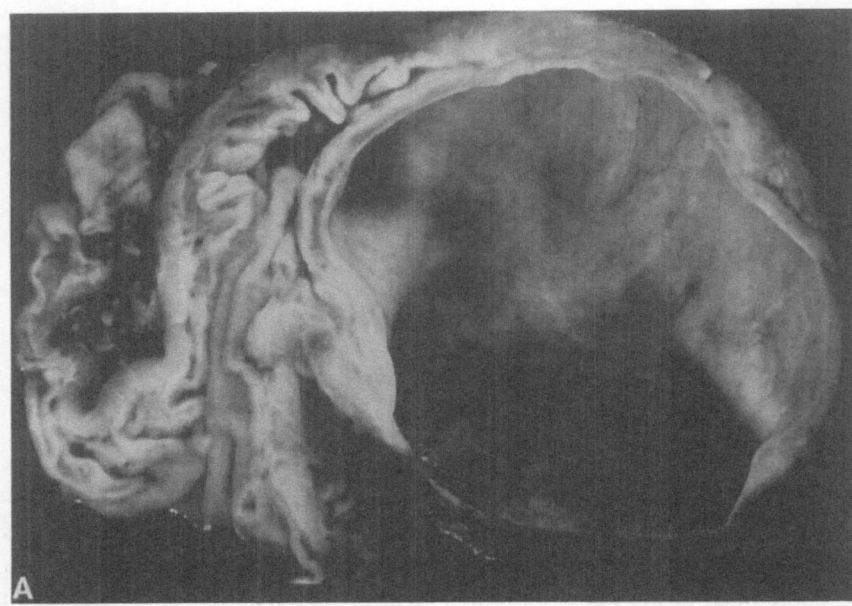

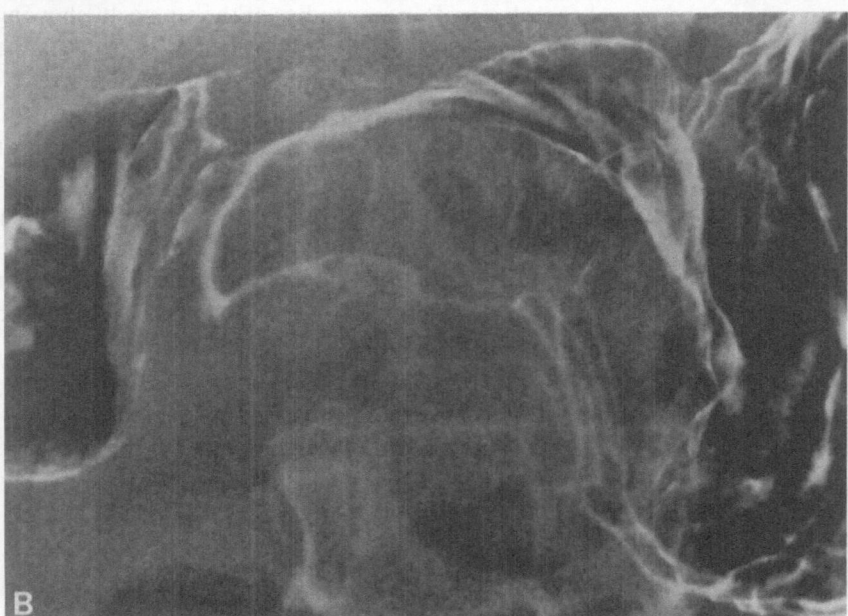

Fig. 1.* Pancreatic pseudocyst (Fig. 1a). Antero posterior radiograph from an upper G.I. series showing extrinsic displacement of the antral stomach by a large mass in the corpus of the pancreas (Fig. 1b). A pseudocyst was found at surgery (Fig. 1a).

* '(Courtesy of Dr. W. Dean Warren). Reproduced with permission from Thomford, N.R.: Current Status of the Warren Shunt, in Najarian, J.S., And Delaney, J.P. (eds.): Advances in Hepatic, Biliary and Pancreatic Surgery. Copyright © 1985 by Year Book Medical Publishers, Inc., Chicago.'

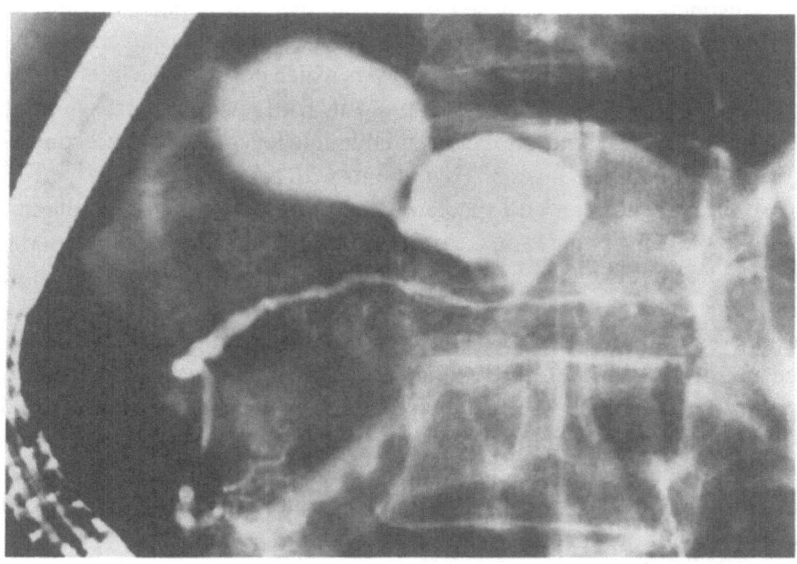

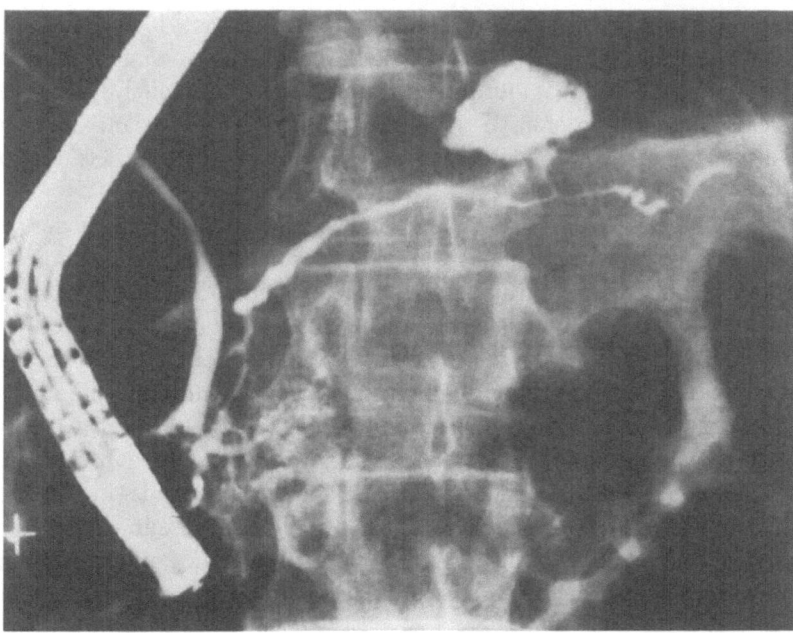

Fig. 2. Film following ERCP shows contrastfilling of two communicating pseudocysts at the pancreatic tail, and irregularity of the main pancreatic duct. Note also irregular filling of multiple side branches distally in the main pancreatic duct.

make a distinction between these causes from the clinical point of view.

During the course of severe pancreatitis abscess formation can occur. These abscesses should be differentiated from cysts which develop in a later phase of the disease. A true pancreatic abscess presents with severe clinical symptoms: abdominal pain, local tenderness, fever, chills and leucocytosis. This condition is rare and may occur in 0.6–2.5% of patients with acute pancreatitis [1, 2]. An increase in incidence can be expected when more patients survive the acute phase of necrotising pancreatitis. The mortality is high when the abscess is not drained (30%) but even after surgical drainage the mortality is approximately 15% [2–6].

A pancreatic abscess should be differentiated from an infected pseudocyst, which can occur in a later phase of acute pancreatitis and has a much better prognosis [7]. In a prospective study of patients with acute pancreatitis 32 out of 413 patients (8%) developed a pseudocyst [8]. Half of the cases resulted from gallstone induced pancreatitis and 15% from alcohol induced disease. It seems likely that cysts smaller than 4 cm in diameter tend to disappear spontaneously [9]. This occurs rarely in patients with larger cysts.

In another series, formation of pseudocysts was the most frequent late complication of acute pancreatitis [10]. Thus patients who survive severe acute pancreatitis should be followed up carefully as in some cases intervention may be indicated. Rupture, sepsis and bleeding are well known complications. In the past it was believed that these complications occurred frequently. In recent years close observation of large series of patients with severe pancreatitis has shown that 'silent' symptomless cysts have a relatively low complication rate [11].

A percentage of 56–66% of pseudocysts which develop during acute pancreatitis may resolve spontaneously [12, 9]. Therefore a distinction should be made between this condition and cysts which develop during chronic pancreatitis, where the damage persists even though the primary cause (alcohol) is suppressed. During the course of chronic pancreatitis dilatation of the pancreatic duct is a constant finding. The primary lesion is the precipitation of a protein plug with secondary calcification in small pancreatic ducts. An obstacle is thus created leading to up-stream dilatation and subsequent formation of cysts which can reach the surface of the gland and spread outside (Fig. 3). Thus in chronic pancreatitis all transitional stages can be present varying from simple acinar dilatation to intra parenchyme cysts whether or not communicating with the main duct, to the voluminous extra pancreatic pseudocysts.

Differential diagnosis

A pancreatic abscess is a surgical emergency, the majority of pseudocysts that develop during the course of acute or chronic pancreatitis should probably not

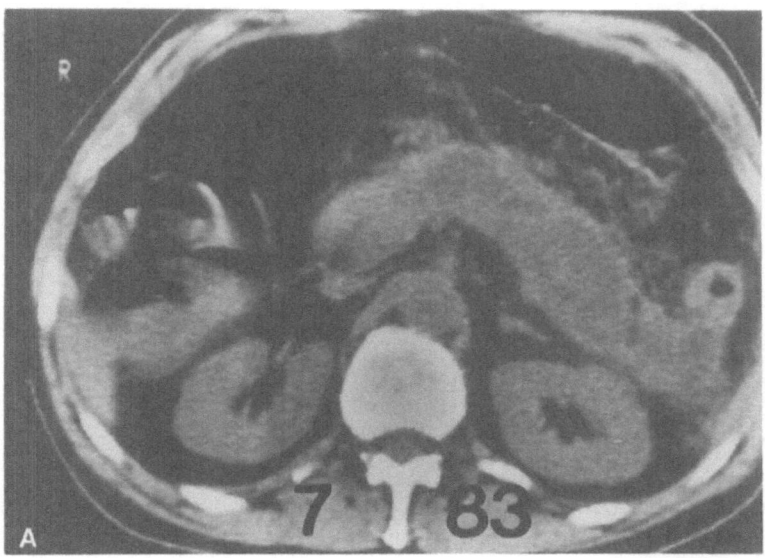

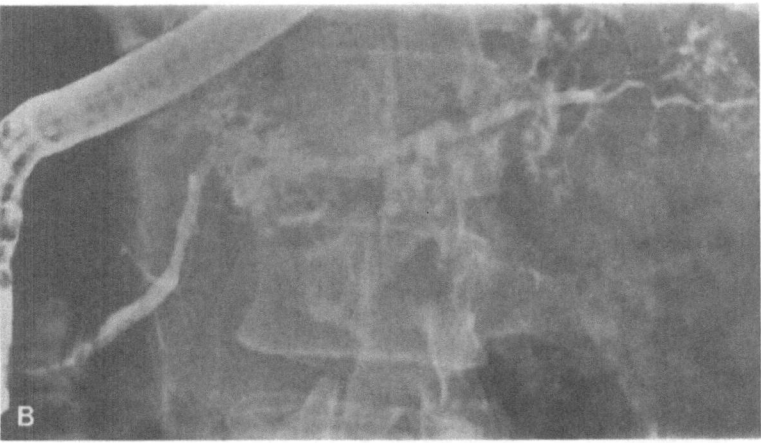

Fig. 3. Computed tomography (CT) (Fig. 3a, c, e) shows the development of an intrapancreatic pseudocyst in the tail during a 3-year-period, as a complication of chronic pancreatitis in a 60-year-old patient. The main pancreatic duct, smoothly narrowed at the corpus pancreatis on ERCP (1983) (Fig. 3b), becomes progressively obstructed by the cyst (1984, 1986) (Fig. 3d, f).

246

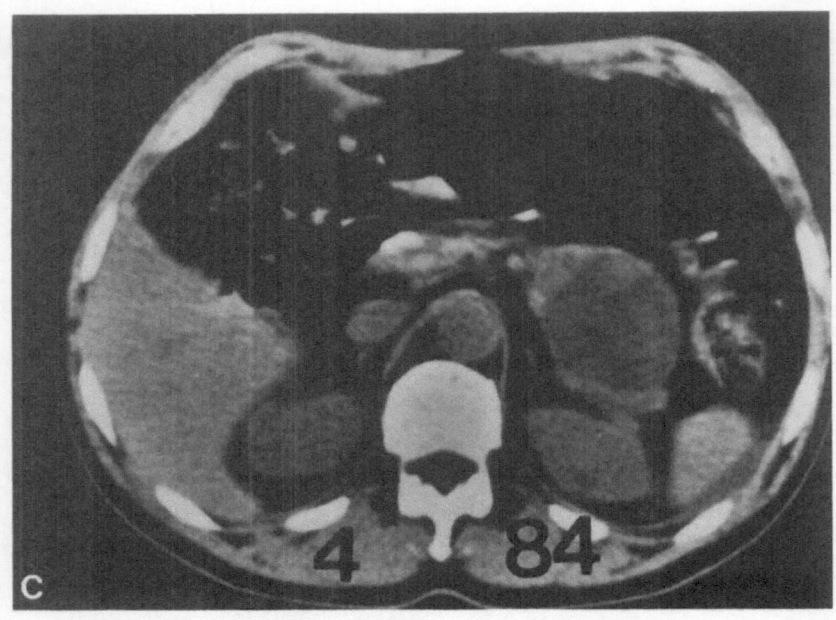

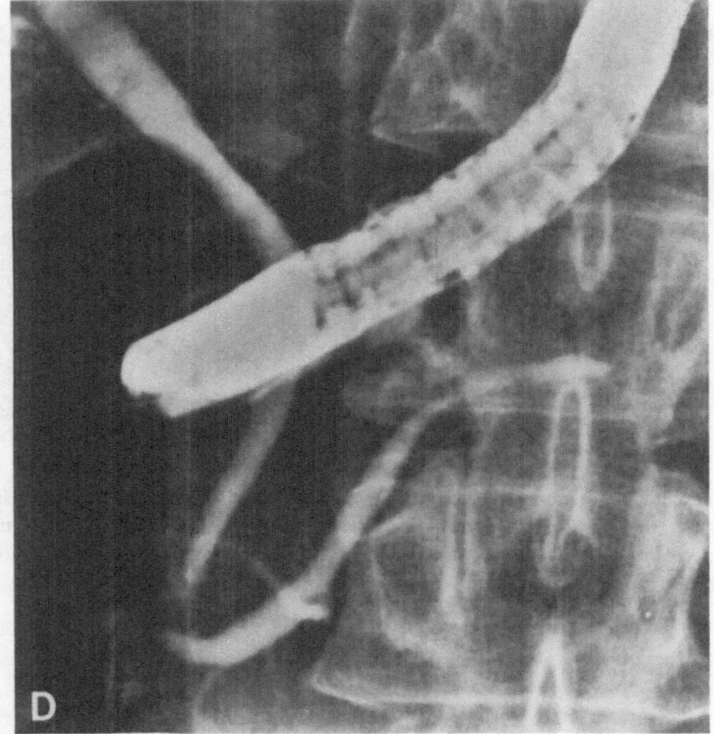

Fig. 3. C, D. for text see page 245.

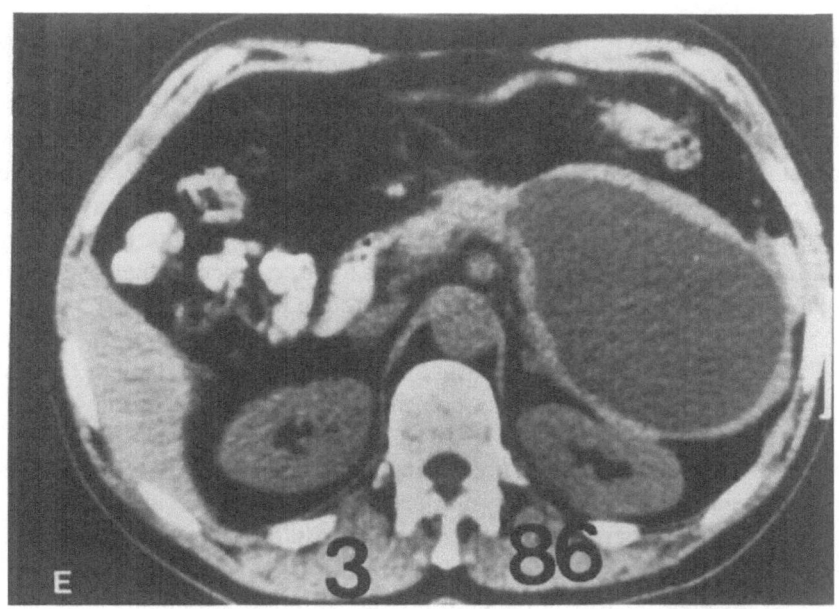

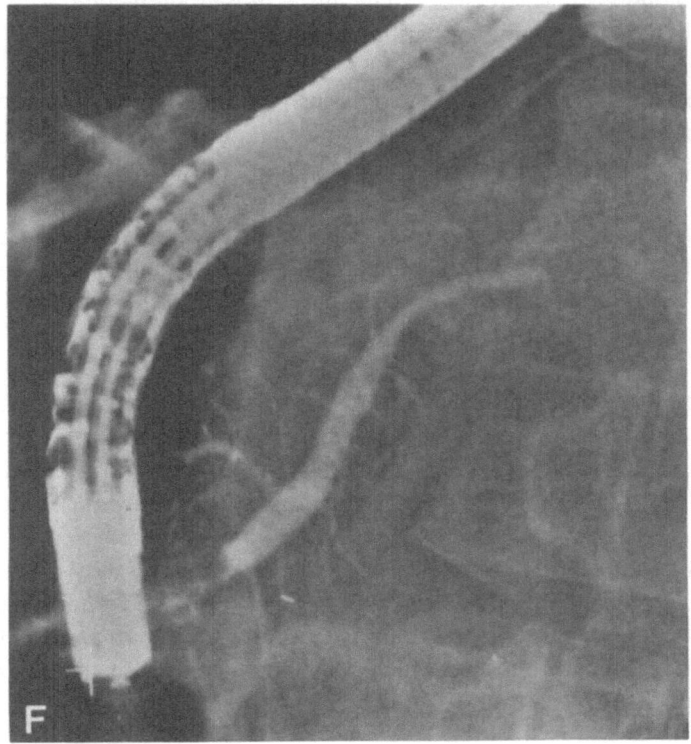

Fig. 3. E, F. for text see page 245.

be treated at all. Therefore a well-founded diagnosis is mandatory in all cases of pseudocysts both in acute and chronic conditions.

The development of an epigastric mass in a patient with pancreatitis suggests the diagnosis of a pseudocyst. In a patient with chronic pancreatitis they may appear at any stage of the disease, whilst in acute pancreatitis they become apparent one to four weeks after onset of the attack. However, it may also be possible that they arise earlier or even appear de novo without premonitory symptoms and signs. Some of the conditions to be considered when establishing the diagnosis of pancreatic pseudocyst are the following.

- Pancreatic abscess: the time course of abscess formation is similar to that of a pseudocyst but the differentiation can usually be made clinically.

- Lesser sac accumulations of fluid should be differentiated from fluid collections inside the pancreas. They may occur in the course of acute pancreatitis or as a result of perforation of a gastric ulcer in the lesser sac.

- Afferent loop obstruction should be kept in mind in patients who have undergone a BII gastrectomy. The initial presentation could be a patient with hyper-amylasemia. A barium meal will reveal the obstructed loop.

- Neoplasm. Cystic pancreatic neoplasms (cystadenoma or cystadenocarcinoma) account for about 5% of cystic pancreatic mass. It may be impossible to distinguish them from pseudocysts except at laparotomy.

- Aneurysms of the peripancreatic visceral arteries may arise de novo or secondary to an attack of acute pancreatitis. Although usually small and detected at ultrasound scanning they may be palpable. Arteriography is the most reliable diagnostic technique.

- The majority of fluid filled cysts appearing in patients with pancreatitis will be pseudocysts. However, when the features are atypical, arteriography or fine-needle biopsy may help to establish the diagnosis. If the clinical features are atypical and other tests inconclusive then laparotomy is indicated.

The development of non-invasive diagnostic procedures has given us the opportunity to gather information about the evolution and natural history of pancreatic pseudocysts. In addition cysts can be detected in patients without complaints. Thus the question which cysts should be treated and how is more important than 15 years ago.

Treatment

A pancreatic pseudocyst can either be punctured or drained. Drainage can be performed endoscopically or surgically. In exceptional cases pancreatic resection may be considered.

Puncture

Previously it has been stated that small pseudocysts which occur during an attack of acute pancreatitis tend to resolve spontaneously. A patient with acute pancreatitis can be followed-up for several weeks. If his general condition is good and if there are no signs of sepsis an occurring cyst should be treated conservatively. Not until it has become obvious that spontaneous resorption is improbable – after waiting for at least six weeks – an uncomplicated cyst should be treated. In these cases percutaneous aspiration without continuous drainage is the treatment of choice. If the cyst recurs after repeated aspiration, a stoma should be considered between the mature cyst wall and the stomach.

In chronic cases the treatment may also be conservative. The cyst can be a sign of a continuing inflammatory process and it should never be treated just because it has been found. When in doubt of the diagnosis, when the cyst is large or the patient is septic, the cyst should be aspirated. If this is not successful, operation may be taken into consideration, keeping in mind the original disease.

Drainage

When a patient develops a pseudocyst in the course of an attack of acute pancreatitis close observation for as long as six weeks is arbitrarily considered admissible. Though pancreatic abscesses may perforate into the intestine, spontaneous disappearance should not be awaited as perforation into the peritoneal cavity is usually lethal. Puncture of pancreatic abscesses is only of diagnostic value, though drainage by means of the percutaneous technique may be useful mostly as a temporary measure. Surgical drainage and wide debridement is the mainstay of the treatment of those abscesses. The friable wall of an abscess cannot be used safely for an anastomosis with the small bowel. In some cases when the abscess is adherent to the gastric wall a transgastric approach may be possible, however, in most cases external surgical drainage is indicated.

Internal drainage is the treatment preferred for unresolving pancreatic pseudocysts. Prolonged observation carries the risk of complications such as rupture, hemorrhage, infection and duodenal obstruction. Internal drainage is usually performed surgically. Recently, an endoscopic drainage procedure has been reported, so far 21 patients have been treated in this way [13]. The procedure is carried out under general anaesthesia. A gastroscope is placed with the tip in the stomach. When the cyst and the stomach have been outlined ultrasonically, a guided puncture is performed. A special tubing set consisting of a polythene double pigtail catheter with a length of 6 cm between the two pigtails is used. The pigtail catheter is mounted on a puncture needle with a stylet together with a pusher. The catheter is passed through the anterior and posterior wall of the stomach into the cyst. Within the stomach the catheter is kept in position by a gastroscopic forceps. Stylet and pusher are removed, whereby the inner pigtail curves up in the cyst and the outer in the stomach.

The procedure was successful in 19 out of the 21 cases. There was no mortality and two complications (dislocation of the catheter and leakage). In all 19 cases the cyst collapsed. At present the catheter is left in place for nine to 12 months after which it is removed endoscopically.

This method seems to be a promising alternative to surgery. Most surgeons, however, use surgical internal drainage to the adjacent stomach or to a small bowel loop. When a pseudocyst which developed in the course of an attack of acute pancreatitis has achieved chronic status, spontaneous resolution is rare [14]. At that stage the cyst-wall is ripe enough to withstand the suture of an anastomosis to either the stomach or the jejunum.

It is very difficult to make the decision for operative treatment in those pseudocysts that develop in the course of chronic pancreatitis: a cyst should not be treated merely because it has been found. When in doubt of the diagnosis, when the cyst is large or when the patient is septic the cyst can be aspirated. If this is not successful operation has to be considered. An operation tailored not only towards the cyst but also towards the chronic pancreatitis. The choice has to be made between drainage and resection. Resection is indicated if the duct of Wirsung is not sufficiently dilated. Sarles reported surgical treatment of 60 patients using the technique mentioned in Table 1.

Table 1. Operative treatment for pancreatic pseudocysts in a series of 60 patients (reported by Sarles).

	no. patients
Cystoductojejunostomy	18
Ductojejunostomy	11
Cystojejunostomy	8
Cystogastrostomy	6
Cystoduodenostomy	2
Whipple procedure	6
Left pancreatectomy	9

It should be borne in mind that occasionally de novo cystic lesions may be detected in patients without a history of acute or chronic pancreatitis. In these cases the presence of a neoplasm should be suspected and a subtotal pancreatic resection should be performed.

Conclusion

The evolution of non-invasive diagnostic procedures has offered the opportunity to learn more about the natural history of pancreatic pseudocysts. This has resulted in a more expectant attitude in the treatment of acute pseudocysts. Puncture of these cysts has been shown to result in cure without surgical intervention. If, however, these cysts have reached a chronic stage, drainage is still the treatment of choice. Even drainage, however, does not automatically mean surgery.

In patients with chronic pancreatitis primary surgery is rarely indicated when one or more cysts are detected. If the cyst bulges into the duodenum an endoscopic cystoduodenotomy is indicated, followed by surgery in case of failure or complications. Cysts can be punctured, in case of rapid recurrence surgery is indicated.

In this group of patients treatment of the cyst should be part of the treatment of the original disease.

References

1. Frey CF, Lindenauer SM, Miller TA: Pancreatic abscess. Surg Gynecol Obstet 149: 723–726, 1979
2. Warshaw AL, Gongliang J: Improved survival in 45 patients with pancreatic abscess. Ann Surg 302: 408–417, 1985
3. Kune GA: Abscesses of the pancreas. Aust NZ J Surg 38: 125–128, 1968
4. Bradley EL, Fulenwider JT: Open treatment of pancreatic abscess. Surg Gynecol Obstet 159: 509–513, 1984
5. Crass RA, Meyer AA, Brooke Jeffrey R, et al.: Pancreatic abscess: Impact of computerized tomography on early diagnosis and surgery. Am J Surg 150: 127–131, 1985
6. Malangoni MA, cotton Shallcross R, Seiler JG, Richardson JD, Polk JR: Factors contributing to fatal outcome after treatment of pancreatic abscess. Ann Surg 203: 605–613, 1986
7. Bradley EL, Gonzalez AC, Clements JL: Acute pancreatic pseudocysts: incidence and implications. Ann Surg 184: 734–737, 1976
8. Shearer MG, Dickson AP, Imrie CW, Mayer AD, McMahon MJ, Corfield AP, Cooper MJ, Williamson RCN: Pancreatic pseudocysts and abscess following acute pancreatitis: Report from a multi-centre study. Digestion 32: 217, 1985
9. Beebe DS, Bubrick MP, Onstad GR, Hitchcock CR: Management of pancreatic pseudocysts. Surg Gynecol Obstet 154: 599–604, 1984
10. Imrie CW: The importance of etiology in respect of outcome of pancreatic pseudocyst. Digestion 30: 126, 1984

252

11. Shatney CH, Lillehei RC: The timing of surgical treatment of pancreatic pseudocysts. Surg Gynecol Obstet 152: 809–812, 1981
12. Banks PA, McLellan PA, Gerzof SG: Mediastinal pancreatic pseudocyst. Dig Dis Sci 29: 664–668, 1984
13. Hancke S, Henriksen FW: Percutaneous pancreatic cystogastrostomy guided by ultrasound scanning and gastroscopy. Br J Surg 72: 916–917, 1985
14. Pollak EW, Michas CA, Wolfman EF: Pancreatic pseudocyst. Management in fifty-four patients. Am J Surg 135: 199–201, 1978

15. Surgical treatment of chronic pancreatitis

E. MORENO GONZÁLEZ

Introduction

Conservative surgery and exeresis for chronic pain-causing pancreatitis refractory to other therapeutic measures have long been considered antagonists.

At present, it is widely accepted that pancreatic tissue alterations, the diameter of the Wirsung duct and the morphologic characteristics of both should be studied by echography, computerized tomography and retrograde cholangiopancreatography to establish the indication for pancreatic drainage surgery or different degrees of exeresis.

The long term results of surgical treatment of this disease depend on careful patient selection, evaluation of the disease stage and the surgical technique chosen.

Sphincterotomy

Section of the papillary sphincters and the distal Wirsung duct was proposed by Doubilet and Mulholland (1958) [2] because the pain of chronic pancreatitis is a consequence of obstruction and of the distal portion of the Wirsung duct followed by its dilation. Papillary obstruction leads to reflux of pancreatic fluids into the biliary tract, to the point of producing cholecystitis, sometimes associated with gallbladder perforation. Surgical sphincterotomy eliminates the obstruction and prevents reflux, alleviating symptoms, especially pain. Of 190 patients operated on by Doubilet (1961) [22], 88% remained symptom-free and gained weight.

Double sphincterotomy was advanced by Jones (1962) [46], who followed a criterion of attempting to attain maximum choledochal caliber. This author affirmed the utility of suturing the duodenal mucosa to the surface of the choledochal section to prevent recurrence of stenosis (Fig. 1).

This procedure can only be indicated in the few patients who have fibrotic

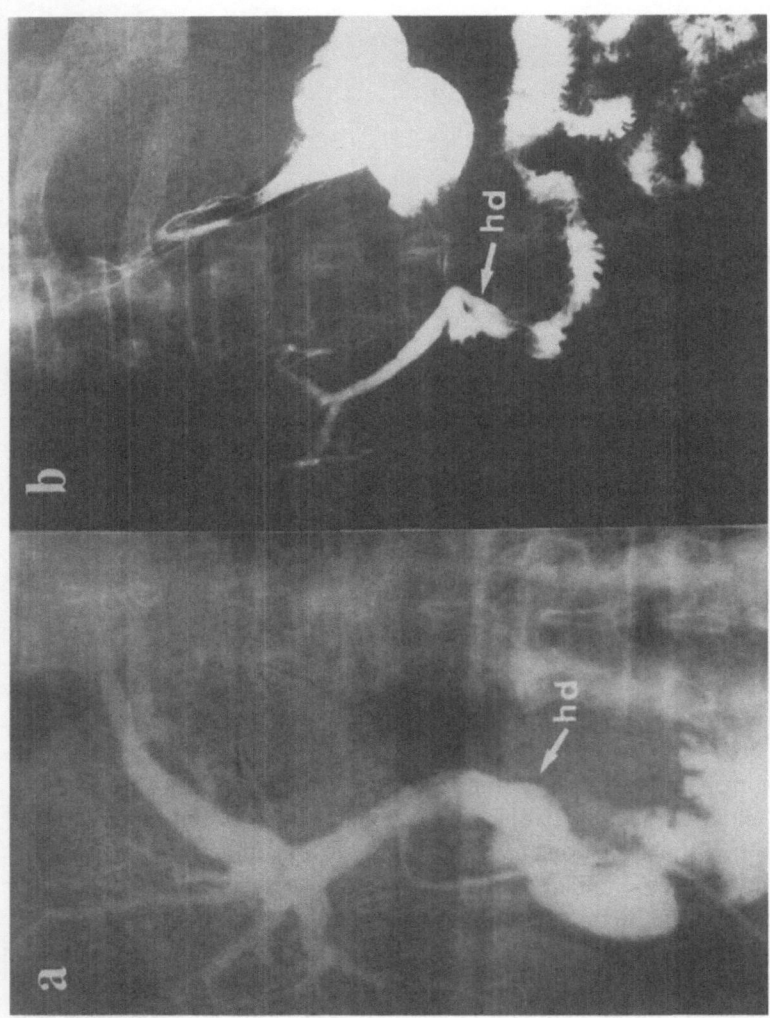

Fig. 1. Comprobation of the diameter of the ampula after Austin-Jones sphincteroplasty. a) Postoperative trastube Kehr cholangiogram. The major diameter of the choledochous continue until the duodenum. hd: common duct. b) Representation of the main duct and intrahepatic biliary branches during barium meal X-Ray examination; barium reflux until the intrahepatic biliary branches using hipotony. hd: main hepatic duct.

changes that affect the Oddi sphincter and medial wall where the Wirsung duct is implanted, with regular dilation of the intrapancreatic duct. Bagley (1981) [5] insisted that only these cases respond favorably and that patients who do not meet these two conditions show no improvement.

In chronic pancreatitis, the intrapancreatic ductal system is not always dilated. If it is, dilation is usually irregular, with successive multiple stenoses and dilations and calculi impacted into the ductal surface. In these case, improved transpapillary drainage does not ameliorate ductal obstruction (Haff 1975 [41], Partington 1966 [72]).

On the other hand, if intracanalicular calculi exist they must be extracted, especially if they obstruct the ductal system. However, through the sectioned sphincter only calculi in the most distal region of the last 20–30 mm of the Wirsung conduct can be removed. It remains to be demonstrated that sphincterotomy and extraction of calculi relieves the pain of chronic pancreatitis, some doubts existing as to its utility (Warren and Catell 1956 [103], Farrel 1963 [25]).

Double sphincterotomy, associated with sphincteroplasty or not, is indicated in pancreatitis secondary to pancreas divisum (Warshaw 1983) [107]. In these cases, pain is attributed to the disproportion between secretion volume and flow in relation to the diameter of the papillary orifice (Warshaw 1983) [107]. This would explain why pain disappears after sectioning the duodenal Santorini orifice, even in patients with a pancreas of normal aspect and morphology.

Although the incidence of pancreas divisum is four times higher in persons with chronic pancreatitis (Cooperman 1982 [17], Warshaw 1983 [107]), special caution should be exercised in attributing chronic abdominal pain to existence of pancreas divisum, especially since the glandular morphological changes typical of chronic pancreatitis are not apparent. In these patients, who exhibit a normal pancreas without ductal dilation, sphincterotomy is especially indicated (Aldrete 1980) [3] (Fig. 2).

It has been demonstrated that the early results of double sphincteroplasty in pancreas divisum do not subsist at long term (Cooperman 1982 [17], Frey 1985 [27], Gregg 1983 [35], Rossi 1985 [83], Warshaw 1983 [107]).

The results obtained with sphincterotomy, including elimination of persistent pain, have not been confirmed by the majority of authors. Still, the utility of this procedure is accepted in selected cases (Blumgart 1982) [12], for some authors more than 60% (Anderson 1985 [4], Moody 1983 [62], Nardi 1983 [67], Traverso 1979 [100]).

In these patients, the etiology of papillary stenosis is debated (Blamey 1983) [9] and patients who suffer lithiasis in any part of the biliary system must be excluded. A possible explanation would be a congenital origin (Frey 1976) [27]. In these patients treatment by double sphincterotomy is reasonable.

The fundamental characteristic to select patients for sphincterotomy is the

256

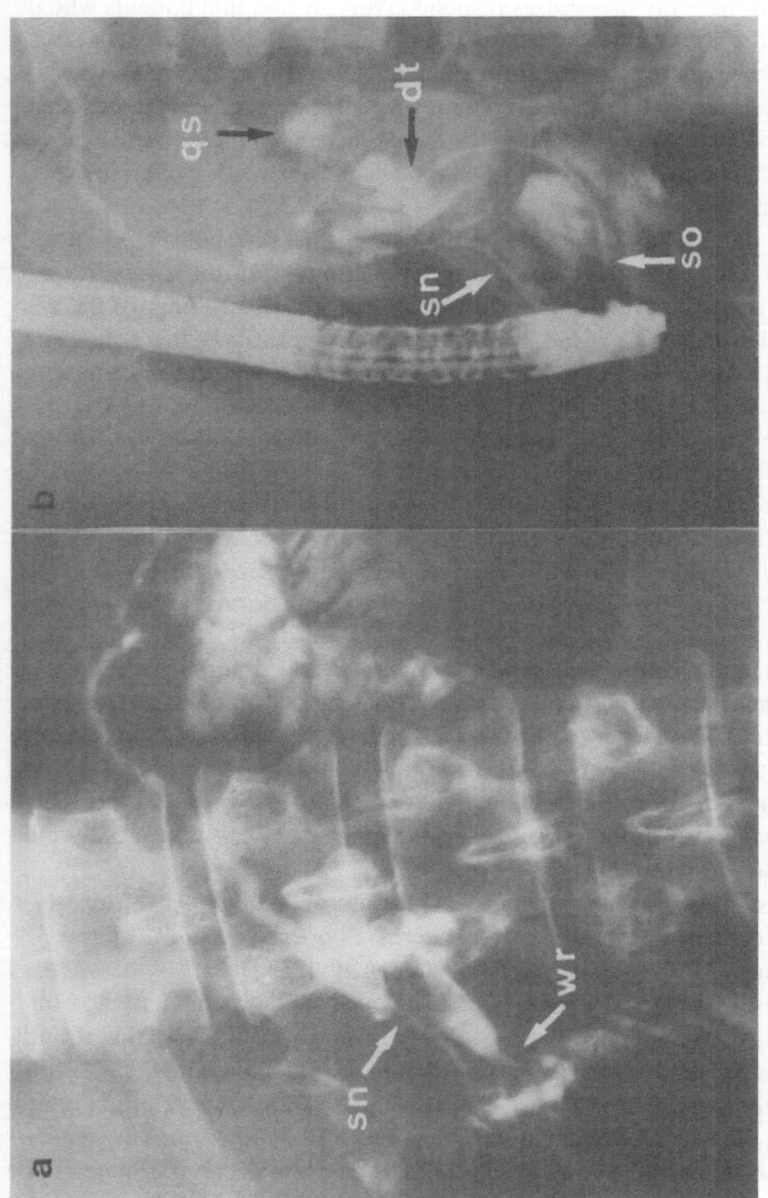

Fig. 2. Endoscopic retrograde pancreatography in pancreas divisum a) sn. Santorini duct. Dilated Wirsung's duct (wr). b) Santorini's duct. The catheter has been introduced into the Wirsung's duct (so) showing dilatation of the pancreatic duct (dt) with a intraparenchimatous cyst (qs).

existence of fibrotic changes affecting the Oddi sphincter. Should the lesions affect only this structure, producing papillary stenosis, response to sphinctero-tomy would be very high, as well as exceptional if there are no fibrotic changes in the Oddi sphincter or if segmental alterations of the pancreatic tree with lith-iasis and parenchymal fibrosis are associated (Bagley 1981) [5]. Another se-lection criterion would be to avoid the procedure in patients who have been previously operated on, due to the poor results obtained in these cases (Moody 1983) [62], or in patients with diarrhea (Nardi 1983) [67].

The need for associating cholecystectomy with papillary section has been discussed. Some authors argue that inflammation and retrograde infection can occur if cholecystectomy is not done (Warshaw 1980) [106], while others sug-gest that this is prevented by the infundibulocystic sphincters, which permit passage of bile to the hepatic and common bile duct and impede its return to the interior of the gallbladder.

At present, in the patients in whom sphincterotomy is considered indicated, this can be performed by endoscopy, avoiding laparotomy. In expert hands, section of the Wirsung duct can be associated using this approach. Nonethe-less, evolution toward recurrence of stenosis is more frequent after endoscopic than surgical sphincterotomy (Frey 1985 [27], Gregg 1984 [34]).

Pancreaticojejunal diversion

McCaugham (1983) [58] published an experimental study on the results of de-compression by distal pancreato-jejunostomy after resecting the tail of the pancreas.

Catell (1947) [24] introduced the concept of pain produced by distension of the intrapancreatic ductal system and alleviated by pancreatico-jejunal diver-sion leading to permanent decompression of the Wirsung duct. This author used it to relieve the pain of certain patients with carcinoma of head of the pan-creas. In 1954, Duval [23] published a study on distal pancreatectomy and end-to-end pancreatojejunostomy in which the utility of retrograde drainage in chronic pancreatitis was demonstrated.

Eleven years later, Puestow (1958) [79] described a decompression tech-nique in chronic pancreatitis that consisted in resection of the head of the pan-creas and spleen, followed by end-to-end telescopic anastomosis of the pan-creatic and ductal section surfaces and drainage into a Roux-en-Y loop (end-to-end pancreatico-jejunostomy).

This procedure, which has been accompanied by a high percentage of ste-noses and anastomotic obstructions, requires pancreato-splenectomy. It is only indicated in patients with a cyst or pseudocyst of the pancreas tail and in-volvement of the splenic hilum or thrombosis of the splenic vein associated with ductal dilation (Gillesby 1961) [30].

The technique has lost popularity because of the large number of failures due to anastomotic fibrosis and obstruction of the pancreatico-jejunal diversion, leading to recurrence of symptoms. These drawbacks in the Duval technique [23] have limited the indication for its realization (Way 1972) [110] to exceptional cases, for instance, in conjunction with surgical sphincterotomy to reduce the elevated number of therapeutic failures that accompany this procedure (Zollinger 1954) [113].

Pancreatico-jejunal diversion. Side-to-side pancreatico-jejunostomy

Partington and Rochele (1960) [71] described side-to-side pancreatico-jejunal diversion without spleno-pancreatic mobilization, insisting that the jejunal section surface should not be sutured to the wall of the Wirsung duct to avoid anastomosis stenosis.

This procedure is technically easy, only entailing section of the gastrocolic ligament and tranverse mesocolon, preparation of a Roux-en-Y loop, and then, side-to-side pancreatico-jejunal anastomosis and end-to-side submesocolic jejuno-jejunal anastomosis (Salembier 1976) [84].

Indications

Longitudinal or side-to-side pancreatico-jejunostomy is indicated in chronic pancreatitis of alcoholic etiology. In a high percentage of patients, refractory pain disappears. Moreover, the insulin dependence produced by resection of 80% or 95% of the pancreas is more difficult to treat in alcoholics or heavy drinkers, leading to numerous complications, while the anarchic life style of these patients makes correct control of diet and insulin needs difficult (Ribet, 1975) [81].

Another indication for side-to-side pancreatico-jejunal diversion is pancreatic ascites when the orifice of the ductal perforation, fistula or pseudocyst can be incorporated into the anastomosis, (Cooperman 1981) [17]. However, in these patients there is no ductal dilation and the pancreatico-jejunal anastomosis frequently becomes obstructed, even after ample longitudinal section of the Wirsung duct, initiating a clinical picture of chronic pancreatitis.

Fundamentally, Wirsung-jejunal diversion is indicated in patients with demonstrated dilation of the Wirsung duct. If ductal dilation is not appreciated, pancreatic resection should be realized. Endoscopic retrograde pancreatography is the best method for making this selection (Blumgart 1982 [12], Cooperman 1981 [17], Moreno 1983 [65], Nogueira 1985 [69], White [112]) (Fig. 3).

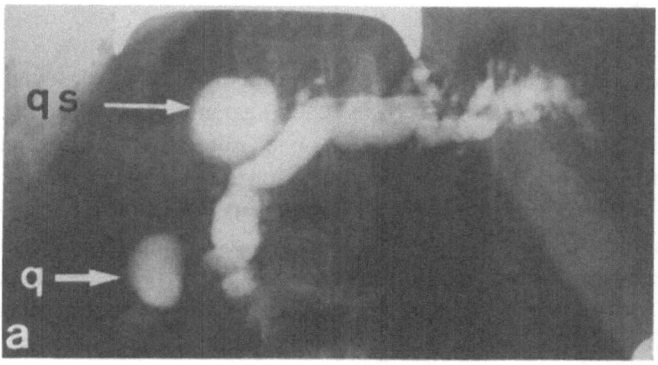

Fig. 3. A. Perioperative pancreatogram by means of transpancreatic puncture, showing diatation of the Wirsung's duct and two cysts (qs, and q).

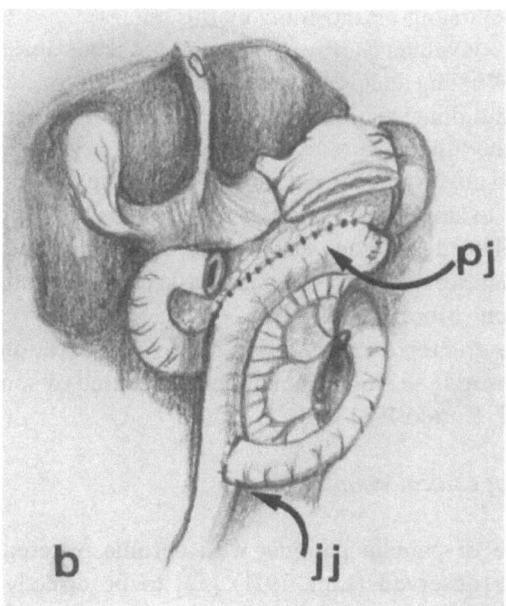

Fig. 3. B. Schema of the pancreato-jejunal side-to-side diversion. pj) pancreato-jejunal anastomosis. jj) jejuno-jejaunal anastomosis.

Stenosis of the pancreatico-jejunal anastomosis

Progressive reduction in the pancreatico-jejunal diameter causes symptoms to recur, in a significant number of cases reaching complete obstruction.

To avoid this reduction in caliber, it has been noted that the most important factor is execution of a wide longitudinal section of the Wirsung duct (Campale 1961) [14], with complete aperture throughout its length (Moreno 1982) [64]. The length of the pancreatico-jejunal anastomosis is apparently directly proportional to patency time and duration of the symptom-free period (Potts 1981) [75]. Most post-pancreato-splenectomy end-to-end Wirsung-jejunal anastomoses become obstructed, producing frequent and rapid reappearance of symptoms (Kugelberg 1976) [52], Warshaw 1980 [105]).

Control of the diameter of the pancreatico-jejunal diversion can be effected more directly by endoscopic retrograde pancreatography (Kusagai 1972 [49], Kugelberg 1976 [52]), although we have found it difficult to estimate the exact diameter of the Wirsung-jejunostomy by this means.

Although the convenience of realizing muco-mucous anastomosis between the jejunal and Wirsung duct section surfaces has been considered, the dimensions of the longitudinal section of the duct are more important (Frey 1976) [27]. Suture of the jejunal section surface to the pancreatic capsule has been recommended to increase the separation between the two jejunal section surfaces. To obtain an ample aperture in the anterior wall of the pancreas, the entire anterior wall of the Wirsung duct should be resected and the edges of the jejunal section anastomosed to the pancreatic capsule along the edge of the pancreatic section (Moreno 1983) [65].

Undoubtedly, greater ductal dilation favors conservation of anastomosis patency (Thompson 1986 [96], although this is debated by some authors (Grodinsky 1980 [38], Kondo 1981 [51]).

Disappearance of clinical symptoms

The appearance of pain in patients with chronic pancreatitis and dilated Wirsung duct is observed (Link 1911) [57] to be directly related to duct diameter, increasing normal intraductal pressure by four times (8–12 cm H_2O) (Frey 1976) [27]. Pain is eliminated in an elevated number of patients, reaching almost 90% when the disease etiology is not related to alcohol abuse (Holmberg 1985) [44]. To prolong the asymptomatic period, it is fundamental that the patient not resume alcohol intake (Cooperman 1981 [17], Grodinsky 1980 [38], Holmberg 1985 [44]). Repeated ingestion reduces the success of pain relief to 50% of the patients operated on (Cooperman 1981) [17]. In calcifying pancreatitis, pancreatico-jejunostomy only partially decreases pain (Way 1972) [110].

Reappearance of pain is frequently related to obstruction of the Wirsung-jejunal anastomosis, although it is difficult to explain how simple obstruction of the Wirsung duct can lead to development of chronic pancreatitis (Grodinsky 1980) [32]. Other factors must contribute to the presentation of symptoms of this disease. As such, pancreatic lesions can continue to evolve in spite of the existence of the Wirsung-jejunal anastomosis and its continued patency (Priestley 1965) [73]. This corroborates the idea that surgical treatment of chronic pancreatitis is always palliative, since parenchymal pancreatic lesions are progressive and irreversible (Nogueira 1985 [69], Prinz 1981 [77], Turcotte 1981 [101], Way 1965 [109], Zollinger 1954 [113]).

Drainage operations produce better results as long as due attention is given to opening not only the main duct, but the smaller branches up to 15 mm from papilla (Warren 1969) [104]. Double transduodenal sphincterotomy should be associated when possible (Moreno 1983 [65], Sato 1983 [89]) to communicate all the saccular dilations in a single cavity with ample opening of the anterior wall. Theoretically, the pain of chronic pancreatitis results from ductal dilation, peripancreatic inflammation and inclusion of nerves proximal to the pancreas in the inflammatory reaction (Block 1983) [11]. Drainage operations only act on ductal dilation, although pancreatic and peripancreatic inflammation can be decreased by extracting calculi impacted in the branches of the Wirsung duct through the longitudinal aperture of its anterior wall. Pancreatic lithotomy is necessary not only for this motive, which is debatable, but because without it sufficient pancreatic drainage cannot be achieved (Moreno 1983 [65], Sato 1983 [89]).

Results of functional endocrine and exocrine study after Wirsung-jejunal diversion in chronic pancreatitis

Because of the scant specificity of pancreatic exocrine function studies and since this function is evidently affected in almost all patients who undergo surgery for chronic pancreatitis, it is difficult to demonstrate significant improvement by objective tests (Block 1983) [11].

Pre- and postoperative studies of pancreatic secretin made in patients submitted to pancreatico-jejunal diversion evidence no manifest changes in most of the patients followed-up. Although a tendency to normalization was observed, the number of patients was insufficient to obtain significant findings.

Control of fat absorption by study of fecal excretion showed improvement in 20–32% of patients and no change in 59–61%. Steatorrhea increased in 6–11% of the patients operated on. The absence of modifications in fat absorption was greater after Wirsung-jejunal diversion.

There are apparently no statistically significant differences in the incidence of steatorrhea between patients who have pancreatectomy and those who have distal pancreatectomy (Frey 1976 [27], Prinz 1981 [77], Warshaw 1980 [106], Way 1972 [110]).

Study of exocrine function using a synthetic peptidase (Sato 1983 [89]) revealed a functional level of 50–74% of normality in 71% of patients who underwent pancreatico-jejunal diversion. These levels were less frequently attained after pancreatic resection.

The glucose tolerance test showed improvement in a number of patients (Moreno 1982) [64], but it was not statistically significant (Sato 1983) [65]. The values for most patients remained unmodified in the first years; reduced tolerance occurred more frequently after 80% pancreatectomy. In the long term, deterioration of tolerance was more frequently observed in relation with continued alcohol abuse (Prinz 1978) [76].

For years, it has been reported that endocrine function improves after sphincterotomy or Wirsung-jejunal drainage (Doubilet) [21]. Still, ductal decompression does not prevent destruction of pancreatic tissue and in the long term the patient's metabolic situation worsens. It has been communicated that pancreatico-jejunal diversion with pancreatic resection (end-to-end) or longitudinal pancreatico-jejunostomy (side-to-side) produces good results in 75% of patients, but 40% of patients later develop diabetes mellitus and 35% intestinal malabsorption (Prinz 1981 [77], Way 1972 [111]).

Association of biliary diversion and Wirsung-jejunostomy in biliary and pancreatic obstruction

At the same time that some authors report that the need for associating biliary and pancreatic diversion is infrequent (Chapuis 1975 [18], Prinz 1978 [74]), others prescribe it so often that it has become routine practice (Mercadier 1974) [60] (Fig. 4).

Papillary fibrosis, when accepted as the primitive cause of obstruction of the Wirsung duct that leads to the tissular alterations typical of chronic pancreatitis, similarly affects the choledochal portion of the papilla and produces progressive obstruction and suprastenotic choledochal dilation (Rossi 1985) [83]. When pancreatic fibrosis and peripancreatic inflammation are established, the progressive stenosis affects the totality of the intrapancreatic choledochal segment and a more extended segment of the Wirsung duct. Then, the typical clinical manifestations of chronic pancreatitis with the corresponding progressive biliary obstruction appear, such as progressive or intermittent jaundice, cholangitis and sepsis (Gregg 1981 [33], Scott, 1977 [91]).

Less frequently, biliary tract obstruction is produced by presentation of a pseudocyst in the cephalic portion of the pancreas, the growth of which progressively compresses the distal common bile duct until obstruction (Frey 1976 [27], Warshaw 1981 [106]).

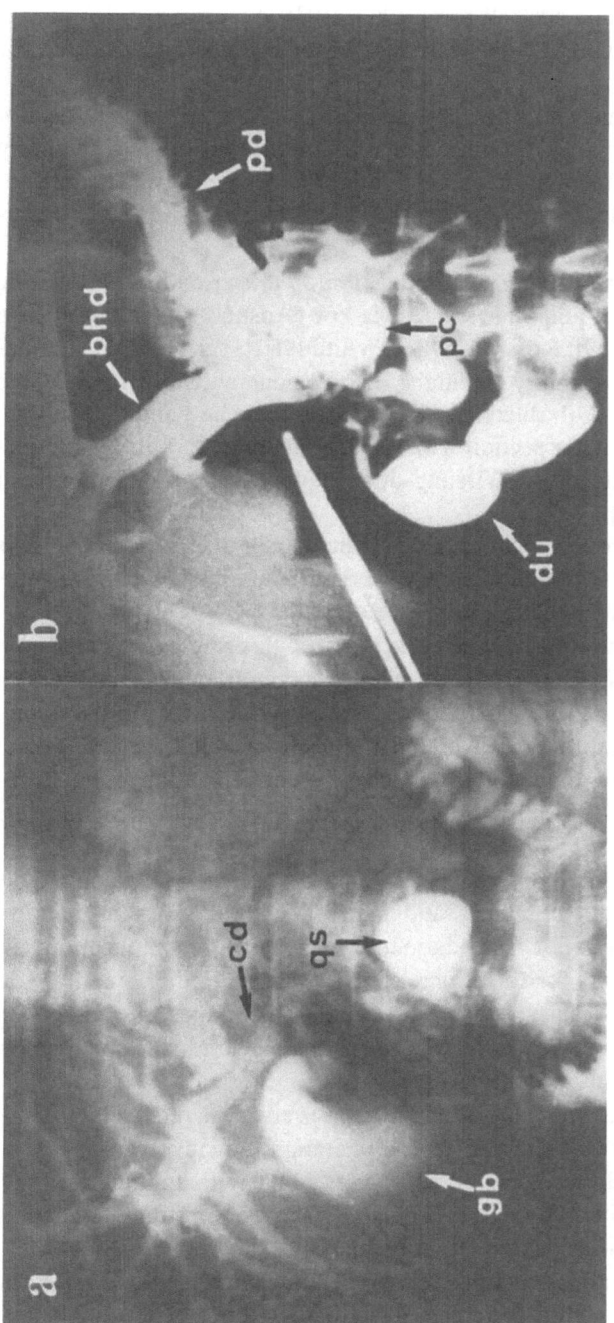

Fig. 4. Obstruction of the choledochous in chronic pancreatitis. a) Perioperative cholangiogram showing dilatation of the common duct (cd), contrast in the gallbladder (gb), an a cys in the head of the pancreas (qs). b) Perioperative cholangio-pancreatogram. Dilatation of the common duct and intrahepatic biliary branches (bhd). Dilatation of the Wirsung's duct (pd) with the presence of a cyst in the head of the pancreas (pc). Duodenum (du).

In chronic alcoholic pancreatitis, biliary tract obstruction takes place in 8% (Afroudakis 1981) [2] and 40% (Warren 1962) [102]. According to the mechanism of production involved, this obstruction can be transitory, recurrent or persistent.

Treatment of patients who suffer chronic pancreatitis with biliary, tract obstruction requires special considerations in relation with the etiology of biliary obstruction and the state of the intrapancreatic ductal system. Biliary and pancreatic diversion are necessary, and less frequently, gastric diversion (Mercadier 1974 [60], Sato 1979 [87]).

a) Papillary stenosis affecting the choledochal sphincter and distal Wirsung duct. The frequency of ampullar stenosis is low (Adson 1979 [1], Frey 1976 [27], Grodinsky 1980 [39], Rossi 1985 [83], White 1980 [112]), as is the number of patients in whom primary papillary involvement with obstruction and secondary dilation of both ducts occurs. If fibrosis of the papilla is demonstrated, papillary sphincter section with or without sphincteroplasty and section of the wall of the distal Wirsung duct may be appropriate treatment (Warshaw 1980) [106].

Although sphincteroplasty continues to control pain in 60% of patients six months after operation, this clinical improvement is maintained for five years in only 40% of patients (Bagley 1981 [5], Rossi 1985 [83]).

b) Distal obstruction of the common bile duct and Wirsung duct with dilation of both, especially the latter. This situation is not common, but when it occurs it can be treated by double pancreatic and biliary diversion (Moreno 1983) [65]. In these patients, the pancreatic diversion is effected by longitudinal Wirsung-jejunostomy and biliary diversion by choledocho-duodenostomy or hepatico-jejunostomy (Warren 1969) [104], preferably into a Roux-en-Y loop and less often, an omega loop.

Double pancreatic and jejunal diversion into a Roux-en-Y loop completely deprives the duodenum of biliary and pancreatic fluid. This logically increments the presentation of gastroduodenal ulcer. For this complication, use of two jejunal segments for the pancreatico-jejunal and bilio-jejunal diversions was conceived, a measure that permits passage of pancreatic and biliary fluids into the duodenum, reestablishing the physiology of this segment (Moreno 1982 [64], Thal 1962 [95]) (Fig. 5).

Another therapeutic possibility in these cases is biliary diversion by side-to-side choledocho-duodenostomy if the duodenum is not involved in the inflammatory process. It is associated with longitudinal Wirsung-jejunostomy, although the possibility of ascendant cholangitis is greater after choledocho-duodenostomy than after hepaticojejunostomy.

In patients with distal obstruction of both ducts and limited affectation of the the cephalic portion of the pancreas, cephalic duodeno-pancreatectomy is sometimes indicated, as a definitive technique with the relatively stable re-

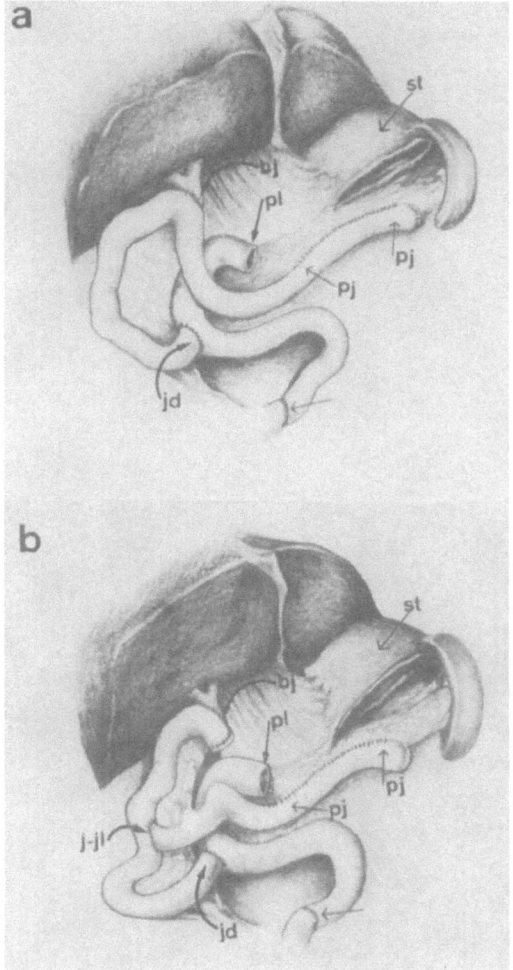

Fig. 5. Double diversion. Pancreato-jejuno-biliary-jejuno-duodenal diversion. a) Utilization of an isolated jejunal loop, st: stomach, pj: pancreato-jejunal diversion, pl: pilorous, bj: biliary-jejunal anastomosis. j-d: jejuno-duodenal anastomosis. b) Utilization of two differents jejunal loops. j-jl: jejuno-jejunal anastomosis.

sults. This procedure achieves both excision of the affected pancreas and pancreatic and gastric biliary diversion (Fig. 6).

c) Cyst located in the cephalic pancreas producing compression of the distal common bile duct. These cases are not uncommon. For their treatment, cephalic duodeno-pancreatectomy can be performed, removing the affected pancreas and reestablishing an outlet for biliary and pancreatic juices by hepatico-jejunostomy and pancreaticojejunostomy.

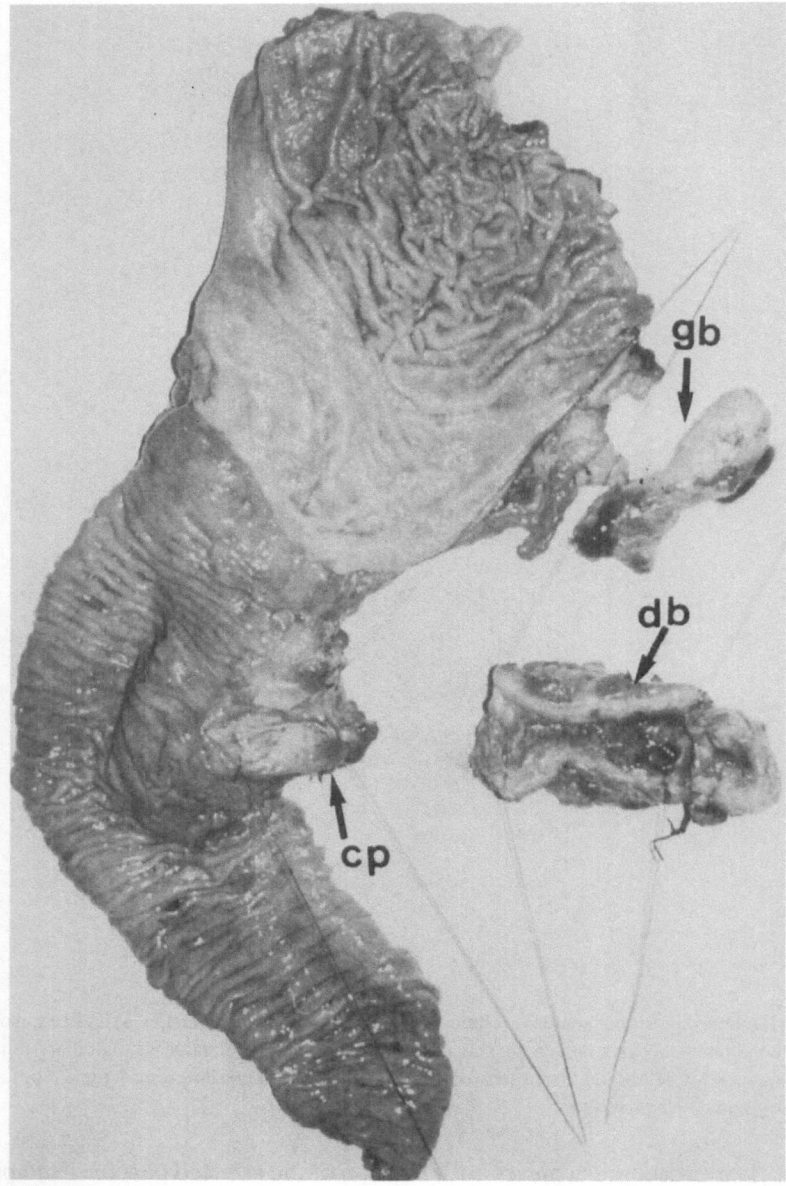

Fig. 6. Specimen of a Subtotal duodeno-pancreatectomy in chronic pancreatitis. The head of the pancreas has been transformen in an inflammatory tumour producing dilatation of the common duct and Wirsung duct. gb: gallbladder, db: dilatated pancreatic duct. cp: head of the pancreas.

The procedure that presents the least risk for the patient and has proven therapeutic efficacy is cysto-duodenostomy with section of the papillary sphincters and sphincteroplasty of the choledochal and Wirsung duct portions. This favors bile and pancreatic drainage and eliminates intracanalicular pressure and peripancreatic inflammation.

The advantage of this operation is its single transduodenal approach, which requires no intestinal loops for diversion.

Association of biliary diversion with pancreatico-jejunostomy is recommended in all cases because most instances of reoperation after diversion surgery for chronic pancreatitis are due to obstruction of the biliary tract. For this reason, whether or not jaundice or cholangitis are present, biliary diversion is recommended whenever pancreatico-jejunostomy is performed (Mercadier 1974) [60], serving to reduce the number of reoperations to 22.6%.

There are still surgeons who prefer cholecysto-jejunostomy because it is the most rapid procedure and does not require cholecystectomy, like other diversion procedures. In this type of diversion, later appearance of cholelithiasis and/or cystic duct obstruction is not uncommon (Nogueira 1985) [69].

Pancreatic resection in chronic pancreatitis

Pancreatic resection can be an elective alternative in distal pancreatic disease (Duval 1954) [23] accompanied or not by the pseudocysts often associated with splenic vein thrombosis (Burbige 1978, Johnston 1973). However, in other patients, total or subtotal resection of the pancreas is a last attempt at alleviating symptoms, especially the pain of chronic pancreatitis (Braasch 1978 [13], Gall 1981 [28], McConnell 1980 [59]) (Fig. 7).

The reason for avoiding total or subtotal pancreatectomy is the serious long term metabolic consequences of exeresis (Dammann 1981 [19], Gebhardt 1981 [29]) and the special lability of the diabetes produced in these patients (Barnes 1976 [6], Tiengo 1982 [97]).

Duval and Zollinger (1954) [23] realized distal pancreatectomy associated with pancreatico-jejunal anastomosis as a necessary preliminary stage before Wirsung-jejunal diversion in patients with macroscopic alterations of chronic pancreatitis and intrapancreatic ductal dilation.

Barret and Bowers (1957) [7] published the first successful 95% pancreatectomy. In 1976, Fry and Child [26] proposed maximum distal pancreatectomy (90–95% of the gland) in patients with chronic diffuse pancreatitis. White (1978) [111] insist on extensive pancreatectomy in patients with intensely painful symptoms refractory to treatment, but no ductal dilation of the pancreas.

Initially, in the medical literature pancreatic resection was performed in 28% of symptomatic patients and pancreatico-jejunal diversion in only 11%.

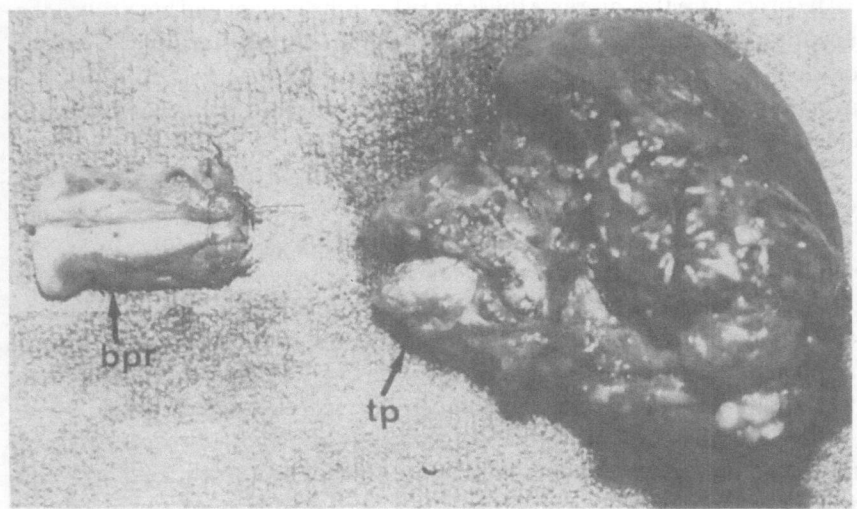

Fig. 7. Specimen of a distal pancreato-splenectomy. On a first step of the operation the spleen and tail of the pancreas were removed with a cyst on the hilium of the spleen. Retrograde pancreatography showed stenosis of the Wirsung's duct in the body of the pancreas. Resection was enlarged to the body of the pancreas (bpr). tp: tail of the pancreas.

In the last ten years, these figures have reversed (Jordan 1977) [47], there now being a preference for diversion over pancreatic resection, which is restricted to specific cases.

Long term analysis of results and demonstration of the serious metabolic consequences that extensive pancreatic resection produces, as well as the introduction in 1970 of retrograde cholangio-pancreatography, have changed the panorama of of the surgical indications for different procedures to treat chronic pancreatitis (Kasugai 1972 [49], Oi 1970 [70]). Wirsung duct morphology is the basis for determining the aggressiveness of the surgical procedure (Block 1983 [11], Grodinsky 1980 [39]).

Pancreatic drainage is indicated in patients with demonstrated dilation of the Wirsung duct. Resection is the procedure of choice for patients in whom endoscopic pancreatography reveals an undilated ductal tree (Cooperman 1981 [17], Keith, White 1980 [112]).

Pain occurs in chronic pancreatitis as a result of any of these mechanisms: a) ductal distension, b) peripancreatic inflammation, c) affectation by proximity of the nervous tracts proximal to the glandular tissue, or the sum of two or more of these factors (Block 1983) [11]. Pancreatic drainage is only indicated when dilation exists. The extension of pancreatic resection varies.

We will analyze criticism of pancreatic resection (mortality and morbidity, recurrence of clinical symptoms and metabolic sequelae) in accordance with the type and extension of pancreatectomy indicated.

Establishment of the indication for pancreatic resection is conditioned by a complex interaction of factors that must be weighed to adequately select candidates for treatment. The most important of these factors are: a) Degree of dilation of the Wirsung duct or cyst formation, b) Extension of pancreatic fibrosis, c) Presence of calculi, their situation, number and extension, e) Presence or absence of diabetes, f) Prior history of alcoholism, present situation, results of follow-up, and g) Psychological or psychiatric study. Generally speaking, the results of surgical treatment are dictated by these parameters (Moreno 1983) [65].

Distal subtotal pancreatectomy

In certain patients with demonstrated diffuse glandular involvement and no evidence of ductal dilation, the pancreas should be removed. To avoid duodenal resection, a small part of the cephalic pancreas proximal to the duodenum is conserved, together with the vessels of the pancreatico-duodenal arcade. This distal pancreatectomy of 90% (Block 1963 [10], Warren 1962 [102]) or 95% (Fry 1965) [26] produces few complications. It is especially effective in treating pain (Mercadier 1974) [60], producing good results in 20% (Taylor 1981), 60% (Frey 1978) [27] and 79% of patients (Braasch 1978) [13].

Recurrence of pain in distal pancreatectomy is probably due to conservation of the small Winslow pancreas. Total pancreatectomy provide better long term results in these patients (Rossi 1985) [83]. Pancreatectomy of 95% includes exeresis of the gland up to the vascular arcade of the duodenum, to about 5 mm of the duodenal surface, with removal of the small Winslow pancreas and retroportal portion of the pancreatic uncinate process, leaving the superior mesenteric vessels apart and preserving only the superior pancreatic vein and its confluence with the vena porta. In these patients, pain can only be attributed to continued alcohol abuse or the presence of duodenal ulcer. Nonetheless, usually no statistically significant difference is found in the effectiveness of pain relief using the different techniques (Nogueira 1985) [69].

Steatorrhea

Presence of steatorrhea means that approximately 90% of the gland has been functionally destroyed by the inflammatory process (Dimagno 1973) [20]. Steatorrhea is frequent in the preoperative period of chronic calcifying pancreatitis and in patients who have previously undergone drainage techniques in whom the disease continued its progressive course.

Steatorrhea, which frequently leads to 20% loss of preoperative body weight (Kiviluoto 1985) [50], is common in patients who undergo pancreatic resection because many surgeons consider this procedure to be indicated only in terminal disease or as a last resort after failure of different drainage techniques.

In the same way that administration of pancreatic enzymes is more effective in previously vagotomized patients, steatorrhea has been shown to be less frequent and intense in patients with a gastric pH above 4. As such, subtotal gastrectomy with or without truncal vagotomy, or proximal gastric vagotomy if gastric resection is not performed, are recommended in patients who must submit to pancreatic resection (Graham 1977 [31], Regan 1977 [82]). In four patients with complementary truncal vagotomy (Kiviluoto 1985) [50], steatorrhea was easily controlled.

Undoubtedly, the incidence of steatorrhea depends on the extension of exeresis, although its severity shows no direct relation. Steatorrhea appears in 15% of patients with 60% pancreatectomy and in 38% of subtotal pancreatectomies (Frey 1978) [27]. It increases to 55% after cephalic duodeno-pancreatectomy and affects all patients who undergo total duodeno-pancreatectomy (Braasch 1978) [13]. Still, it is accepted that the incidence of steatorrhea is higher after pancreatectomy than after diversion, but this difference statistical significance (Nogueira 1985) [69].

It is evident that duodenal resection with subtotal gastrectomy and end-to-side gastro-jejunostomy favors intestinal absorption disorders (Ralphs 1978) [80]. Steatorrhea is more frequent when extensive pancreatic resection is associated with excision of the duodenum and 20 cm of proximal jejunum. In patients who undergo duodeno-pancreatectomy, 22–76% of ingested fat is excreted in stool (Frey 1976 [27], Prinz 1981 [77], Sato 1981 [88], Way 1965 [109]).

Diabetes

The major problem of total or subtotal pancreatic resection is immediate appearance of diabetes. However, insulin needs are less in pancreatectomy patients than in type I diabetes and they are more sensitive to insulin (Barnes 1977) [7]. Diabetes produced by pancreatic resection is fairly easy to control by insulin administration (Moosa), generally requiring a dosage of 25 IU of insulin retard in 24 hours. The fact that post-pancreatectomy diabetes responds well to insulin administration is due in large measure to the reduction in glucagon production that accompanies pancreatectomy, which reduces hyperglycemic phenomena (Miyata 1974). However, it has been reported that acinar tissue can hypertrophy after subtotal pancreatectomy (Block and Paloyan 1963) [10].

Insulin needs increase with time because of enhanced appetite and increased intake and carbohydrate absorption (Griffin 1971) [36], aside from the fact that administration of pancreatic enzymes can increase insulin requirements (Warren 1969) [104].

We should remember that 30–40% of patients with chronic pancreatitis have untreatable pain and were diabetic in the preoperative period. As for the rest of the patients, only 25–30% of those who undergo surgery will need a special oral diet or administration of insulin or antidiabetics (Clot 1976 [15], Griffin 1971 [36], Grossidier 1974 [40], Hollender 1979 [43]).

In any case, the most frequent motive for repeated postoperative hospitalization in the experience of most authors is poor diabetes control, weight loss or the impossibility of weight gain (Kiviluoto 1985) [50]. Glycemia instability can be so serious that artificial pancreas treatment (Cavallo-Perin 1983) is the only means to improve the metabolic situation.

Mortality from postoperative diabetic coma reaches 20% (Kiviluoto 1985) [50] and is significantly higher in patients who continue alcohol abuse.

In an attempt to reduce the incidence of postoperative diabetes, two procedures have been described and are presently used, even though cumulative experience has not been sufficient to evaluate their complete therapeutic possibilities.

a) Subtotal (near-total) pancreatectomy and pancreatic autograft of cell islets. Although transplantation of pancreatic cell islets injected into the vena porta or superior mesenteric vein do not make diabetes disappear in the human (Lillehei 1972) [56], in the last twenty years the work of a group of researchers continues in an attempt to obtain clinically useful results from islet transplantation for treatment of human diabetes (Sutherland 1982) [93].

This procedure is used to avoid the serious metabolic consequences of 95% pancreatectomy in the treatment of chronic pancreatitis (Merrell 1985 [61], Kiviluoto 1985 [50], Najarian 1980).

The procedure is interesting and continues to be realized because of its scant patient morbidity, although more frequently on an experimental basis. Reports have been compiled of 159 diabetics treated by hepatic or splenic embolization of cell islets with sufficient pre- and postoperative data for evaluation (Sutherland 1984) [94]. None of these patients has attained insulin independence.

In contrast, embolization of cell islets was associated in 69 patients treated by subtotal pancreatic resection for chronic pancreatitis or cancer of the pancreas. In this group, 50% needed no insulin administration in the immediate and long-term postoperative period. This observation is difficult to understand since it shows that there is a highly significant difference with treated diabetics (Sutherland 1984) [94].

At present, autograft of cell islets has not been proved useful in the prophylaxis of diabetes produced by total or near-total pancreatectomy in patients with chronic pancreatitis. Nonetheless, the results cited, although they must still be confirmed, are sufficient motive for a prospective study with exhaustive analysis of the pre- and postoperative metabolic status to establish this method's utility.

One of the most important drawbacks to this procedure is the method used to prepare the cell islets and the techniques of tissular digestion and islet preservation. The methods are extremely elaborated but require processing a large amount of pancreatic tissue to obtain a sufficient cell mass (Scharp 1984) [90].

Besides, thrombosis of the vena porta and splenic vein and splenic infarct have been reported in a significant number of patients, complications that would seriously deteriorate the patient's general situation.

b) Total or near-total pancreatectomy with autotransplantation of the distal half of the pancreas. The mortality of total or near-total pancreatic ablation of the pancreas is higher in alcoholics with calcifying pancreatitis, death frequently occurring in the early years of follow-up (Leger 1973 [55], Prinz 1978 [76], White 1980 [112]). The greatest risk of mortality in patients who undergo pancreatectomy is considered to be severe post-resection pancreatic insufficiency.

To avoid the immediate metabolic and long-distance complications produced by total pancreatectomy, an autograft of the body and tail of the pancreas is moved to the left inguinocrural region (Rossi 1985) [83]. The splenic artery of the organ is anastomosed to the external iliac artery or femoral and the splenic vein to the common femoral or primitive external iliac vein. The transplanted organ is thus extraabdominal. The surface of the pancreatic section is closed by manual suture (interrupted nonabsorbible sutures).

Two factors are important for the success of the autograft: a) Sealing the excretor system of the pancreas by injecting neoprene and occlusion of the surface of the Wirsung duct by double ligature, avoiding pancreatico-jejunal diversion, b) Arterio-venous anastomosis between the splenic vein and splenic artery to avoid obstruction and later thrombosis of the splenic axis. Realization of this anastomosis with the precise diameter, not so small as to lead to thrombosis or so large as to produce high debit arteriovenous fistula, is very important for optimal evolution of the transplanted organ (Land, 1980) [54].

The situation and caliber of the vascular anastomoses are evaluated by angiography. The functional status of the transplanted organ is controlled by studying plasma insulin levels in blood from both iliac veins to compare levels. Graft biopsies demonstrate acinar atrophy, generalized glandular fibrosis, inflammatory infiltrates and acinar obstruction by the polymer (Rossi 1985) [83], evidencing the progressive nature of these histologic changes.

However, functional graft capacity was sufficient to maintain six of seven patients controlled without exogenous insulin supply (Rossi 1985) [83]. At present, this procedure has been used in thirteen patients with similar results (Rossi 1985) [83].

The clinical results of near-total pancreatectomy and autograft of the body and tail of the pancreas obtained in the Lahey Clinic surpass all other known experiences. This practice should therefore be continued to prospectively analyze the evolution of the gland as regards insulin production and the histologic changes that ensue during follow-up.

Near-total or 95% pancreatectomy is a very useful procedure for treating resistant pain in chronic pancreatitis. The starting-point for contemplating this surgery is existence of diffuse disease affecting the pancreatic body, tail and head. To select candidates for this procedure, the following diagnostic tests can be used: echography, axial tomography, retrograde endoscopic cholangio-pancreatography, angiographic study (celiac arteriography and arterial or per-cutaneous splenoportography) and evaluation of exocrine and endocrine function.

Special attention must be paid to patients' habits. In drug addicts, psychiatric patients and a number of alcoholics, pancreatic resection may be contraindicated (Ammann 1979).

For pancreatic resection, pain should be sustained and refractory to treatment by other methods. There should also be manifest endocrine and exocrine insufficiency and evidence of chronic pancreatitis. Three elective indications are accepted for this operation: a) Presence of pseudocysts associated with generalized glandular changes, b) Negative results with previous diversion operations, c) Demonstration of the presence of pseudoaneurysms, and d) Absence of intrapancreatic ductal dilation which would permit pancreatico-jejunal diversion.

Cephalic or subtotal duodenopancreatectomy in the treatment of chronic pancreatitis

Duodeno-pancreatectomy is indicated when the glandular affectation, although diffuse, is preferentially located in the head of the pancreas, moreso if there are intraglandular cysts, pseudocysts or intraparenchymal lithiasis at this level.

Duodeno-pancreatectomy in chronic pancreatitis is not easily executed due to the peripancreatic inflammatory reaction typical of the disease, which is more accentuated in patients with cysts of pancreas head and even more intense if extensive portal thrombosis has occurred, less frequently affecting the splenomesenteric axis. The presence of portal hypertension with thick fragile phlebectasias not only makes duodeno-pancreatic resection difficult, but risky (Nogueira 1985) [69]. In these patients, postoperative mortality is higher than that produced in pancreatic cancer.

Little more than 10 years ago, the indication for duodeno-pancreatectomy in chronic pancreatitis represented 10% of the techniques utilized (Leger 1974). Although operative mortality was scant in some experienced groups (6.3%, Leger 1973) [55], it reached 20% in less expert hands (Gall 1981) [28].

In 334 cases compiled by Cohen (1983) of duodeno-pancreatectomy performed for chronic pancreatitis, sixteen patients (4.7%) died in the immediate postoperative period. These are excellent results if we compare them with other statistics, particularly those of patients with cephalic cysts, cystoadenoma, pseudoaneurysm and calcifying pancreatitis (Cohen 1983) [16].

In relation with pancreatico-jejunal diversion, duodeno-pancreatectomy has 3 to 5 times higher mortality (Hollender 1969) [43]. This difference would probably decline if we considered deaths produced by reoperation of patients who undergo diversion.

Cephalic duodeno-pancreatectomy allows us to leave the distal pancreas intact, which may suffice to maintain an adequate endogenous insulin supply to avoid appearance of diabetes. It has been communicated that this can be achieved by leaving 10–15% of the gland (Traverso 1979) [100].

The section surface of the pancreatic tail can be anastomosed end-to-end or end-to-side to the proximal end of the jejunum. Indications for this anastomosis depend on the diameter of the Wirsung duct, its central situation and the consistency of pancreatic parenchyma, which should be sufficient to enable suture without breaking under pressure. In patients with a soft-consistency distal pancreas and nondilated peripheral Wirsung duct, obstruction of the acinar system using a polymer (Gall 1981) [28] or by suture-ligature (Hutson 1979) [45] is better. This avoids the risks of pancreatitis, fistula of the anastomosis and hemorrhage that can appear in the immediate and short term postoperative period (Jordan 1975) [48].

Although conservation of the distal pancreas initially prevents appearance of diabetes, in the long term the progressive evolution of fistular pancreatic lesions frequently produces endocrine insufficiency with the same metabolic connotations for the patient as total or near-total pancreatectomy.

Pain disappears with a frequency similar to that of near-total resection or side-to-side pancreatico-jejunal diversion, varying between 30% and 85%. (Frey 1976 [27], Hivet 1976 [42], Leger 1974 [55], Proctor 1979 [78], Sarles 1977 [85], Sato 1979 [87], Taylor 1981, White 1978 [111]). In spite of improved knowledge of the disease, the clinical success rate of diversion and extensive resection does not exceed 50% of the patients treated (Coopermann 1981) [17]. Cephalic duodeno-pancreatectomy is one of the procedures with the best long term results (Gall 1981 [28], Hivet 1976 [42], Nogueira 1985 [69]).

As was mentioned at the beginning of this paper, steatorrhea, malabsorption and gastro-jejunal anastomotic ulcer appear with an approximate incidence of 8–32% due to gastric resection with loss of the antropyloric mechanism and duodenum and the absence of capacity for mixing biliary and pancreatic juices with intestinal contents. The frequency and seriousness of these complications has been reported to decrease when bilateral or selective truncal vagotomy is associated with the duodeno-pancreatectomy (Grant, 1979) [32].

Exeresis of the cephalic pancreas has specific indications that make its substitution with another surgical procedure difficult. Although diabetes mellitus appears less often if the distal pancreas is conserved, fat excretion in stool reaches 22–76% of intake. To reduce the malabsorption that results from resection of the stomach, duodenum and first jejunal loop, two procedures have been described. As of yet, the acquired experience is insufficient to judge them:

a) Duodeno-pancreatectomy with preservation of the pylorus. The duodeno-cephalo-pancreatic block can be resected with preservation of the first duodenal portion, gastrohepatic ligament and greater omentum. The pyloric artery and vein and the first segment of the gastroduodenal artery have to be conserved, together with the origin of the right gastroepiploic artery and vein and its confluence with the superior mesenteric vein by way of the Henle venous collector (Fig. 8).

Duodeno-pancreatectomy without gastric resection, which maintains pyloric integrity (Traverso 1978) [98], has steadily gained acceptance. It now constitutes the technique of choice in patients in whom there is an indication for excision of the cephalic pancreas for chronic pancreatitis (Moosa 1981 [63], Newman 1983 [66]).

The most important advantage of preserving the antropyloric mechanism is that it reduces the frequency and gravity of postoperative diarrhea, more frequently maintaining body weight above the levels achieved by duodeno-pancreatectomy with distal gastrectomy (Ralphs 1978) [80]. The influence of gastric emptying time in these patients has been reported (Warshaw 1985) [108] and the difference between pyloric conservation and two thirds gastrectomy in these patients has been demonstrated. In a certain measure, one of the differences between them is the possibility of tolerating a wider diet range with pyloric conservation.

Gastric acid production is conserved, which means that when the contents of this viscus pass to the jejunum they are not always neutralized, since elimination of the bile through the hepatico-jejunal anastomosis, while permanent, is limited and pancreatico-jejunal juice is scant because of affectation of the pancreatic parenchyma. Moreover, this secretion can eventually disappear due to progression of glandular fibrosis (Traverso 1980) [99].

All this can contribute to the presentation of jejunal ulcers. Although exceptional, reports exist (Warshaw 1985) [108] and these ulcers are generally serious because they tend to hemorrhage or perforation. To avoid this complication, proximal gastric vagotomy, which does not excessively complicate the operation, can be performed.

At present, there is little experience of duodeno-pancreatectomy with antropyloric conservation because the procedure is relatively new and the number of patients in whom it is indicated is small. However, its postulates are interesting (Newman 1983) [66].

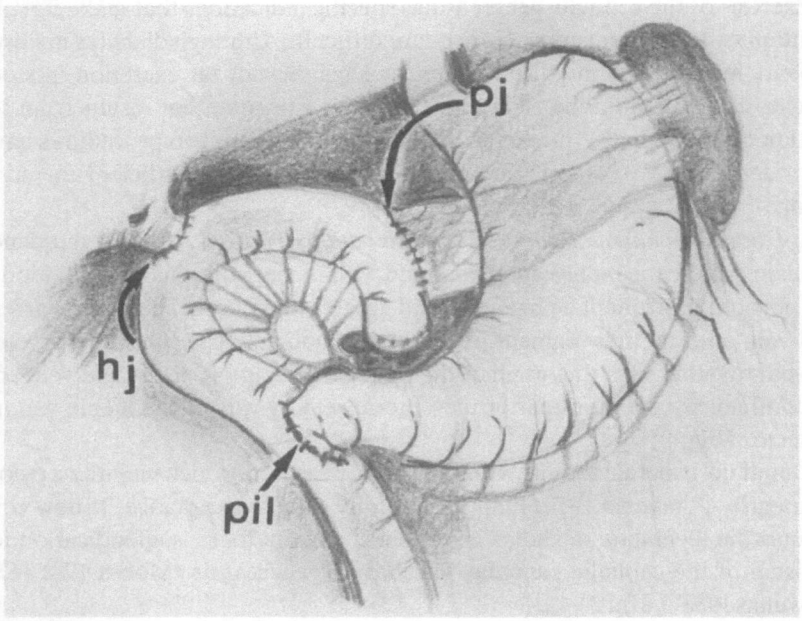

Fig. 8. Schema of the Pilorous preserving operation after cephalic duodenopancreatectomy. pj: pancreato-jejunostomy. hj): hepatico-jejunostomy. pil): pilorous.

b) Cephalic or total pancreatectomy with gastroduodenal conservation. Duodenal resection requires papillary excision and bilio-jejunal anastomosis, together with a new pyloric situation or creation of a gastric reservoir, leading to morbidity in the long term postoperative period (Lambert 1987) [53]. In an attempt to respect gastro-duodenal physiology while eliminating all the pancreas possible, Beger (1985) [8] conceived dissection of the internal duodenal surface with occlusion and section the branches of the duodeno-pancreatic arcade close to the duodenal surface while conserving a small part of glandular parenchyma. Fourteen percent of these patients later suffered episodes of pancreatitis (Beger 1985) [8].

Conservation of the duodenum leaving a minimum part of pancreatic parenchyma on its surface is a technique that has been described in children with nesidioblastosis (Gough 1984) [37]. No complications affecting the integrity of the duodenal wall were observed.

However, to avoid recurrence of pancreatitis in the small piece of pancreas left on the duodenum, total pancreatectomy with conservation of duodenal and antropyloric integrity has been proposed (Lambert 1987) [53]. This procedure has been practiced in fourteen patients without producing any death, although one patient had hematemesis in the immediate postoperative period and another had distal choledochal stenosis and required hepatico-jejunal diversion six months later. This study is of special value because all fourteen patients had been previously operated on from one to seven times. Although this increased the difficulties of operation, it established total pancreatectomy as the only possibility to eliminate recurrent pain in these patients (McConnell 1980 [59], White 1980 [112]).

References

1. Adson MA: Surgical treatment of pancreatitis. Review of a series Mayo Clinic Proc 54: 443–448, 1979
2. Afroudakis A, Kaplowitz N: Liver histopathology in chronic common bile duct stenosis due to chronic alcoholic pancreatitis. Hepatologi 1: 65–72, 1981
3. Aldrete JS, Jimenez H, Halpern MB: Evaluation and treatment of acute and chronic pancreatitis: A review of 380 cases. Ann Surg 191: 664, 1980
4. Ammann RW: Largiader F, Akovbiantz A: Pain relief by surgery in chronic pancreatitis? Scand J Gastroenterol 14: 209–215, 1979
5. Bagley FH, Braasch JW, Taylor RH, Warren KV: Sphinterotomy or sphinteroplasty in the treatment of pathologically mild chronic pancreatitis. Am J Surg 141: 418, 1981
6. Barnes AJ, Bloom SR: Pancreatetomized man: a model for diabetes without glucagon. Lancet 1: 219–221, 1976
7. Barret O, Bowers WF: Total pancreatectomy for end-stage chronic pancreatitis. V.S. Armed Forces Med J 83: 1037–1041, 1957
8. Beger HG, Krautzberg W, Bittner R, et al.: Duodenum-preserving resection of the head of the pancreas in patients with severe pancreatitis. Surgery 97: 467–473, 1985
9. Blamey SL, Osborne DH, Gilmour WH, et al.: The early identification of patients with Gallstone associated pancreatitis using clinical and biochemical factors only. Ann Surg 198: 574–578, 1983
10. Block GE, Paloyan D: Operation for pancreatitis. Surg Clin, North Am 43: 1, 1963
11. Block G: Selection of the appropiate operation for chronic pancreatitis. In: Delaney and Vasco Editors Controversies in Surgery. Saunder WB: 319–325, 1983
12. Blumgart LH, Imrie CW, NcKay AJ: Surgical management of chronic pancreatitis. J Clin Surg 1: 229, 1982
13. Braasch JW, Vito L, Nugent FW: Total pancreatectomy for end stage chronic pancreatitis. Ann Surg 3: 317–322, 1978
14. Campanale RP, Gardner B: 'Fore ans aft' split pancreaticojejunostomy for chronic pancreatitis. Surgery 50: 618, 1961
15. Clot JP, Richard JP, Mercadier M: La pancreatectomie presque totale dans le traitement des pancreatites chroniques. Ann Surg 30: 827–828, 1976
16. Cohen JR, Kuchta N, Geller N, et al.: Pancreaticoduodenectomy for benign disease. Ann Surg 197: 68–71, 1983
17. Cooperman AM: Chronic pancreatitis. Surg Clin North Am 61: 71–83, 1981
18. Chapuis Y: Les interventions de deribation dans le traitement de la pancreatite chronique. Ann Chir 30: 828–830, 1975
19. Damman HG, Besterman HS, Bloom SR, Schreiber HW: GUT-hormone profile in totally pancreatectomized patients. Gut 22: 103–107, 1981
20. Dimagno EP, Go ULM, Summerrskill WHJ: Relations between pancreatic enzymes out-

278

puts and malabsortion in severe pancreatic insuficiency. N Engl J Med 228: 813–815, 1973
21. Doubilet H, Mulholland JH: Sphincterotomy. JAMA 100: 521, 1956
22. Doubilet H, Mulholland JA: Surgical treatment of chronic pancreatitis. JAMA 175: 177, 1961
23. Duval MK: Caudal pancreaticojejunostomy for chronic pancreatitis. Ann Surg 140: 775–785, 1954
24. Catell RB: Anastomosis of the duct of Wirsung: its use in palliative operations for cancer of the head of the pancreas. Surg Clin North Am 27: 636, 1947
25. Farrell JJ, Richmon KC, Morgan MM: Transduodenal pancreatic duct dilatation and curetage in chronic relapsing pancreatitis. Am J Surg 105: 30, 1963
26. Fry WJ, Child CG: Ninety-five percent distal pancreatectomy for chronic pancreatitis. Ann Surg 162: 543, 1965
27. Frey CF, Child CG, Fry W: Pancreatectomy for chronic pancreatitis. Ann Surg 184: 403–414, 1976
28. Gall FP, Mühe E, Gebhardt C: Results of partial and total pancreaticoduodenostomy in 117 patients with chronic pancreatitis. World J Surg 5: 269–275, 1981
29. Gebhardt Ch, Gall FP, Mühe E, Lauterwald: Ist die totale pancreatektomie zur behandlung der chronichen pankreatitis noch zu verantworten. Langebech Arch Chir 350: 129–137, 1979
30. Gillesby WJ, Puestow CB: Pancreaticojejunostomy for chronic relapsing pancreatitis: An evaluation. Surgery 50: 618, 1961
31. Graham DY: Enzyme replacement therapy of exocrine pancreatic insufficiency in man: relation between *in vitro* enzyme activiries *in vivo* patency in commercial pancreatic extracts. N Engl J Med 296: 1314, 1977
32. Grant CS, Vanherden JA: Anastomotic ulceration following subtotal and total pancreatectomy. Ann Surg 190: 1–5, 1979
33. Gregg JA, Carr-Locke DL, Gallagher MM: Importance of common bile duct stricture associated with chronic pancreatitis: Diagnosis by endoscopic retrograde cholangiopancreatography. Am J Surg 141: 199–203, 1981
34. Gregg JA, Carr-Locke DL: Endoscopic pancreatic and biliary manometry in pancreatic, biliary and papillary disease an after endoscopic sphinterectomy and surgical sphinteroplasty. GOT 25: 1247–1252, 1984
35. Gregg JA, Nonaco AP, McDermott WV: Pancreas divisum. Results of surgical intervention. Am J Surg 145: 488–492, 1983
36. Griffin JM, Starkloff GB: Surgery of chronic pancreatitis. Am J Surg 122: 18–21, 1971
37. Gough MH: The surgical treatment of hyperinsulinism in infancy and chilhood. Br J Surg 71: 75–78, 1984
38. Grodinsky C, Shuman BM, Block MA: Absence of pancreatic duct dilatation in chronic pancreatitis. Arch Surg 112: 444, 1977
39. Grodinsky C: Surgical treatment of chronic pancreatitis. A review after a ten-years experience. Arch Surg 115: 545–551, 1980
40. Grosdidier J, Boissel P, Richaume B, *et al.*: Le traitement chirurgicale des pancreatites chroniques primitives. Lyon Chir 70: 7–10, 1974
41. Haff RC, Torma MJ: Oddi sphinteroplasty in the management of complicated biliary and pancreatic disease. Am J Surg 129: 509, 1975
42. Hivet M, Paullet-Audy JC, Poilleux J: Bilan de 56 duodenopancreatectomies cephaliques pour pancreatite chronique. Ann Chir 30: 371–376, 1976
43. Hollender LF, Meyer C, Marrie A, *et al.*: Etude 'comparative' des resections et des operations de derivation dans le traitement de la pancreatite chronique. J Chir 116: 401–406, 1969
44. Holmberg JT, Isaksson G, Ihse I: Long term results of pancreaticojejunostomy in chronic pancreatitis. Surg Gynecol Obstet 5–160: 339–346, 1985

45. Hutson DG, Levi JV, Livingston A, Zeppar R: Pancreatic duct ligation in therapy of chronic pancreatitis. Am Surg 45: 449–456, 1979
46. Jones SA, Steedman RA, Keller TB, Smith LL: Transduodenal sphinteroplasty (not sphinterostomy) for biliary and pancreatic disease. Am J Surg 118: 292, 1969
47. Jordan JL, Strug BS, Crowder WF: Current status of pancreaticojejunostomy in the management of chronic pancreatitis. Am J Surg 133: 46, 1977
48. Jordan PH, Grossman MI: Pancreaticoduodenectomy for chronic relapsing pancreatitis. Arch Surg 74: 871–880, 1975
49. Kasugay T, Kuno K, Kobayashi S, Hattori K: Endoscopic pancreaticocholangiography I and II. Gastroenterology 63: 217–234, 1972
50. Kiviluoto T, Schröeder T, Lempinen M: Total pancreatectomy for chronic pancreatitis. Surg Ginecol and Obstet 3–160: 223–227, 1985
51. Kondo T, Hayakawa T, Noda A, et al.: Follow-up study of chronic pancreatitis. Gastroent Jpn 16: 46–53, 1981
52. Kugelberg Ch, Wehlin L, Arnesjo B, Tylen V: Endoscopic pancreatography in evaluating results of pancreaticojejunostomy. GUT 17: 267–272, 1976
53. Lambert MA, Limeham IP, Rusell RCS: Duodenum-preserving total pancreatectomy for end stage chronic pancreatitis. Br J Surg 74: 35–39, 1987
54. Land W, Gebhardt C, Gall FP: Pancreatic duct obstruction with prolamine solution. Transplantation of the pancreas. New York Grune & Stratton: 72–75, 1980
55. Leger L, Lenriot JP, LeMaigre G: Five to 20 year follow-up after surgery for chronic pancreatitis in 148 patients. Ann Surg 180: 185, 1973
56. Lillehea RC, Ruiz JO: Pancreas. In: Najarian JS, Simons BL (eds) Transplantations. Philadelphia. Lea & Febiguer 1972, 627
57. Link G: The treatment of chronic pancreatitis by pancreatostomy. Am Surg 53: 768–782, 1911
58. MacCaugham JM: Experimental pancreatic fistula. Am J Dig Dis 6: 392, 1939
59. MacConell DB, Sasaki TM, Garnjobet W, Vetto RM: Experience with total pancreatectomy. Am J Surg 139: 646–649, 1980
60. Mercadier M, Clot JP, Colmat A: Le probleme des reintervention dans les pancreatities chroniques. Ann Chir 28: 473–476, 1974
61. Merrell RC, Marincola F, Maeda M, et al.: The metabolic response of intrasplenic islet autografts. Surg Gynecol Obstet 160: 552–556, 1985
62. Moody FG, Becker JM, Potts JR: Transduodenal sphinteroplasty and transampullary septectomy for postcholecystectomy pain. Ann Surg 197: 627–636, 1983
63. Moosa AR, Dimagno EP, Warshaw AL: Symposium on chronic pancreatitis. Contemp Surg 19: 51, 1981
64. Moreno Gonzalez E, Garcia-Blanch G, Garcia Garcia I, et al.: Biliary and pancreato duodenal diversion by means of an isolated jejunal loop. Br J Surg 69: 254–256, 1982
65. Moreno Gonzalez E, Garcia-Blanch G, Hidalgo Pascual M, et al.: Deriva cion pancreato-bilio-yeyuno-duodenal en pancreatitis cronica. In: Moreno Gonzalez E (ed) Actualizacion en Cirugia de Aparato Digestivo. Vol II: 314–321, 1983
66. Newman KD, Braasch JW, Rossi RL, et al.: Pyloric ans gastric preservation with pancreaticoduodenectomy. Am J Surg 145: 152–156, 1983
67. Nardi GL, Michelassi F, Zanini P: Transduodenal sphinteroplasty. Ann Surg 198: 453–461, 1983
68. Nogueira CED, Dani R: Tratamento cirurgico da pancreatite crônica. Rev Assoc Med Minas Gerais 22: 77–96, 1971
69. Nogueira CED, Dani R: Evaluation of the surgical treatment of chronic calcifying pancreatitis. Sur Gynecol & Obstet 8–161: 117–128, 1985

70. Oi I, Kobayashi S, Kondo T: Endoscopic pancreaticocholangiography. 4th World Congress of Gastroenterology. Copenhagen 1970.
71. Partington PF, Rochell REL: Modified Puestow procedure for retrograde drainage of the pancreatic duct. Ann Surg 152: 1037, 1960
72. Partington P: Sphinterotomy for stenosis of the sphincter of oddi. Surg Gynecol & Obstet 123: 282, 1966
73. Priestley JT, ReMine WH, Barber Jr KW, et al.: Chronic relapsing pancreatitis: Treatment by surgical drainage of pancreas. Ann Surg 161: 838, 1965
74. Prinz RA, Kaufman BH, Folk FA, et al.: Pancreaticojejunostomy for chronic pancreatitis: two to 20 years follow-up. Arch Surg 113: 520, 1978
75. Potts JR, Moody FG: Surgical therapy for chronic pancreatitis selecting the appropiate approach. Am J Surg 142: 654–659, 1981
76. Prinz RA, Kaufman BH, Folk FA, et al.: Pancreaticojejunostomy for chronic pancreatitis. Two-to-21-years follow-up. Arch Surg 113: 520–525, 1978
77. Prinz RA, Greenlee HB: Pancreatic duct drainage in 100 patients with chronic pancreatitis. Ann Surg 194: 313–320, 1981
78. Proctor HJ, Mendes OC, Thomas CG, Herbst CA: Surgery for chronic pancreatitis, Drainage versus resection. Ann Surg 189: 664–671, 1979
79. Puestow CB, Gillesby WJ: Retrograde surgical drainage of pancreas for chronic relapsing pancreatitis. Arch Surg 76: 898, 1958
80. Ralphs DNL, Thompson JPS, Haynes S, et al.: The relationship between the rate of gastric emptying and the dumping syndrome. Br J Surg 65: 637–641, 1978
81. Ribet M, Prost M, Quandalle P, Wurtz A: Traitement chirurgical des pancreatites chroniques autonomes (A propos de 147 observations). J Chir 110: 25–38, 1975
82. Regan PT, Malagelada JR, Dimagnos EP: Comparative effects of antiacids, cimetidine, and enteric coating of the therapeutic response to oral enzymes in severe pancreatic insufficiency. N Engl J Med 297: 854–858, 1977
83. Rossi LR, Meiss WF, Braasch IW: Surgical Treatment of chronic pancreatitis. Surg Clin North Am 65–1: 79–101, 1985
84. Salembier V: Traitement de la pancreatite chronique par la derivation totale (pancreaticobilio-digestive). Dix annes d'experience. Act Gastroent Belg 39: 603–610, 1976
85. Sarles JC, Delacourt P, Castelo H: Le traitement chirurgical des pancreatites chroniques calcifiantes. Arq Gastroenterol 14: 83–88, 1977
86. Sarles J, Nachiero M, Garani F, Salasc B: Surgical treatment of chronic pancreatitis. Am J Surg 144: 317, 1982
87. Sato T, Saitoh Y, Noto M, Matsuno K: Apraisal of operative treatment for chronic pancreatitis. With special reference to side pancreaticojejunostomy. A J Surg 129: 209–215, 1979
88. Sato T, Noto N, Matsuno S, Miyakawa K: Follow-up results of surgical treatment for chronic pancreatitis-Present status in Japan. Am J Surg 142: 317, 1981
89. Sato T: Pancreatitis cronica. Fisiopatologia, tratamiento quirurgico. Resultados. In: Moreno Gonzalez E (ed) Actualizacion de Cirugia de Aparato Digestivo II: 306–313, 1983
90. Scharp DW: Isolation and transplantation of islet tissue. World J Surg 8: 143–151, 1984
91. Scott J, Summerfield JA, Elias E: Chronic pancreatitis. A cause of cholestais. Gnt 18: 195–201, 1977
93. Sutherland DER, Goetz FC, Najarian JS: Pancreas and islet transplantation in man. In: 'Islet-Pancreas-Transplantation and artificial pancreas. Hormone and metabolic research'. Supplement Series Vol 12 Georg Thieme Verlag Ed: 81–87, 1982
94. Sutherland DER: Pancreas and islet transplant registry date. World J Surg 8: 270–275, 1984
95. Thal AP: A technique for the drainage of the obstructed pancreatic duct. Surgery 51: 313, 1962

96. Thompson IC: Year Book of surgery, 1986
97. Tiengo A, Bessiond M, Valverde I, *et al.*: Absence of islet alpha cell function in pan-createctomized patients. Diabetologia 22: 25–32, 1982
98. Traverso LW, Longmire Jr WP: Preservation of the pylorus during pancreaticoduodenecto-my. Surg Gynecol & Obstet 146: 959–962, 1978
99. Traverso LW, Longmire Jr WP: Preservation of the pylorus in pancreaticojejunostomy. A follow-up evaluation. Ann Surg 192: 306–310, 1980
100. Traverso LV, Tompkins RK, Urrea PT, Longmire Jr WP: Surgical treatment of chronic pan-creatitis (22 years experience). Ann Surg 190: 312, 1979
101. Turcotte JG, Eckhauser EF: Total pancreatectomy for chronic pancreatitis. In: Dent LT, Eckhauser EF, Vinik IA, Turcotte GS (eds) Pancreatic Disease. Diagnosis and Therapy. Grune & Straton 1981, pp 353–359
102. Warren KV, Veidenheimer M: Pathological consideration in choice of operation for chronic pancreatitis. N Engl J med 266: 323, 1962
103. Warren KV, Catell RB: Basic techniques in pancreatic surgery. Surg Clin North Am 36: 704, 1956
104. Warren KV: Surgical management of chronic relapsing pancreatitis. Am J Surg 117: 24–32, 1969
105. Warshaw AL, Popp JW, Shapiro RH: Long term patency, pancreatic function and pain re-lief after lateral pancreaticojejunostomy for chronic pancreatitis. Gastroenterology 79: 189, 1980
106. Warshaw AL, Rattner DW: Facts and fallacies of common bile duct obstruction by pan-creatic pseudoquiste. Ann Surg 192: 33–37, 1980
107. Warshaw AL, Richter JM, Scharpiro RH: The cause ane treatment of pancreatitis associ-ated with pancreas divisum. Ann Surg 198: 443–452, 1983
108. Warshaw AL, Torchiana DL: Delayed gastric emptying after pylorus-preserving pan-creaticoduodenectomy. Surgery 160–1: 1–2, 1985
109. Way LW, Gadacz T, Goldman L: Surgical treatment of chronic pancreatitis. Am J Surg 161: 838, 1965
110. Way LV, Dunphy JE: Biliary stricture. Am J Surg 124: 287–295, 1972
111. White TT, Hart MJ: Pancreaticojejunostomy versus resection in the treatment of chronic pancreatitis. Am J Surg 138: 129, 1978
112. White TT, Slavotinek AH: Results of surgical treatment of chronic pancreatitis. Ann Surg 189: 217–224, 1980
113. Zollinger R: Pancreatitis. N Engl J Med 251: 497–501, 1954

16. Management of pancreatic cancer

H. OBERTOP

Most patients with adenocarcinoma of the exocrine pancreas have incurable disease at the time of diagnosis. Only 30% of the patients will undergo resection for a potentially curable tumor and only one third of these tumors is found to be localized [1–4]. Thus, about 10% of patients with pancreatic cancer will have hope of cure by surgery. Although the incidence of pancreatic cancer is increasing and a relation with certain life styles such as smoking is shown [5–7] no population group at risk from the disease has been delineated sofar. Therefore, there is little hope that screening procedures will lead to earlier diagnosis and treatment. Resection for pancreatic cancer is a formidable procedure with an operative mortality of around 20% [8, 9], although figures of well below 10% have been reported more recently [10, 11]. Five year survival after resection is not much more than 5% [9, 12–14] and not better than survival after palliative procedures, according to some authors [15, 16]. Therefore many doctors have a nihilistic therapeutic attitude toward pancreatic cancer. For them extensive diagnostic and staging procedures are superfluous since palliative treatment should be initiated for all patients. Although palliation is all that can be achieved for most patients, many physicians pursue curative treatment for a small minority.

To select the patients that may benefit from resection, to give them the best treatment with minimal morbidity and mortality and to give optimal palliation to all others are the mainstays of our own approach. This approach will be illustrated with the report of the work-up and treatment of a hypothetical patient with obstructive jaundiced referred to our service.

History and physical examination

Our patient is a male heavy smoker of 60 years of age. He is progressively jaundiced, has lost 4 kilograms of weight, and complains of vague upper abdominal non-colicky pain since 3 months. He has no history of biliary or other disease. At physical examination a large distended non-tender gall-bladder is palpated. Otherwise there are no abnormalities.

Initial symptoms are present for more than 3 months in 40% of the patients with pancreatic cancer. Although jaundice is an alarming sign it can be ignored by patient and doctor, especially when concomitant benign biliary or pancreatic disease is present [3]. Jaundice is a relatively early symptom and resectability in jaundiced patients with pancreatic cancer is higher than in non-jaundiced patients [3, 17]. Jaundice is only infrequently seen as a sole symptom, but is usually accompanied by other symptoms as pain and weightloss. Pain was a symptom in only 33% of the patients with a localized tumor but in 72% of the patients with advanced or metastatic disease in our study [17].

Like jaundice, the Courvoisier phenomenon was a relative good prognostic sign in this study [17].

Diagnosis (First step)

Ultrasound reveals dilation of the intra- and extrahepatic bile ducts and gallbladder. No stones, no tumor and no liver metastases are shown.

Ultrasonography is the best non-invasive test and should be employed in the first line of non-invasive investigation for obstructive jaundice [18–20]. CT-scanning can also be employed as a complementary investigation and is probably more suitable in obese and non-jaundiced patients and more sensitive in detection of liver metastasis [21, 22]. The visibility of a pancreatic 'tumor' on ultrasound has its significance with regard to therapy and prognosis. Only 6 out of 26 (23%) localized periampullary and pancreatic head cancers were shown by US, whereas 12 out of 20 (60%) locally advanced and 11 out of 15 (75%) metastasized tumors were shown in our series [17]. It is also known that these small 'invisible' tumors (<2 cm) have a good prognosis after resection; five-year survival of more than 30% has been reported in a multicenter study in Japan [23]. Liver metastasis detected by US or CT should be confirmed by fine needle aspiration or biopsy. Since curative resection is impossible in these patients exploratory laparotomy for diagnostic purpose only can be prevented and non-surgical biliary drainage can be applied for palliation of obstructive jaundice [24–26]. The frequency of exploratory laparotomy decreased over the years from 28% to 5% of all surgery for pancreatic cancer in a recent report [12].

Operative risk

Age: 60 years.
Laboratory examination: Serum bilirubin $= 250\,\mu$mol/L.

Elderly and frail patients are no candidates for pancreatic resection since operative mortality can be as high as 40% in patients over 70 years of age [27]. Therefore no further diagnostic and staging procedures are necessary in these patients and only palliation should be provided. Postoperative mortality is high in patients with obstructive jaundice [12, 28], although this was not evident in our series [27]. It has been reported that a serum bilirubin of more than $200\,\mu$mol/L, combined with a hematocrit of less than 30% and the presence of malignancy is associated with a 60% operative mortality, whereas mortality is only 5% when these three factors are absent [29]. Biliary obstruction leads to hepatocellular dysfunction and impaired function of the hepatic Kupfer cells [30]. Clearance of gut-derived endotoxins by the reticulo-endothelial system is impaired. Since the bile salts, that can bind endotoxins are absent in the gut during biliary obstruction, absorption of endotoxins is elevated. This two factors lead to an increased endotoxaemia in obstructive jaundice. The high postoperative mortality rate and the high number of complications, such as renal failure, coagulation disorders, impaired wound healing and gastrointestinal hemorrhage are thought to be due to endotoxaemia. Impaired specific cell-mediated immunity was shown in rats with experimental biliary obstruction [31]. Although little is known about the immunological status of patients with obstructive jaundice, impairment of host immunity may be one of the reasons for the high incidence of septic complication in patients with obstructive jaundice. In an excellent review Pain, Cahill and Bailey [29] mention several ways to diminish the number of endotoxin associated complications: oral administration of bile salts (sodium desoxycholate), preoperative bowel preparation or whole bowel irrigation and oral administration of lactulose. By these therapies the amount of endotoxin absorpted by the bowel will be lower. Preoperative biliary drainage is another way to decrease mortality after surgery in patients with biliary obstruction. The beneficial effect of this procedure has been shown in retrospective clinical studies [32, 33]. However, in three prospective studies the postoperative morbidity and mortality were not decreased in patients treated with percutaneous transhepatic biliary drainage as compared with non-drained control patients [34–36]. In experiments in rats, after internal biliary drainage a beneficial effect on survival after peritonitis [37] and a decrease of endotoxaemia estimated by the limulus lysate test (portal and systemic) was found, whereas external biliary drainage had no such effect (Fig. 1). Serum bilirubin returned to normal after both internal and external drainage [38]. In most patients studied sofar in retro- and prospective

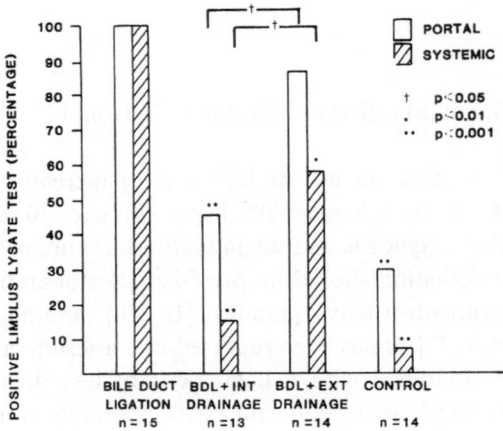

Fig. 1. Results of the limulus lysate test on portal and systemic blood after bile duct ligation (BDL) and internal and external drainage. Asterisks indicate values significantly different from those of the animals with bile duct ligation only. The dagger indicates the significant difference between the animals with internal drainage and those with external drainage.
(Reproduced with permission from the American Journal of Surgery 1986).

studies external biliary drainage was carried out and therefore endotoxin levels and endotoxin-related complications were not affected as much as could be expected after internal biliary drainage [39].

Furthermore the PTD technique had its own severe complications [35]. Although it has not been studied in a prospective randomized trial (and probably will never be studied that way), on basis of the experimental data [31, 37, 38] preoperative internal drainage can be advised in patients with severe obstructive jaundice. Transpapillary introduction of an endoprosthesis offers a way of internal drainage, that is safe in experienced hands [24, 25]. Although this procedure carries a risk of inducing cholangitis drainage should last more than two weeks according to experimental and clinical studies [40] to allow normalisation of serum bilirubin and improvement of various other parameters. When transpapillary introduction of an endoprosthesis fails, other preoperative measures as advised by Pain *et al.*, can be taken [29].

Deterioration of the nutritional status in obstructive jaundice has been reported in man and experimental animal [41, 42]. Hyperalimentation during at least 12 days after relief of biliary obstruction by means of percutaneous drainage lowered the percentage of postoperative complications significantly when compared with patients that underwent drainage without hyperalimentation in a randomized clinical trial (17.8% vs 46.8%). Preoperative biliary drainage together with hyperalimentation was advocated for malnourished and severely jaundiced patients [41].

Tumor markers

> CA 19-9 = 300 U/ml (normal <75 U/ml) [43]
> CEA =   3 ng/ml (normal <5 ng/ml)

Sensitivity and specificity of the new serum assay CA 19-9 in detecting adeno-carcinoma of the pancreas have been studied and compared with the results of those of the serum assay to carcinoembryonic antigen (CEA) [43]. The carbo-hydrate cancer-associated antigen CA 19-9 is defined by the monoclonal antibody that was developed using a human colon cancer cell line. The CA 19-9 antibody was demonstrated to bind more often to pancreatic and gastric cancers than to colon cancer.

Although the expression of the CA 19-9 antigen by cells of the duct of normal pancreas was demonstrated [44], in well to moderately differentiated ductal adenocarcinomas positive tissue staining was associated with an elevated serum Ca 19-9 concentration [45].

The sensitivity of CA 19-9 was 78.6% in resectable and 91.3% in unresectable cancer [43]. Together with CEA, CA 19-9 will be helpful in the diagnosis and follow-up of pancreatic disease. Because of the low sensitivity of CA 19-9 in small pancreatic cancers [23], the role of the assay in the detection of early pancreatic cancer will be limited.

Further diagnostic procedures

> ERCP is performed, showing a normal papilla, partial obstruction of the distal pancreatic duct and total obstruction of the common bile duct 1 cm proximal to the papilla. Diameter of the tumor is estimated 2.5 cm. Pancreatic juice obtained after i.v. injection of Secretin, does not reveal malignant cells. Tumor markers are not tested in the pancreatic juice. Papillotomy is performed and a polyethylene endoprosthesis is introduced. Antibiotics are given for 24 hours.

Visualization of the bile ducts is usually the next step in the work-up of patients with suspected pancreatic cancer. In distal biliary obstruction ERCP is the method of choice [46]. The procedure has a low failure rate and low morbidity when performed by an experienced endoscopist. The diagnostic accuracy of ERCP can be as high as 90% [47]. Pancreatic juice collected during ERCP after an i.v. injection of Secretin can be used for estimation of CEA and cytology. A correct diagnosis of malignancy can be made in 86.4% by combination of these tests [48]. This combination may prove to be the best discriminating investigation [18]. The diagnostic value of CA 19-9 in pancreatic juice is low since high levels were found both in controls and patients with benign and malignant pancreatic disease [49].

Transpapillary introduction of an endoprosthesis can be performed in patients with severe obstructive jaundice as a preoperative measure to decrease postoperative complication rate, or as a palliative procedure in elderly patients and in patients with incurable disease [25], as long as no gastrointestinal obstruction is present. In these cases laparotomy is indicated.

Tissue diagnosis

No further attempt is made in our patient to obtain cytological or histological confirmation of malignancy.

Preoperative tissue diagnosis is important for the further approach, although the problem of differentiation between benign or malignant pancreatic disease should not be overestimated. Ultrasound, CT-scan, angiography and cholangiography can be used as guidance for fine needle aspiration of the primary tumor or metastasis with a low complication rate and high success rate [50–52]. There is but little chance of tumor seeding along the needle track. Histological confirmation is essential when palliative aggressive treatment, such as radiotherapy or chemotherapy are being considered. But in small, potentially resectable tumors invasive diagnostic techniques will have a low yield and will not alter the therapeutic approach anyhow. Laparoscopy may have its role in staging and planning of therapy. Warshaw and co-workers [53] reported that positive findings during laparoscopy altered the course of therapy in 14 out of 40 patients with pancreatic cancer examined that way. Since non-surgical palliative procedures were available unnecessary laparotomies could be prevented.

Angiography as a staging procedure

Selective coeliac and superior mesenteric arteriography reveals 'normal' anatomy and no malignant changes in larger arteries and veins.

Selective arteriography of the coeliac axis and superior mesenteric artery is advocated more as a staging procedure than for diagnostic purposes [1–3]. The procedure also gives a roadmap for future surgery. Excellent arteriographies can be used for diagnosis [54]. The procedure should be performed in patients that are candidates for pancreatic resection. Encasement, tortuosity and amputation of the larger arteries are signs of irresectability. These signs were absent in arteriographies in 14 patients with a localized cancer, but were present in 17 out of 29 patients with locally advanced or metastatic disease in one series. Transhepatic portography can be used to visualize the portal vein, splenic vein, superior and inferior mesenteric vein [55, 56], although the portographic phase of the arteriography will usually suffice.

Laparotomy

Four weeks after the biliary drainage procedure, laparotomy is performed. A tumor is palpated in the head of the pancreas. Inspection of the abdominal cavity does not reveal liver or peritoneal metastasis, invasion of lymphnodes of the second grade or invasion of larger blood vessels. Two transduodenal needle biopsies are negative.

Patients that have potentially resectable pancreatic cancer after preoperative work-up should be operated by a surgeon who is experienced in pancreatic surgery and can do the resection with a mortality of not more than 10% [2]. When a safe resection is not possible a T-tube should be brought in the common bile duct and patients should be referred to a specialist centre [1]. Resectability rate of pancreatic cancer is usually not much over 20%. Even a referral center does not report a higher rate than 40% [3]. Resectability rate of operated patients is higher especially after extensive work-up and in case of small tumors. In 104 patients with a small carcinoma of the pancreas (<2 cm) only one patient underwent a palliative procedure because of her age. All other tumors were resected (99%) [23].

Histological proof should be obtained before resection. However, because of sampling error and difficulties in interpretation of the biopsies the number of false negative biopsies can be as high as 30% (15% sampling-error, 15% error of interpretation) [57]. Type and number of biopsies did not make much difference in that study. Intraoperative fine needle aspiration especially under US-guidance will most likely be helpful in obtaining tissue diagnosis [58, 59]. In case of one or two negative biopsies the decision whether to proceed with the resection should be made on clinical judgement. It is most likely that this problem occurs more frequently with small tumors, that have the best prognosis. Also intraoperative assessment of tumor stage and resectability is not simple. Peritoneal seeding and large liver metastases can usually be diagnosed, but local invasion in bloodvessels is hard to assess, and preoperative studies, such as arteriography are probably more helpful. Extensive lymphnode sampling in the peripancreatic fat is not advised [3, 10]. The presence of regional lymphnode metastases have but little effect on the outcome of surgery, especially in small tumors in one study [22]. However, others have reported

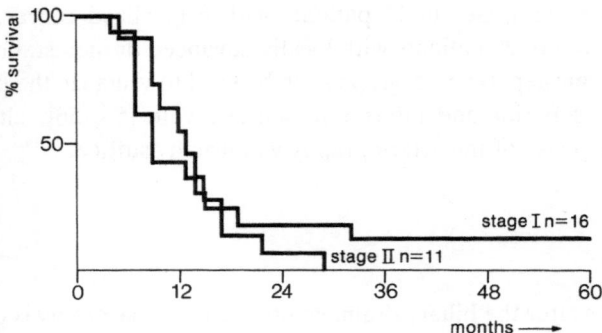

Fig. 2. Survival after resection for pancreatic adenocarcinoma with (Stage II) and without (Stage I) regional lymphnode metastasis excluding postoperative morbidity.

important prognostic significance of lymphnode metastases even for small tumors [4]. In a series of pancreatic cancer resected by us estimated 3-year survival was similar for localized tumors with or without regional lymphnode metastasis. (Fig. 2, Obertop *et al.*, unpublished observation). Therefore, when major vessels can be kept in tact and lymphnodes of the second stage are not involved resection can be carried out [3, 10].

Resection of pancreatic cancer

Pancreatoduodenectomy is performed, gallbladder and common bile duct are removed. Antrectomy and truncal vagotomy are performed. Frozen section of resection margins of common hepatic duct and pancreas are negative.

Much has been said about the superiority of total pancreatectomy over pancreatoduodenectomy (Whipple's operation) and four reasons have been put forward [60].
1. Total pancreatectomy allows better radicality by dissection of the peripancreatic lymphnodes at places that are not reached by pancreatoduodenectomy [61].
2. Pancreatic cancers are multifocal in as much as 30% [62] and tumor growth is frequently found beyond the line of the Whipple's operation [13].
3. Since no pancreatoenterostomy has to be made operative risk is lower than after Whipple's operation.
4. Since a great number of patients with pancreatic cancer has insulin-dependent diabetes, endocrine insufficiency after total pancreatectomy is not much of a problem.

However, no significant longer survival has been reported after total pancreatectomy sofar [9, 12, 14, 63]. Operative mortality is certainly not lower [9, 63] and a higher complication rate has been reported [64]. Furthermore, hypoglycaemia is a dangerous sequella of total pancreatectomy. Therefore, total pancreatectomy is only indicated when tumor growth is found at the resection margin for the Whipple's operation [14].

Regional pancreatectomy with wide lymphnode dissection and excision of adjacent and involved larger vessels, such as the pancreatic segment of the portal vein has been performed by Fortner and coworkers with considerable mortality [65]. The validity of this approach has not proven as yet. In some cases resection of the pancreatic segment of the portal vein can be indicated for practical reasons when invasion is found at an advanced stage of the operation. The pylorus preserving pancreatoduodenectomy has been advocated by Traverso and Longmire [66]. This operation leads less frequently to postoperative problems, such as the postgastrectomy syndrome. The procedure is the operation of choice for small periampullary cancers and benign disease [67]. Since the field of resection is reduced, Moossa feels that the procedure should be reserved for these indications [3]. However, it has been shown that also cancer of the head of the pancreas can be treated by this method. The 5-year survival was similar after this procedure as compared with the conventional Whipple's operation [11]. Common bile duct, gallbladder and lymphnodes should be removed together with the specimen and when less than 60% of the stomach is resected truncal vagotomy should be added to prevent marginal ulcers [3].

Reconstruction

Pancreatojejunostomy is performed by using a row of staples on the soft pancreatic remnant at the line of transection of the pancreas. A few staples are removed to open the pancreatic duct. The pancreatic remnant is invaginated into a Roux-loop. Hepaticojejunostomy is performed with the same loop and a T-tube is left to splint the biliodigestive anastomosis and to decompress the loop. Gastrojejunostomy and jejunojejunostomy are made next.

Operative mortality after pancreatoduodenectomy is mainly due to problems with the anastomosis between pancreas and the digestive tract. Various surgical techniques have been developed to prevent leakage of activated pancreatic juice leading to an abdominal catastrophe. Some authors prefer a mucosa to mucosa anastomosis [28], a technique that has most complications in the non-obstructed pancreas [67], others use invagination of the stump into a jejunal loop. Splints in the anastomosis have been advocated [28]. Drainage of

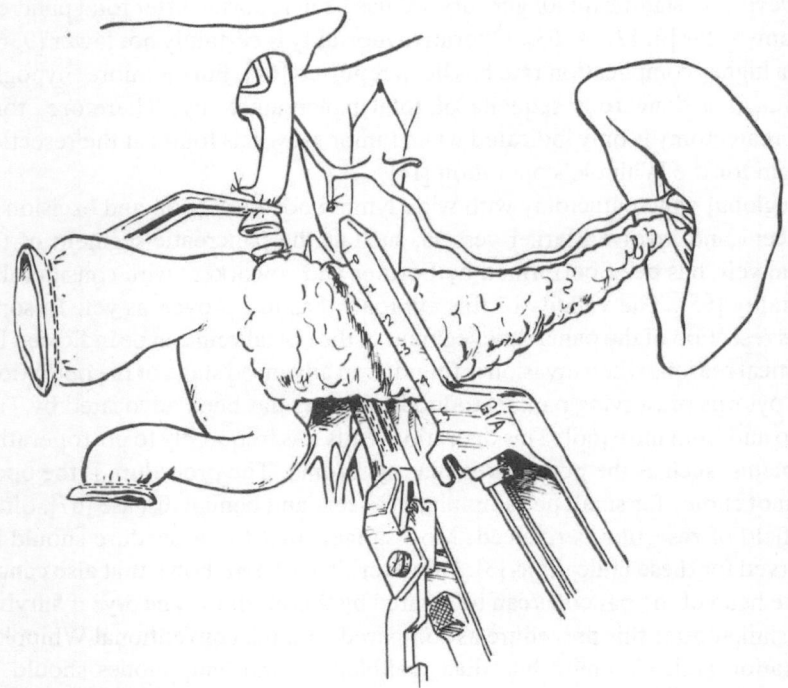

Fig. 3. The neck of the pancreas is transected over the superior mesenteric vein using an automatic Stapling and cutting instrument (GIA).
(Reproduced with permission from the Journal Surgery Gynecology and Obstetrics 1984).

the jejunal loop by a T-tube has been claimed to lead to uneventful healing [15]. Ligation of the pancreatic duct, duct obliteration with Ethibloc [12] double Roux-Y-loop to separate bile from pancreatic juice and pancreato-gastrostomy have all been reported with variable success. It is claimed that with these techniques leakage will simply result in a non-activated pancreatic fistulas that can be successfully treated by conservative means, such as TPN and Somatostatin [69].

A method using a GIA-Stapler and invagination of the stump into a jejunal loop has been described by us [70] (Figs. 3, 4, 5, and 6). The method was applied since 1980 in 38 patients, with a soft and friable pancreas. Post-

Table 1. Mortality after Whipple operation. The influence of surgical technique.

No staples	(1977–1984)	5/32 (15%)
Staples	(1980–1986)	3/38 (7%)

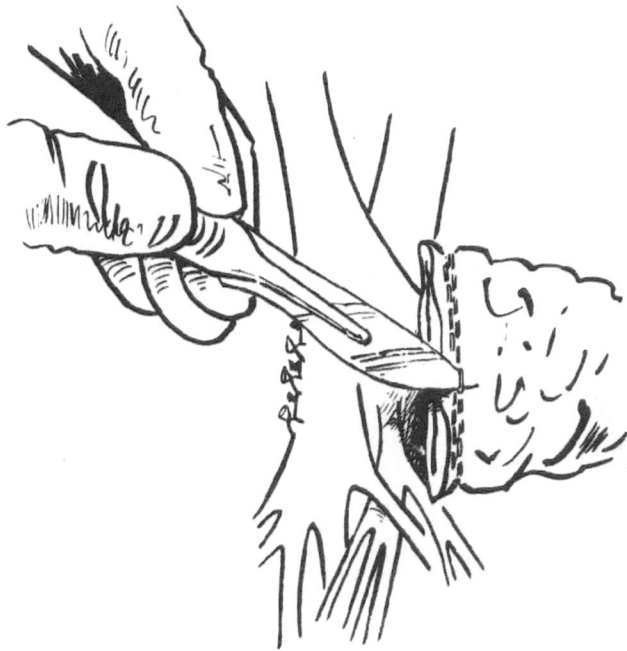

Fig. 4. Three or four staples are removed from the staple line at the site where the compressed pancreatic duct can be seen.
(Reproduced with permission from the Journal Surgery Gynecology and Obstetrics 1984).

operative mortality was studied in a group treated with this technique and a group who underwent pancreatojejunostomy by simple invagination of the pancreatic remnant. Postoperative mortality was lower when the staple-technique was used (Table 1). Postoperative mortality was found when advanced age and preoperative jaundice were present as risk factors (Table 2).

Table 2. Mortality after 'stapled' pancreatojejunostomy. The influence of preoperative jaundice and age.

	Age		Total
	<70	>70	
Normal	0/16 (0%)	0/2 (0%)	0/18 (0%)
Jaundice	0/14 (0%)	3/6 (50%)	3/20 (15%)
Total	0/30 (0%)	3/8 (37%)	3/38 (7%)

294

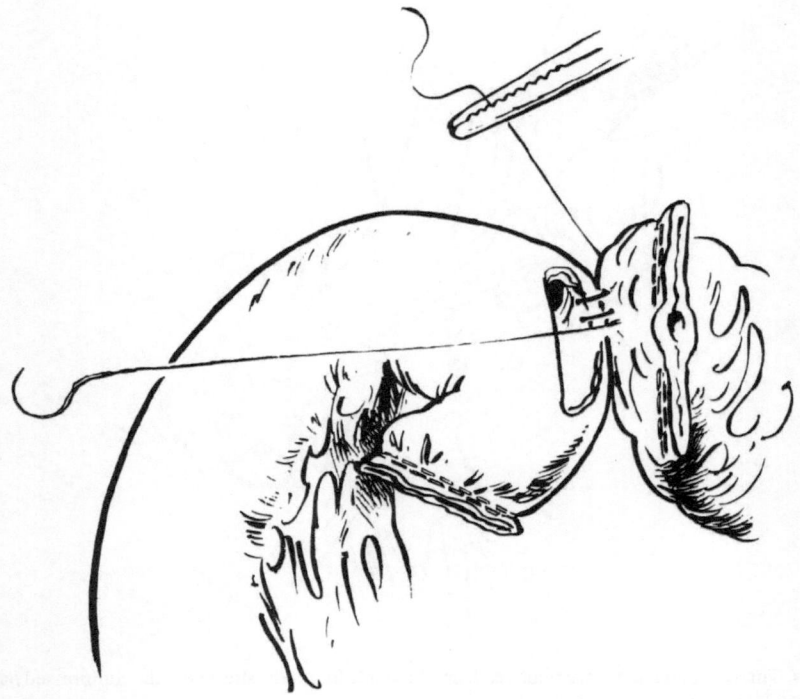

Fig. 5. The end of the jejunum is closed by an automatic stapler and brought under the mesenteric root and the pancreas is invaginated in the lateral wall of the jejunum with a one layer running No. 2-0 chromic catgut suture.
(Reproduced with permission from Journal Surgery Gynecology and Obstetrics 1984).

Palliative treatment

In patients with incurable pancreatic cancer palliation can be given for obstructive jaundice, gastrointestinal obstruction and pain. Palliative surgery has a considerable morbidity and the postoperative mortality is 18% in a collective review [71], although mortality lower than 10% has been reported [17]. Mortality was high in elderly patients. In these patients and in patients with incurable disease proven before laparotomy non-surgical means of biliary drainage, such as transpapillary [24, 25, 72, 73] or percutaneous transhepatic introduction of an endoprosthesis [26] can be performed with a high chance of success. Mortality related to these procedures is usually low especially after the endoscopic technique.

But in a prospective randomized study of palliative surgery and percutaneous transhepatic endoprosthesis (PTE) [74], postprocedural complications and mortality were similar after both treatments, whereas recurrent jaundice

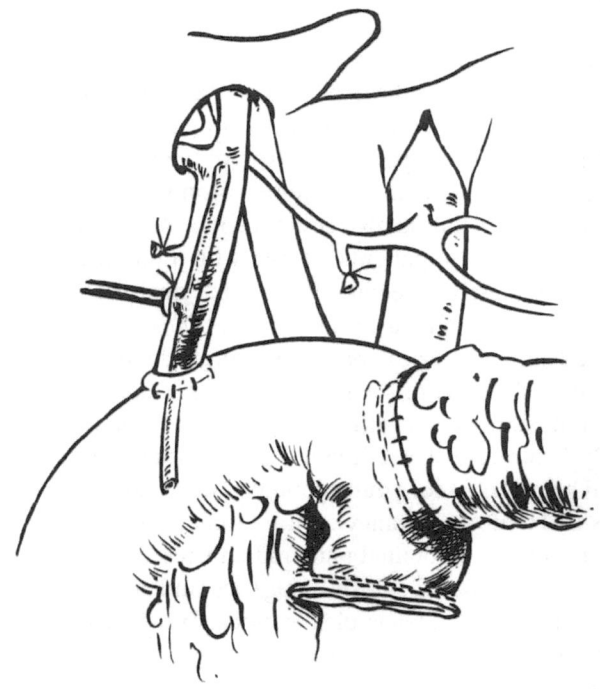

Fig. 6. A choledochojejunostomy is made end-to-side and an anastomosis is splinted with a T-tube brought out through the wall of the bile duct.
(Reproduced with permission from Journal Surgery Gynecology and Obstetrics 1984).

occurred more frequently after PTE. Although the initial postprocedural hospital stay was shorter in the PTE group, difference was no longer significant when readmission for blocked an endoprosthesis and gastric obstruction were taken into account [74]. A higher number of readmissions after non-surgical biliary drainage than after surgical bypass has also been reported by others [75]. The results of transpapillary introduction of an endoprosthesis in 200 patients with incurable pancreatic cancer are excellent in the hands of Huybregtse and co-workers [72, 73]. This procedure was feasible in one session in 147 patients (73.5%), in two sessions in 45 patients and in three sessions in 8 patients. Mortality related to the procedure was 2%. Cholangitis was the most frequent complication occurring in 8%, but was only 2.7% in the patients who were treated in one session [42]. Recurrent jaundice was seen in 75 patients (37.5%), 42 patients (21%) underwent reintervention because of blockade of the prosthesis. In 33 (other) patients no evaluation of the jaundice was carried out, because of their terminals stage. Only 7.5% of their patients had to be operated for gastric obstruction. Therefore the procedure is worthwhile considering as palliation when this can be performed by an experienced endoscopist. Patients with obstructive jaundice undergoing laparotomy should have a form of biliodigestive bypass.

Choledochojejunostomy is the bypass of choice with lower chance of recurrent jaundice [71] but a higher mortality than non-surgical procedures [72–75]. Because gastric obstruction can occur in 16% of the patients undergoing only biliary bypass [71], prophylactic gastroenterostomy is advocated [76]. However gastroenterostomy has its own complication. In a study of Wongsuwanporn and co-workers of 26 patients treated with a biliodigestive bypass and gastrojejunostomy massive bleeding from a marginal ulcer was seen in four patients and perforation of an ulcer in one [77]. Thus, addition of a vagotomy to the combined biliary enteric bypass procedure is advocated [78]. Complications of marginal ulcers were seen in patients that underwent radiotherapy after gastrojejunostomy even with vagotomy, also when the bypass was prophylactic [79]. Therefore it is a general feeling that a prophylactic enteric bypass should be reserved for young patients (<60 years) with no evidence of liver deposits and a life expectancy of more than 3 months [71].

Patients with severe abdominal pain and an irresectable pancreatic cancer are often difficult to manage with analgetics and narcotics. They can be succesfully palliated by a coeliac plexus block with 50 or 75% alcohol [80]. Coeliac plexus blockade can be performed during laparotomy, but outcome of the block appeared unrelated to previous surgery [80]. The injection can be given under radiological control [80] or ultrasound guidance [81]. Because coeliac plexus blockade can have serious neurological complications the technique should only be used in patients with severe pain and terminal pancreatic cancer.

Chemotherapy [82] and radiotherapy [83] have been given to patients with irresectable pancreatic cancer with very little, if any, benefit. Several prospective randomized studies have shown a low response rate after combination chemotherapy [84]. Survival was prolonged in only one study [85]. Patients treated with a combination chemotherapy (5F U, CTx, MTx, Vcr, MitoC) had a median survival of 44 weeks whereas non-treated patients had a median survival of 10 weeks. The combination of radiotherapy and Fluorouracil lead to longer survival of patients with advanced pancreatic cancer than radiotherapy alone [86]. There was no non-treated control group in that study. Intraoperative radiotherapy in combination with external radiation for locally advanced pancreatic cancer may have a future, especially when Misonidazole is used as a radiosensitizer [87]. Further data should be awaited of this interesting therapy. The beneficial effect of implantation of radioactive seeds into a locally advanced pancreatic cancer has not been proven as yet [88].

Postoperative staging and prognosis

Pathological examination shows a moderately differentiated adenocarcinoma of the pancreatic head without invasion in the duodenum. Lymphnodes and resection margin are free of tumor.

Different staging systems for pancreatic cancer are being used and no one is generally accepted [89, 90]. The rather simple staging system of Hermreck and coworkers [91] recognizes four stages: I = localized tumor, II = with invasion of the duodenum, III = with invasion in larger blood vessel or lymphnode metastasis, IV = with distant spread. Survival after resection for pancreatic cancer has shown a correlation with this staging system [13, 14, 91]. In one study 2-years survival after total pancreatectomy for Stage I was 34%, for Stage II 11%, and for Stage III 4% [13]. Localized tumors are relatively infrequent but have a good prognosis. Also patients with tumors less than 2 cm in diameter can do very well after resection. Using a stage classification as suggested by the Japanese Pancreatic Society, cumulative five-year survival rate was 37% in Stage I and 26,2% in Stage II (lymphnode metastasis and/or invasion) [23]. Another publication from Japan showed less favourable results also for small tumors, especially with lymphnode metastasis and pancreatic capsular invasion [4].

Postoperative adjunctive therapy

After an uneventful recovery the patient is given radiotherapy in two courses of 20 Gy each, separated by an interval of two weeks. Fluorouracil is administered for three consecutive days at the beginning of each RT course and will be continued on a weekly basis for two years. The daily dose is 50 mg/sqm body surface area, given by an intravenous bolus.

Because of the poor results of resection for pancreatic cancer adjunctive therapy has been given. Since combination therapy with Fluorouracil, Adriamycin and Mitomycin (FAM) had response rate of 37% in one Phase II study [92], this modality was as adjunctive therapy used by ourselves in a pilot-study in 9 patients who underwent 'curative' resection for pancreatic cancer. Cumulative 3-year survival was 34% and similar to the survival of 18 non-treated patients operated by the same team (Obertop *et al.* unpublished observation, Fig. 7). Radiation therapy in combination with Fluorouracil has proven its efficacy over radiotherapy alone in patients with locally advanced pancreatic cancer [86]. In the first and sofar only published prospective randomized trial on adjuvant treatment after resection for pancreatic cancer the effect of

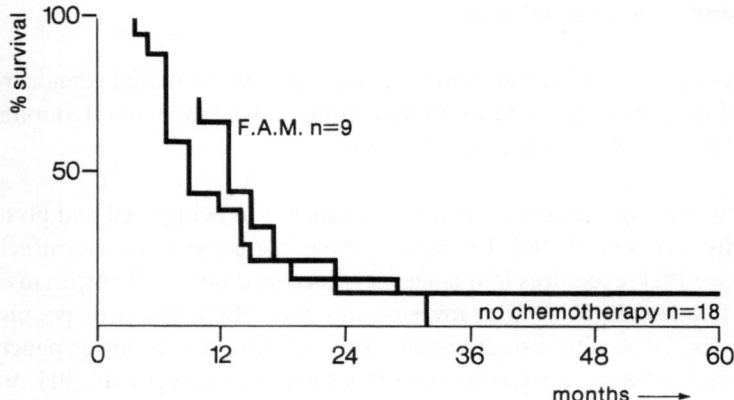

Fig. 7. Survival after resection for pancreatic cancer with and without adjunctive chemotherapy (FAM).

combination radiotherapy and 5 FU was studied [93]. Median survival was 20 months in the treated group and significantly longer than 11 months in the control group. Therefore this treatment seems promising for selected patients.

Conclusion

For only a small percentage of patients with adenocarcinoma of the pancreas (10%) there is hope for cure. More research should be initiated to find the aetiology of pancreatic cancer in order to decrease the incidence of this dismal disease or to find a population group at risk so that an early diagnosis and treatment can be possible. At the present time our efforts should be directed to select patients that may benefit from extensive treatment. Surgery should be performed by surgeons experienced in pancreatic surgery. Only then optimal treatment with low morbidity and mortality can be given. Internal biliary drainage or other measures should be applied preoperatively in patients with severe obstructive jaundice to minimize the number of complications. Pancreatoduodenectomy is still the operation of choice, especially the pylorus preserving modification. A safe anastomosis between pancreatic remnant and the small bowel is crucial for the Whipple procedure. The surgeon must be able to perform a total pancreatectomy or resection of the portal vein when this is indicated because of tumor growth. Radiotherapy in combination with chemotherapy has proven its efficacy as adjunctive therapy for selected patients. For elderly patients and patients with incurable disease, good palliation should be provided. The transpapillary introduction of an endoprosthesis by an experienced endoscopist should always be considered.

For incurable patients undergoing laparotomy choledochojejunostomy and gastrostomy are performed when indicated. A prophylactic gastroenterostomy and vagotomy should be performed in young patients with a relative long life expectancy. Coeliac plexus block is indicated for patients with otherwise untreatable pain. The value of palliative chemo- and radiotherapy is still not established.

References

1. Carter DC: Surgery for pancreatic cancer. Br Med J 1: 744–6, 1980
2. Malt RA: Treatment of pancreatic cancer. JAMA 250: 1433–7, 1983
3. Moossa AR: Pancreatic cancer: Approach to diagnosis, selection for surgery and choice of operation. Cancer 50: 2689–98, 1982
4. Matsuno S, Sato T: Surgical treatment for carcinoma of the pancreas. Am J of Surg 152: 499–504, 1986
5. Wormsley KG: Aetiology of pancreatic cancer. Ital J Gastroenterology 17: 102–8, 1985
6. Gordis L, Gold EB: Epidemiology of pancreatic cancer. World J Surg 8: 808–21, 1984
7. Mack TM, Yu MC, Hanisch P, et al.: Pancreas cancer and smoking, beverage consumption and past medical history. JNCI 76: 49–60, 1986
8. Levin B, ReMine WH, Herrmann RE, et al.: Panel: Cancer of the pancreas. Am J Surg 135: 185–91, 1978
9. Longmire WP: Cancer of the pancreas: Palliative operation, Whipple procedure or total pancreatectomy. World J Surg 8: 872–9, 1984
10. Trede M: The surgical treatment of pancreatic carcinoma. Surgery 97: 28–35, 1985
11. Grace PA, Pitt HA, Longmire WP: Pancreatoduodenectomy with pylorus preservation for adenocarcinoma of the head of the pancreas. Br J Surg 73: 647–50, 1986
12. Kümmerle F, Rückert K: Surgical treatment of pancreatic cancer. World J Surg 8: 889–94, 1984
13. Andrén-Sandberg A, Ihse I: Factors influencing survival after total pancreatectomy in patients with pancreatic cancer. Ann Surg 198: 605–10, 1983
14. Edis AJ, Kiernan PD, Taylor WF: Attempted curative resection of ductal carcinoma of the pancreas. Mayo Clin Proc 55: 531–36, 1980
15. Crile Jr G: The advantages of bypass operations over radical pancreatico-duodenectomy in the treatment of pancreatic carcinoma. Surg Gynecol Obstet 130: 1049–53, 1970
16. Shapiro TM: Adenocarcioma of the pancreas: A statistical analysis of biliary bypass vs Whipple resection in good risk patients. Ann Surg 182: 715–21, 1975
17. Obertop H, Bruining HA, Eeftinck Schattenkerk M, et al.: Operative approach to cancer of the head of the pancreas and the periampullary region. Br J Surg 69: 573–6, 1982
18. Mackie CR, Cooper MJ, Lewis MB, et al.: Non-operative differentiation between pancreatic cancer and chronic pancreatitis. Ann Surg 189: 480–7, 1979
19. Pollock D, Taylor KJW: Ultrasound scanning in patients with clinical suspicion of pancreatic cancer: A retrospective study. Cancer 47: 1662–5, 1981
20. Silverstein MD, Richter JM, Podolsky DK, et al.: Suspected pancreatic cancer presenting as pain or weight loss: Analysis of diagnostic strategies. World J Surg 8: 839–45, 1984
21. Redman HC: Standard radiologic diagnosis and CT-scanning in pancreatic cancer. Cancer 47: 1656–61, 1981
22. Wittenberg J, Ferrucci JT, Warshaw AL: Contribution of computed tomography to patients

with pancreatic adenocarcinoma. World J Surg 8: 831–8, 1984

23. Tsuchiya R, Noda T, Harada, *et al.*: Collective review of small carcinomas of the pancreas. Ann Surg 203: 77–81, 1986

24. Huibregtse K, Tytgat GN: Palliative treatment of obstructive jaundice by transpapillary introduction of a large bore bile duct endoprosthesis. Gut 23: 371–75, 1982

25. Cotton PB: Endoscopic methods for relief of malignant obstructive jaundice. World J Surg 8: 854–61, 1984

26. Gouma DJ, Wesdorp RIC, Oostenbroek RJ, *et al.*: Percutaneous transhepatic drainage and insertion of an endoprosthesis for obstructive jaundice. Am J Surg 145: 763–8, 1983

27. Snellen JP, Obertop H, Bruining HA, *et al.*: The influence of preoperative jaundice biliary drainage and age on postoperative morbidity and mortality after pancreatoduodenectomy and total pancreatectomy. Neth J Surg 37: 83–6, 1985

28. Pitt HA, Cameron JL, Postier RG, *et al.*: Factors affecting mortality in biliary tract surgery. Am J Surg 141: 66–72, 1981

29. Pain JA, Cahill CJ, Bailey ME: Perioperative complications in obstructive jaundice: therapeutic considerations. Br J Surg 72: 942–45, 1985

30. Benjamin IS: The obstructed biliary tract. In: Blumgart LH (ed) The Biliary Tract. Edinburg: Churchill Livingstone 1982, pp 157–82

31. Roughneen PT, Gouma DJ, Kulkarni AD, *et al.*: Impaired specific cell-mediated immunity in experimental biliary obstruction and its reversibility by internal biliary drainage. J of Surg Res 41: 113–25, 1986

32. Ellison EC, Van Aman ME, Carey LC: Preoperative transhepatic biliary decompression in pancreatic and periampullary cancer. World J Surg 8: 862–71, 1984

33. Gundry SR, Strodel WE, Knol JA, *et al.*: Efficacy of preoperative biliary tract decompression in patients with obstructive jaundice. Arch Surg 119: 703–8, 1984

34. Hatfield ARW, Terblanche J, Fataar S, *et al.*: Preoperative external biliary drainage in obstructive jaundice. Lancet 2: 896–9, 1982

35. McPherson GAD, Benjamin IS, Hodgson HFJ, *et al.*: Preoperative percutaneous transhepatic drainage: the results of a controlled trial. Br J Surg 71: 371–5, 1984

36. Pitt HA, Gomes AS, Lois JF, *et al.*: Does preoperative percutaneous biliary drainage reduce operative risk or increase hospital costs? Ann Surg 201: 545–53, 1985

37. Gouma DJ, Coelho JCU, Schlegel JF, *et al.*: The effect of preoperative internal and external biliary drainage on mortality of jaundiced rats. Arch Surg 122: 731–4, 1987

38. Gouma DJ, Coelho JCU, Fisher JD, *et al.*: Endotoxaemia after relief of biliary obstruction by internal and external drainage in rats. Am J Surg 151: 476–9, 1986

39. Gouma DJ, Moody FG: Preoperative percutaneous transhepatic drainage: Use or abuse. Surg Gastroenterol 3: 74–80, 1984

40. Koyama K, Takagi Y, Ito K, *et al.*: Experimental and clinical studies on the effect of biliary drainage in obstructive jaundice. Am J Surg 142: 293–9, 1981

41. Foschi D, Cavagna G, Callioni F, *et al.*: Hyperalimentation of jaundiced patients on percutaneous transhepatic biliary drainage. Br J Surg 73: 716–9, 1986

42. Gouma DJ, Roughneen PT, Kumar S, *et al.*: Changes in nutritional status associated with obstructive jaundice and biliary drainage in rats. Am J Clin Nutr 44: 362–9, 1986

43. Steinberg WM, Gelfand R, Anderson KK, *et al.*: Comparison of the sensitivity and specificity of the CA 19-9 and carcinoembryonic antigen assays in detecting cancer of the pancreas. Gastroenterology 90: 343–9, 1986

44. Arends JW, Verstynen C, Bosman FT, *et al.*: Distribution of monoclonal antibody-defined monosialogangliosise in normal and cancerous human tissues: an immunoperoxidase study. Hybridoma 2: 219–229, 1983

45. Haglund C, Lindgren J, Roberts PJ, *et al.*: Gastrointestinal cancer-associated antigen CA

19-9 in histological specimens of pancreatic tumours and pancreatitis. Br J Cancer 53: 189–95, 1986

46. Freeny PC, Ball TJ: Endoscopic retrograde cholangiopancreatography (ERCP) and percutaneous transhepatic cholangiography (PTC) in the evaluation of suspected pancreatic carcinoma: Diagnostic limitations and contemporary roles. Cancer 47: 1666–78, 1981

47. Nix GAJJ, Schmitz PIM, Wilson JHP, et al.: Carcinoma of the head of the pancreas. Gastroenterology 87: 37–43, 1984

48. Tatsuta M, Yamamura H, Yamamoto R, et al.: Significance of carcinoembryonic antigen levels and cytology of pure pancreatic juice in diagnosis of pancreatic cancer. Cancer 52: 1880–5, 1983

49. Schmiegel WH, Kreiker C, Eberl W: Monoclonal antibody defines CA 19-9 in pancreatic juices and sera. Gut 26: 456–460, 1985

50. Beazly RM: Needle biopsy diagnosis of pancreatic cancer. Cancer 47: 1685–1687, 1981

51. Evander A, Ihse I, Lunderquist A, et al.: Percutaneous cytodiagnosis of carcinoma of the pancreas and bile duct. Ann Surg 88: 90–92, 1978

52. Hancke S, Holm HH, Koch F: Ultrasonically guided percutaneous fine needle biopsy of the pancreas. Surg Gynecol Obstet 140: 361–4, 1975

53. Warshaw AL, Tepper JE, Shipley WU: Laparoscopy in the staging and planning of therapy for pancreatic cancer. Am J Surg 151: 76–80, 1984

54. Suszuki T, Imamura M, Matsuoka K, et al.: Surgical importance of oblique projection in arteriography for carcinoma of the pancreas. Surg Gynecol Obstet 148: 847–54, 1979

55. Russell E, LePage R, Viamonte M, et al.: An angiographic approach to hepatobiliary disease. Surg Gynecol Obstet 143: 414–24, 1976

56. Rosch J, Keller FS: Pancreatic arteriography, transhepatic pancreatic venography and pancreatic venous sampling in diagnosis of pancreatic cancer. Cancer 47: 1679–84, 1981

57. Campanale RP, Frey CF, Farias R, et al.: Reliability and sensitivity of frozen-section pancreatic biopsy. Arch Surg 120: 283–8, 1985

58. Keighley MRB, Moore J, Thompson H: The place of fine needle aspiration cytology for the intraoperative diagnosis of pancreatic malignancy. Ann R Coll Surg Engl 66: 405–8, 1984

59. Sigel B, Coelho JCU, Nyhus LM, et al.: Detection of pancreatic tumors by ultrasound during surgery. Arch Surg 117: 1058–61, 1982

60. Moossa AR, Scott MH, Lavelle-Jones M: The place of total and extended total pancreatectomy in pancreatic cancer. World J Surg 8: 895–9, 1984

61. Cubilla AL, Fitzgerald PJ: Pancreas cancer: Duct cell adenocarcinoma. In: Pathology Annual, part 1 New York: Appleton-Century Crofts I: 241–55, 1978

62. Brooks JR: The case for total pancreatectomy. In: Delaney JP, Varco RL (eds) Controversies in Surgery II. Philadelphia WB Saunders Co 1983, pp 327–35

63. Van Heerden JA: Pancreatic resection for carcinoma of the pancreas: Whipple versus total pancreatectomy. An institutional perspective. World J Surg 8: 880–8, 1984

64. Grace PA, Pitt HA, Tompkins RK, et al.: Decreased morbidity and mortality after pancreatoduodenectomy. Am J Surgery 151: 141–8, 1986

65. Fortner JG: Regional pancreatectomy for cancer of the pancreas, ampulla and other related sites. Tumor staging and results. Ann Surg 199: 418–25, 1984

66. Traverso WL, Longmire WP: Preservation of the pylorus in pancreaticoduodenectomy. Ann Surg 192: 306–9, 1980

67. Braasch JW, Deziel DJ, Rossi RL, et al.: Pyloric and gastric preserving pancreatic resection. Ann Surg 204: 411–8, 1986

68. Lerut JP, Gianello PR, Otte JB, et al.: Pancreaticoduodenal resection. Surgical experience and evaluation of risk factors in 103 patients. Ann Surg 199: 432–7, 1984

69. Pederzoli P, Bassi C, Falconi M, et al.: Conservative treatment of external pancreatic fistulas with parenteral nutrition alone or in combination with continuous intravenous infusion of

somatostatin, glucagon or calcitonin. Surg Gynecol Obstet 163: 428–32, 1986

70. Obertop H, van Houten H: A new technique for pancreatojejunostomy. Surg Gynecol Obstet 159: 88–90, 1984

71. Sarr MG, Cameron JL: Surgical palliation of unresectable carcinoma of the pancreas. World J Surg 8: 906–18, 1984

72. Tytgat GNJ, Huibregtse K, Bartelsman JFWM, et al.: Endoscopic palliative therapy of gastrointestinal and biliary tumours with prostheses. Clinics in Gastroenterology 15: 249–71, 1986

73. Huibregtse K, Coene PP, Tytgat GNJ: Endoscopische behandeling van patienten met een pancreaskopcarcinoom. Ned Tijdschr Geneesk 130: 120–123, 1986

74. Bornmann PC, Harries-Jones-Jones EP, Tobias R, et al.: Prospective controlled trial of transhepatic biliary endoprosthesis versus bypass surgery for incurable carcinoma of head of pancreas. Lancet I: 69–71, 1986

75. Leung JWC, Emery R, Cotton PB, et al.: Management of malignant obstructive jaundice at the Middlesex Hospital. Br J Surg 70: 584–86, 1983

76. Blievernicht SW, Neifield JP, Terz JJ, et al.: The role of prophylactic gastrojejunostomy for unresectable periampullary carcinoma. Surg Gynecol Obstet 151: 794–6, 1980

77. Wongsuwanporn T, Basse E: Palliative surgical treatment of sixty-eight patients with carcinoma of the head of the pancreas. Surg Gynecol Obstet 156: 73–5, 1983

78. Scott Jr HW, Dean RH, Parker T, et al.: The role of vagotomy in pancreaticoduodenectomy. Ann Surg 191: 688–96, 1980

79. Skibber JM, Weiss SM, Mohiuddin M, et al.: Impact of radiotherapy on palliative gastroenterostomy in pancreatic cancer. Ann Surg 202: 725–8, 1985

80. Leung JWC, Bowenwright M, Aveling W, et al.: Coeliac plexus block for pain in pancreatic cancer and chronic pancreatitis. Br J Surg 70: 730–2, 1983

81. Greiner L: Punktionssonographische alkoholneurolyse der Coeliakalganglien. Dtsch Med Wochenschr 110: 883–6, 1985

82. Harvey JH, Schein PS: Chemotherapy of pancreatic carcinoma. World J Surg 8: 935–9, 1984

83. Dobelbouwer RR, Milligan AJ: Treatment of pancreatic cancer by radiation therapy. World J Surg 8: 919–28, 1984

84. Bukowski RM, Balcerzak SP, O'Bryan RM, et al.: Randomized trial of 5-Fluorouracil and Mitomycin C with or without streptozotocin for advanced pancreatic cancer. Cancer 52: 1577–82, 1983

85. Mallinson CN, Rake MO, Cocking JB, et al.: Chemotherapy in pancreatic cancer: results of a controlled prospective, randomised, multicentre trial. Br Med J 281: 1589–91, 1980

86. GITSG: A multi-institutional comparative trial of radiation therapy alone and in combination with 5-fluorouracil for locally unresectable pancreatic carcinoma. Ann Surg 189: 205–8, 1979

87. Shipley WU, Wood WC, Tepper JE, et al.: Intraoperative electron beam irradiation for patients with unresectable pancreatic carcinoma. Ann Surg 200: 289–96, 1984

88. Morrow M, Hilaris B, Brennan MF: Comparison of conventional surgical resection, radioactive implantation and bypass procedures for exocrine carcinoma of the pancreas 1975–80. Ann Surg 199: 1–5, 1984

89. Cancer of the pancreas task force. Staging of cancer in the pancreas. Cancer 47: 1631–7, 1981

90. Dietzen CD, Cohn Jr I: The future in treatment of pancreatic cancer. World J Surg 8: 952–5, 1984

91. Hermreck AS, Thomas CY, Friesen SR: Importance of pathologic staging in the surgical management of adenocarcinoma of the exocrine pancreas. Am J Surg 127: 653–7, 1974

92. Smith FP, Hoth DF, Levin B, et al.: 5-Fluorouracil, Adriamycin and Mitomycin-C (FAM) chemotherapy for advanced adenocarcinoma of the pancreas. Cancer 46: 2014–8, 1980

93. Kalser MH, Ellenberg SS: Pancreatic cancer: Adjuvant combined radiation and chemotherapy following curative resection. Arch Surg 120: 899–903, 1985

17. Identification and treatment of common bile duct stones before cholecystectomy

B. LANGER

Introduction

The classical management of common duct stones associated with gall bladder stones is cholecystectomy and common bile duct exploration. This approach gives excellent results, but is associated with a mortality rate in the 2% range [1] and an incidence of recurrent or residual stones of 4% to 10% [2, 3]. This incidence is higher in the more aged population and in patients with complications of stones such as cholangitis or jaundice. The last two decades have seen the development of new technology which has called into question the appropriateness of this classical approach. Improved methods are now available for pre and intraoperative identification of common bile duct stones and the capability now exists for carrying out stone extraction via endoscopic means without laparotomy. These procedures are however associated with their own risks and complications. How has this affected the clinical indications for common bile duct exploration? This paper will review some of the current literature on the subject as well as presenting a synopsis of three papers given at the first World Congress of Hepato Pancreato Biliary Surgery in Sweden in June 1986 and then attempt to answer the following questions:

1. How vigorously should one pursue the investigation for common bile duct stones in patients with known gall stones?
2. When coincidental common bile duct and gall bladder stones are identified, what is the preferred approach
    a) preliminary ERCP and papillotomy and removal of stones only?
    b) ERCP, papillotomy, removal of stones followed by elective cholecystectomy?
    c) operative cholecystectomy and common bile duct exploration?

Preoperative investigation for common bile duct stones

Some patients present with clinical manifestations of common bile duct stones, ie. jaundice, cholangitis, pancreatitis. In such patients there is increasing use of preoperative endoscopic cholangiography (ERC) to identify whether and how many stones remain in the bile duct, and also to allow papillotomy and stone extraction in those situations where it may be indicated. Intravenous cholangiography is little used now in most centres, because its accuracy is much less than ERC. Preoperative liver function tests are used as screening for common bile duct stones, but accuracy and predictability are low when other manifestations of common bile duct stones are absent.

Risks and benefits of endoscopic cholangiography and papillotomy

Endoscopic cholangiography is now widely available and success rates are reported over 90%. It is agreed that success varies with a number of factors including operator experience, quality of equipment and pattern of referral. Also as Cotton has pointed out [4], when reporting on success rates, one must be careful to specify whether the rate reported is of successful endoscopic cholangiography only, cholangiography plus papillotomy, or cholangiography, papillotomy and complete stone removal. Cotton's own overall success rate including stone extraction was 87%. The cumulative stone extraction rate in 14 British centres [5] however reported an overall success rate of only 76%. A review from nine West German centres of 1499 patients similarly revealed a success stone removal rate of 80.5% [6]. The common reasons for failure of the combination of cannulation, sphincterotomy and stone extract include stone size, duct shape, presence of duodenal diverticulae, and previous Billroth II gastric resection. The major determinant in achieving success rates closer to 90% rather than 75% is operator experience. Very few achieve 90%; most (especially those who neither publish nor audit their results) can be expected to achieve 75% or lower.

The complications which follow ERC and EP include bleeding, perforation, pancreatitis, cholangitis, and late sphincter stenosis. As with success rates, operator experience is an important determinant. Overall, 8–10% of patients having endoscopic papillotomy will develop one or more complications, urgent surgery is required in 1–2%, and overall mortality is around 1% [4].

Risk and benefits of operative common bile duct exploration and stone clearance

There is an extensive literature on complication rates and mortality rates following common bile duct exploration, and in this there is less variation from centre to centre, and in fact from surgeon to surgeon, assuming that the operations are done by fully trained surgeons. The mortality rate in good risk patients under 60 years of age is less than 1% [7]. In older high risk patients, mortality varies with risk factors, but including all ages, recent mortality rates are still only in the 2% range [1]. Recurrent or residual stone rates also vary depending mainly on patient selection and duration of follow-up, but most rates are between 4 and 10% [2, 3].

Comparison of the results of surgical and endoscopic common bile duct stone removal is currently not possible because of lack of control of population selected for therapy. In most centres, however, endoscopic papillotomy and stone removal is usually used in the population of patients at highest risk for complications of laparotomy, the assemption that it is a more benign procedure, even though this too is not proven. The extension of endoscopic papillotomy to young, healthy patients is an approach which is currently experimental, considering the risk of endoscopic papillotomy. Finally the question remains as to the management of the residual gall bladder in patients who have had endoscopic papillotomy and stone removal. What is the risk of elective cholecystectomy versus the risk of leaving a gall bladder containing stones in place? There is data accumulating to suggest that short term (1–5 years) the incidence of gall bladder symptoms requiring cholecystectomy is only 10 to 20% [4]. One can expect that this figure will increase with time, however suggesting that the younger the patient, the stronger the indication for elective cholecystectomy both on the grounds of safety of the operation and likelihood of subsequent trouble from the gall stones.

Definitive answers to the questions posed are not yet available, and will likely require carefully controlled prospective trials. In addition there is a need to carefully audit current practice, since results of standard therapy vary somewhat from centre to centre and are dependent on factors including operator experience, and the presence of specific protocols. The following are three abstracts of papers presented at the First World Congress of Hepatopancreatobility Surgery outlining three approaches to this issue.

Biliary lithiasis – surgical therapy

J.J. Jakimowicz, Eindhoven, The Netherlands. We have evaluated the classical surgical approach to biliary lithiasis in a prospective study. Preoperative assessment is limited to the minimum necessary to diagnose cholelithiasis and establish the indication for operative therapy. It includes ultrasound of gall-bladder, liver, common bile duct and pancreas, liver function tests and, when indicated, x-ray examination of the GI-tract. The decision to carry out common bile duct exploration is based upon intraoperative diagnostic procedures and the presence of clinical criteria.

Table 1. Surgical therapy for biliary lithiasis (Jakimowicz).

	All patients in study	Patients having both ultrasound and cholangiography
No. of patients	615	449
Mean age	55.5 yrs.	54.3 yrs.
Cholecystectomy only	411	301
Cholecystectomy + CBD	202	146
CBD exploration only	5	2
Papilloplasty	6	5
Choledochoduodenostomy	12	9
Choledochojejunostomy	2	1
Positive CBD exploration	141 (70%)	112 (76.7%)
Jaundice	40	34
Acute cholecystitis	71	27
Acute cholangitis	13	8
Retained stones	1 (0.5%)	1 (0.7%)
Unexpected stones		23 (7%)

Table 2. A comparison of preoperative diagnostic procedures (Jakimowicz).

	Ultrasonography n = 449	Cholangiography n = 449
True negative	333	311
True positive	104	93
False negative	7	15
False positive	4	14
Technically unsatisfactory	1	16
Sensitivity	93.7%	86.1%
Specificity	98.8%	95.6%
Accuracy	97.5%	94.4%
Predictive value of a negative test	97.9%	95.3%
Predictive value of a positive test	96.3%	86.9%
Prevalence	24.7%	24.1%

Since April 1982, 615 patients have undergone operative treatment for common bile duct stones according to the study protocol. Both operative ultrasound and cholangiography were carried out in 449 patients. In the remaining patients, only one or other test was able to be carried out because of technician or equipment availability. The data is evaluated to assess the relative efficacy of operative ultrasound and operative cholangiography, and the overall results of the primary operative approach to management of common bile duct stones.

Table 1 shows the patients' data and in Table 2 the results of a comparison of operative cholangiography and operative ultrasonography are presented, previously reported in detail [8]. If an operative diagnostic procedure is used, it results in a relatively high percentage of positive common bile duct explorations (76.6%) although in the trial situation exploration of the common bile duct was also undertaken when there were clinical indications, even if the intraoperative tests were negative. Unexpected 'silent stones' were detected in 23 (7%) of cholecystectomized patients. The current study data suggests that intraoperative ultrasonography alone could reduce the rate of negative common duct explorations to 3%.

The results show that a common bile duct exploration, slightly increases the morbidity rate (13.8% vs 8.3%) over cholecystectomy alone, but the mortality rate of CBD exploration in the current experience is 0.9%, the same as the mortality of cholecystectomy. In our previous retrospective study of 1007 patients, we reported an overall operative mortality of 0.9% for patients under 70, 2.6% for those 70–79 and 9.5% for those over 80 years [12].

Conclusions

1. The routine use of an intraoperative diagnostic procedure to indicate whether or not the common bile duct should be explored is recommended. Intraoperative ultrasound is at least as accurate as intraoperative cholangiography, and with experience may be more accurate.
2. Performing surgical common bile duct exploration with current surgical techniques and expertise in this study did not cause an increase in the mortality rate, as compared to cholecystectomy alone. Surgical exploration of the common bile duct is a safe effective therapy for common duct stones and at the present time should remain the treatment of choice.

Comment. This report of a classical approach demonstrates a very respectable morbidity and mortality rate but does not give data regarding longterm recurrent stone rates. It is however a model of what can be achieved in skilled hands. The larger retrospective review quoted is probably more representative of mortality rates to be expected in good hands when taking all comers with common bile duct stones. This kind of data is the standard against which endoscopic papillotomy and stone extraction will need to prove itself.

Combined use of endoscopy and surgery in treatment of bile duct stone disease

O. Boeckl, M. Heinerman, W. Satzburg, Austria. In biliary surgery retained bile duct stones and negative duct explorations as well as mortality from interventions on the bile duct system remain a major problem. The incidence of negative duct exploration and retained stones is 18.5% and 4.5% respectively, and the mortality rate may be as high as 4.4% when cholecystectomy is combined with duct exploration (World J of Surgery, Vol. 10, 1: 116–112).

We have carried out a prospective study of patients with stone disease to evaluate the additional routine use of preoperative bile duct endoscopy, and endoscopic papillotomy and stone extraction, where possible.

Method and patients

480 patients with cholecystolithiasis or bile duct stones were entered in this study. All patients underwent examination by ultrasonography and other routine clinical and biochemical tests other than oral or i.v. cholecystocholangiograms. During cholecystectomy in every case a routine examination of the bile duct and the papilla was carried out by cholangiography and manometry. Patients with either clinical or biochemical evidence suggesting common bile duct stones had preoperative endoscopy, plus papillotomy where stones were identified, and attempted stone extraction.

Results

Group A (n = 305): Elective cholecystectomy in patients in whom no bile duct disease was suspected by preoperative screening. Intraoperative cholangiography revealed in 27 patients (9%) stones of the common bile duct system not suspected preoperatively. In 20 patients they were removed surgically, in 7 patients by postoperative endoscopy. A second surgical procedure was necessary in one of these. No surgical negative duct exploration, one postoperative death (pancreatitis due to surgical complication).

Group B (n = 99): Patients with cholecystolithiasis in whom common bile duct disease was suspected by preoperative screening. This group includes patients with biliary pancreatitis (n = 8). Preoperative endoscopic examination

(ERCP) of the bile duct, was carried out and endoscopic papillotomy (ES) and stone extraction where possible. Subsequent cholecystectomy with intraoperative examination of the common bile duct system and operative revision if necessary.

In 38 patients common bile duct disease suspected by preoperative screening could not be proved by ERC. In 61 patients common bile duct stones were found, in 46 (62%) they were removed by endoscopy and in 15 patients surgically during cholecystectomy. No negative duct exploration, postoperative deaths, or reoperation.

Group C (n = 61): Patients who had a previous cholecystectomy. Preoperative ERC and stone extraction (ES). Subsequent operative revision when endoscopic procedure failed.

In 59 patients common bile duct stones were removed by endoscopy, 2 patients had to undergo surgery. One post procedural death of a 87 year old patient due to myocardial infarction. No surgical reintervention.

Group D (n = 15): Old patients (mean age = 78.8 years) unfit for surgery and suffering from cholecystolithiasis and common bile duct stones which were removed by endoscopy. No subsequent cholecystectomy.

All patients had common bile duct stones which were removed only by endoscopy. The gall bladder with stones was left. No post-endoscopic death, no reintervention. Mean observation time after ES 6.5 months.

Conclusion

By the routine use of endoscopy a precise diagnosis of the bile duct can be achieved preoperatively and negative surgical duct exploration can usually be avoided. The combined use of endoscopy and surgery in patients with common bile duct stones revealed a mortality rate in this series of 1.36% (2 of 146) which compares favourably with the recently published figure of 4.4% after surgical treatment.

Comment. This approach uses selective ERCP and preoperative stone removal and reports a respectable overall morbidity and mortality rate, although only 62% of stones identified preoperatively were removed endoscopically. This study does not make clear what age it is safe to leave a diseased gall bladder in after endoscopic removal of common bile duct stones.

A controlled trial of endoscopic papillotomy and stone removal

Anders Evander, Lund, Sweden. The management of patients with or without stones in the gallbladder and the suspicion of stones in the common bile duct

(CBD) includes two steps. The first is to identify or exclude CBD-stones and the second step is if and how to remove present stones and to decide what to do with the gallbladder. This presentation briefly describes the management as we generally advocate and practice in Lund.

Identification

Preoperative identification

The non-jaundiced patient with signs and symptoms indicating gallbladder stones is investigated with ultrasonography (US) of the gallbladder, liver, biliary tract and pancreatic region. US is very accurate in identifying or excluding stones in the gallbladder but its accuracy in diagnosing CBD-stones is low. In non-jaundiced patients with a history suggesting CBD-stones we perform intravenous infusion cholangiography in patients under 55 years, and endoscopic retrograde cholangiography (ERC), in patients 55 years or older. The former is cheaper, and less invasive, but ERC has a higher accuracy and allows immediate treatment by papillotomy, which is our policy in the older age group. In the jaundiced patient with intact gallbladder US is our first radiologic procedure, followed by ERC, which will discriminate between malignant obstruction or CBD-stones as the cause for jaundice in most of the patients. Should ERC be unsuccessful, the patient undergoes a fine-needle percutaneous transhepatic cholangiography (PTC).

In patients with acute pancreatitis due to gallstone disease ERCP is done within 24–48 hours, and papillotomy is done if CBD stones are found. In patients with acute cholangitis we advocate ERC and papillotomy as an emergency procedure.

Treatment

Our general policy is to recommend every patient younger than 55 years with stones in the gallbladder and with symptoms to undergo an elective cholecystectomy preceeded by infusion cholangiography. Operative cholangiography is done routinely. If CBD stones are found preoperatively, they are removed by CBD exploration at operation.

In patients older than 55 years of age with their gallbladder in place and identified CBD-stones the options are surgical treatment, i.e. cholecystectomy and choledocholithectomy, or ES and stone extraction with or without elective cholecystectomy. In the hands of experts as represented by Drs Jacimowitz and Boekl both options are excellent and competitive.

One year ago we initiated a study in patients aged 55–85 years who were good operative risks. The patients with intact gallbladder and CBD-stones are randomized first to surgical or endoscopic treatment. Those patients allocated to the endoscopic group, and who consequently have their gallbladder still in place, are randomized to elective cholecystectomy within 2 months or observation only. The number included into the study is too low to permit any conclusions so far.

Comment. This is a report on a trial in progress with good study design in patients over 55 years of age to answer the question regarding operative versus endoscopic approach to common duct stones, and the role of elective cholecystectomy. This will require very large numbers to provide answers, since differences in morbidity and mortality in the best hands appear to be similar from non-randomized data. It is however, only from studies such as these that the answers to the questions posed will come.

Overall conclusions

Definitive answers to the questions posed can not be provided at the present time, however, there is enough data to allow individual surgeons to develop an approach based on availability of local expertise and an understanding of the results obtainable at the present time.
1. All patients with gallstone disease should have preoperative screening for common bile duct stones. The minimum is routine liver function tests and ultrasound. The patients with clinical symptoms and signs suggestive of common bile duct stones (jaundice, cholangitis, pancreatitis, or abnormal liver function tests) should have preoperative cholangiography providing that it can be done by an expert with a high success rate (over 90%).
2. Cholecystectomy alone, or combined with common bile duct exploration when carried out by trained surgeons, and including intraoperative cholangiography or ultrasound, or choledochoscopy, carries a low morbidity and mortality except in the very aged or infirm. For the present time the practice of routine cholecystectomy and common bile duct exploration in fit patients is acceptable therapy.
3. Endoscopic papillotomy and stone removal is a legitimate option to operative bile duct exploration, but the risk of this procedure does not appear to differ significantly from bile duct exploration, except in the very bad risk patient. Also, in from 13–25% of patients the procedure fails, and those patients are subjected to both the risk of attempted ERCP and papillotomy, and the subsequent bile duct exploration. The success rate of ERCP and stone removal is more operator dependant than operative common bile

duct exploration, and currently surgical expertise is more widely available than endoscopic expertise.

4. In patients where the increased risk of operation is well documented, (very old patients, serious cardiorespiratory or other disease) ERCP and endoscopic stone removal alone without cholecystectomy is a reasonable approach. The incidence of subsequent gallbladder symptoms requiring operation on such patients is at least 10–20% at three years and is expected to increase with time.

5. Any more definitive guidelines with regard to age of patient or advantage for endoscopic papillotomy over operative bile duct exploration will require carefully controlled prospective randomized trials.

References

1. Pitt HA: Is endoscopic sphincterotomy a safe and effective method for management of stones in the distal bile duct? In: Gitnick G (ed) Negative in controversies in gastroenterology. Churchill, Livingston, N.Y., 1984
2. Glenn F: Retained calculi within the biliary ductal system. Ann Surg 179: 528–39, 1974
3. Way LW, Amirand WH: Dunphey Management of choledocholithiasis. Ann Surg 176: 347–59, 1972
4. Cotton PB: Endoscopic management of bile duct stones; (apples and oranges). Gut 25: 587–597, 1984
5. Cotton PB, Vallon AG: British experience with duodenoscopic sphincterotomy for removal of bile duct stones. Br J Surg 68: 373–5, 1981
6. Jurgen J, Reiter MD, Hans P, et al.: Results of Endoscopic Papillotomy: A Collective Experience from Nine Endoscopic Centers in West Germany. World J Surg 2: 505–511, 1978
7. McSherry CK, Glenn F: The incidence and causes of death following surgery for nonmalignant biliary tract disease. Ann Surg 191: 271–5, 1980
8. Jakimowicz JJ, Rutten H, Jurgens Ph J, Carol EJ: Comparison of operative ultrasonography to contrast radiography in screening of the CBD for stones. World Journ of Surg. In press
9. Jakimowicz JJ, Carol EJ, Jurgens Ph J: The preoperative use of real-time B-mode ultrasound imaging in biliary and pancreatic surgery. Dig Surg 1: 55–60, 1984
10. Jakimowicz JJ: Operative ultrasonography in biliary and pancreatic surgery. In: Hess W, Cireni A, Rohner A, Akowbiantz A (eds) Biliopankreatische Chirurgie. PICCIN, Padova, 1985
11. Jakimowicz JJ: Intraoperative ultrasound-biliary disease. In: Blumgart L (ed) Surgery of the liver and biliary tract. Churchill and Livingstone. In press
12. Roukema JA, Carol EJ, Liem F, Jakimowicz JJ: A retrospective study of surgical common bile duct exploration: ten years experience. Neth J Surg 381: 11–13, 1986

18. Does preoperative transhepatic biliary decompression improve surgical results?

P.J. FABRI

For decades surgeons have feared the complications of surgical procedures on patients with obstructive jaundice. A high incidence of renal failure, septic complications, and even liver failure are described. In his early procedures, Whipple performed a preliminary decompressive procedure followed later after relief of jaundice by definitive pancreaticoduodenectomy. Clinical evidence seemed to indicate that biliary decompression prior to a high risk, major procedure was advantageous.

With the development of appropriate catheters and guidewires and the courage of aggressive radiologists, the technique of transhepatic percutaneous catheterization of the bile duct was introduced. First described by Molnar and Stockum [12] in the United States, this procedure has slowly gained acceptance as a contributor to decreased surgical morbidity and mortality in complicated surgical procedures for the relief or treatment of biliary obstruction. In Molnar's original report, 11 patients were described in which 2 were preoperative. Indications for treatment of strictures were described. The authors suggested that the procedure was most beneficial in those who were beyond surgical help. Fever was described as a common abnormality. Hemobilia requiring transfusion occurred in 2 patients. Removal of the tube occurred in 2 patients requiring reinsertion. Overall, significant complications (excluding fever) occurred in 4 of 11.

Early noncontrolled studies

Several groups have published series in which percutaneous transhepatic cholangiography was performed in preoperative patients. Mori *et al.* [13] in 1977 presented 13 patients with obstructive jaundice and concluded that the results of preoperative decompression were favorable and improved the morbidity and mortality of surgery. There were no historical or concurrent controls. Tylen *et al.* [19] also demonstrated in 1977 that transhepatic decompression could be performed but described the need for emergency surgery in 6 of 83 patients and a death in an additional patient with hemorrhage who was not operated upon. These authors concluded that decompression was effective in relieving jaundice and improved preoperative condition. A high complication rate was noted in the decompressed patient but was not greater than the complications occurring in the patient who did not undergo decompression.

Pollock et al. [16] in 1978 presented a series of 41 patients with obstructive jaundice who underwent PTD. The procedure was performed preoperatively in several patients and the authors concluded that it was of benefit in preoperative preparation of patients but provided no controls. Hansson et al. [8] in 1979 extended the previous experience from Lund, Sweden in a series of 105 patients of which 68 were preoperative. Emergency surgery was required in approximately 3% and significant complications were identified at the time of surgery in 6 additional patients. 12% of patients undergoing subsequent surgery developed significant cholangitis. Based on this larger series, these authors concluded that the complication rate from percutaneous transhepatic biliary drainage is much higher if patients are followed for a longer period of time. The procedure was still recommended for preparation of patients as being less morbid than a surgical decompression.

Wong et al. [20] in 1984 presented a noncontrolled series of 30 consecutive patients who underwent percutaneous drainage. 3 of 10 patients having preoperative drainage had major complications. 7 of 30 patients died within 15 days of the procedure. The authors concluded that percutaneous drainage was a useful alternative in patients not suitable for bypass but did not comment on its specific role in the preoperative preparation of the patient. Josef et al. [10] in 1986 presented a series of 81 patients with attempted PTBD with 90% success rate. 42 patients underwent drainage in anticipation of a definitive surgical procedure. 5 of 40 preoperative patients required emergency surgery. The direct mortality of the procedure itself was 5% which increased to 8.6% if death from continuing sepsis was included. The authors felt that additional trails were needed to define the role of percutaneous drainage because of the very high complication rate and no evidence of preoperative benefit.

Nonrandomized controlled trials

None of these studies had the advantage of controls for comparison but the controversy was deeply entrenched just from the reports of these varied noncontrolled studies. Gobien et al. [6] compared their patients to a series of historical controls from the same institution prior to the institution of PTDB. On the basis of their study, they showed a decreased surgical complication rate from 44% to 15% and a decreased mortality from 30% to 12%. On the basis of these results, they concluded that the complication rate and mortality were decreased and the long term survival of patients was increased. Denning *et al.* [3] looked at a nonrandomized series of patients and compared those who underwent decompression with those who did not. While they showed no decrease in mortality, they showed a significant decrease in complications which they attributed to the preoperative decompression. These authors suggested that preoperative decompression of the bile ducts was advantageous in preparing the patient for surgery.

Shortly after, Norlander [14] looked at a consecutive series of patients, some of whom underwent percutaneous drainage. His group was unable to identify a significant difference in morbidity and mortality and suggested that external drainage may be detrimental because it diverts the bile from the enterohepatic circulation and delays relief of jaundice. They could not support the use of preoperative decompression based on their experience.

Gundry *et al.* [7] looked at patients who were concurrently treated but not randomized. Patients who underwent percutaneous decompression had a decreased length of overall hospital stay and decreased morbidity and mortality of their subsequent surgical procedures. There is no mention of patients who might have undergone decompression but did not subsequently undergo surgery because of complications, etc. These authors strongly recommended preoperative decompression based on their clinical experience. Ellison *et al.* [5] in 1984 extended the series of Denning to include 44 patients of which 17 had radical resection and 27 a palliative operation only. This study was unable to demonstrate any benefit in the palliative group but did show that there was a significant reduction in morbidity from 70% to 40% and in mortality from 60% to 28% in the group undergoing radical surgery. They concluded that preoperative decompression has an important role in preparation of the patient who has 'probably resectable' disease.

Prospective randomized trials

The introduction of prospective randomized trials has clarified many of the controversies arising from the early studies. Hatfield *et al.* [9] from the University of Capetown, South Africa entered 57 patients who were prospectively randomized to preoperative external biliary drainage versus no drainage. 47 patients ultimately underwent surgery. Perioperative mortality was no different in the two groups. The authors noted no advantage and also commented on the numerous complications which were associated with drainage. In particular, 2 patients had major bile leaks, 2 patients developed renal failure, 5 patients developed severe electrolyte imbalance, and many developed minor respiratory problems. This group of investigators could not substantiate a decrease in complications and in fact felt that the major risks, renal failure and sepsis, were actually increased by the procedure.

McPherson et al. [11] from the Hammersmith Hospital in London prospectively evaluated 37 patients. 3 patients required early laparotomy. Sepsis incidence rose during drainage and led specifically to 2 deaths. The authors felt that evidence for a staged approach to the treatment of obstructive jaundice in the ill patient was theoretically supportable but that percutaneous transhepatic drainage carried excessive hazards to justify its use.

Pitt et al. [15] in 1985 presented a prospective, randomized study of 79 patients. Preoperative decompression averaged 8.3 days and did not result in a decreased length in postoperative hospital stay. There was no improvement in morbidity or mortality. The authors concluded that the increased hospital stay due to preoperative decompression unnecessarily increased the cost of the hospital stay without resulting in a significant decrease in complications.

Smith et al. [17] from Australia presented an interesting series in 1985 which on the surface tends to support preoperative decompression. In this randomized, controlled, prospective trial, patients having decompression had fewer surgical complications than those undergoing immediate surgery, but this difference disappeared when the complications of drainage were included. While there was no evidence of difference in gross renal function as measured by creatinine clearance, etc., the authors noted less interference with renal function as measured by plasma urea concentration, plasma B_2-microglobulin, phosphate clearance, etc. They felt that there was some objective biochemical evidence of benefit after an average of 13.8 days of percutaneous decompression. Unfortunately, this biochemical benefit did not appear to translate to an overall decrease in morbidity or mortality.

As if to go back and reassess the original premise, Thomas et al. [18] presented an interesting series in which 34 consecutive patients with periampullary carcinoma were evaluated prospectively but without randomization. 10 patients underwent surgical biliary decompression before a subsequent definitive surgical procedure. 13 patients with comparable jaundice had a single operative procedure. The authors showed no difference in operative complications between the two groups and concluded that preoperative surgical decompression did not appear to be beneficial.

Bitzer [1] looked specifically at the complication rate of percutaneous transhepatic biliary drainage in a series of 18 consecutive patients. Serious complications occurred in 28% with 2 deaths. This group concluded that the complication rate from the procedure was excessive and therefore the procedure should not be used.

Blenkharn [2], addressing the sepsis problem, suggested that the incidences of sepsis could be decreased by modifications in the external collecting system. They showed a 100% incidence of positive bile cultures by 20 days in the system having standard drainage as compared with 40% at the time of initial decompression. An antiseptic barrier (the addition of antiseptic solution to the collection bag) decreased the positive culture incidence to 50%. At the time of definitive surgery, fewer patients had positive bile cultures and fewer complications occurred. Additional reductions in bile cultures were obtained by addition of a closed drainage system. Only 1 patient had bacteria in the bile that had not been present at the initial study. This investigative group felt that perhaps the complication rate associated with percutaneous decompression could be decreased by appropriate attention to the external drainage system which appeared to be the source of the infections.

Summary

The evidence to date is clearly controversial but can be summarized into some meaningful conclusions. It is apparent from the early, noncontrolled studies that clinicians felt that there was significant benefit to be achieved by preoperative decompression of the bile duct. Technical ability to perform the procedure was clearly evident and relief of jaundice was obvious. As studies continued, an increasing complication rate was noted. Prospective, randomized trials would suggest that the intrinsic complication rate of the procedure due to bleeding, hemobilia, sepsis, etc. when added to the operative mortality of the procedure results in no net benefit of the combination procedure and a significant increase in cost because of the prolongation of hospital stay. At the present time, we must conclude that there is probably no benefit of *percutaneous* preoperative decompression, at least as assessed by prospective randomized trials [4].

Nevertheless, we must be reminded of the clinical inferences of the early groups who felt that there was a significant benefit to be obtained. It appears clear that the transhepatic route is not ideal. It is possible that other approaches to biliary decompression, such as endoscopic sphincterotomy with transampullary decompression may decrease the risks of surgery without introducing intrinsic risks of the procedure. We await the results of appropriate, prospective studies of this technique to evaluate its role in the preparation of the patient for relief of biliary obstruction.

References

1. Bitzer LG, Rypins EB, Sarfeh IJ, Juler GL, Conroy RM: The Role of percutaneous transhepatic biliary drainage (PTD) in preoperative patients with obstructive jaundice. Gastroenterology 88: 1326, 1985

318

2. Blenkharn JI, McPherson GA, Blumgart LH: Septic complications of percutaneous transhepatic biliary drainage. Evaluation of a new closed drainage system. Amer J Surg 147: 318–321, 1984

3. Denning DA, Ellison EC, Carey LC: Preoperative percutaneous transhepatic biliary decompression lowers operative morbidity in patients with obstructive jaundice. Amer J Surg 141: 61–65, 1981

4. Elias E: Clinical and experimental aspects of jaundice. Current Opinions in Gastroenterology 2: 365–372, 1986

5. Ellison EC, VanAman ME, Carey LC: Preoperative transhepatic biliary decompression in pancreatic and periampullary cancer. World J Surg 8: 862–871, 1984

6. Gobien RP, Stanley JH, Soucek CD, Anderson MC, Vujic I, Gobien BS: Routine preoperative biliary drainage: Effect on management of obstructive jaundice. Radiology 152: 353–356, 1984

7. Gundry SR, Strodel WE, Knol JA, Eckhauser FE, Thompson NW: Efficacy of preoperative biliary tract decompression in patients with obstructive jaundice. Arch Surg 119: 703–708, 1984

8. Hansson JA, Hoevels J, Simert G, Tylen U, Vang J: Clinical aspects of nonsurgical percutaneous transhepatic bile drainage in obstructive lesions of the extrahepatic bile ducts. Ann Surg 189: 58–61, 1979

9. Hatfield ARW, Terblanche J, Fataar S, Kernoff L, Tobias R, Girdwood AH, Harries-Jones R, Marks IN: Preoperative external biliary drainage in obstructive jaundice. Lancet: 896–899, 1982

10. Joseph PK, Bizer LS, Sprayregen SS, Gliedman ML: Percutaneous transhepatic biliary drainage. JAMA 255: 2763–2767, 1986

11. McPherson GAD, Benjamin IS, Habib NA, Bowley NB, Blumgart LH: Percutaneous transhepatic drainage in obstructive jaundice: Advantages and problems. Brit J Surg 69: 261–264, 1982

12. Molnar W, Stockum AE: Relief of obstructive jaundice through percutaneous transhepatic catheter-a new therapeutic method. Am J Roentgenol 122: 356–367, 1974

13. Mori K, Misumi A, Sugiyama M, Okabe M, Matsouka T, Ishii J, Akagi M: Percutaneous transhepatic bile drainage. Ann Surg 185: 111–115, 1977

14. Norlander A, Kalin B, Sundblad R: Effect of percutaneous transhepatic drainage upon liver function and postoperative mortality. Surg Gynecol & Obstet 155: 161–166, 1982

15. Pitt HA, Gomes AS, Lois JF, Mann LL, Deutsch LS, Longmire WP: Does Preoperative percutaneous biliary drainage reduce operative risk or increase hospital cost? Ann Surg 201: 545–553, 1985

16. Pollock TW, Ring ER, Oleaga JA, Freiman DB, Mullen JL, Rosato EF: Percutaneous decompression of benign and malignant biliary obstruction. Arch Surg 114: 148–151, 1979

17. Smith RC, Pooley M, George CRP, Faithful GR: Preoperative percutaneous transhepatic internal drainage in obstructive jaundice: A randomized, controlled trial examining renal function. Surg 97: 641–648, 1985

18. Thomas JH, Connor CS, Pierce GE, MacArthur RI, Iliopoulos JI, Hermreck AS: Effect of biliary decompression on morbidity and mortality of pancreatoduodenectomy. Amer J Surg 148: 727–731, 1984

19. Tylen U, Hoevels J, Vang J: Percutaneous transhepatic cholangiography with external drainage of obstructive biliary lesions. Surg Gynecol & Obstet 144: 13–18, 1977

20. Wong IH, Krippaehne WW, Fletcher WS: Percutaneous transhepatic biliary decompression – results and complications in 30 patients. Amer J Surg 147: 615–617, 1984

19. Problems in surgery of cirrhotic patients

G.W. JOHNSTON

Introduction

Cirrhosis of the liver is not a single entity but embraces a wide variety of differing pathologies with differing prognoses. The term 'cirrhosis' strictly requires the presence of diffuse destruction of parenchyma, replacement by fibrosis with destruction of the lobular architecture and associated liver cell regeneration. I propose to widén the discussion to include intrahepatic causes of portal hypertension which do not exactly fit this pathological description but nevertheless give rise to similar clinical problems. In doing so I am well aware of the risk of translating the results of treatments too easily from one aetiological group to another or from one society to another. Indeed we would wish to emphasize the differences that the different aetiologies make, not only in the management of these patients but also in their prognosis. If one looked only at the end stage alcoholic cirrhotic with jaundice, ascites, encephalopathy and muscle wasting, it might be justified to take the attitude of a recent editorial suggesting that limited transfusion and sedation are all that is justified [1]. By contrast patients with non-cirrhotic fibrosis or schistosomiasis which carry a good prognosis if bleeding is controlled, must not be subjected to any form of therapy which produces an unacceptable quality of survival. This chapter looks at the problems of surgery in the cirrhotic patient under two headings:
1. Management of variceal bleeding problems in the cirrhotic patient,
2. Management of non-variceal problems in the cirrhotic patient,

Management of variceal bleeding problems in the cirrhotic patient

Centralisation of therapy

The technical revolution in fibre-optics has allowed vast numbers of clinicians to become experts in endoscopy. Consequently, doctors who may see only one

320

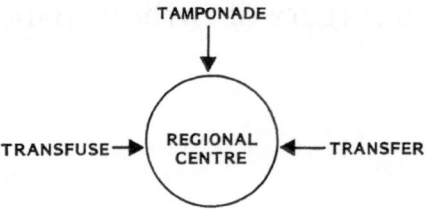

Fig. 1. Transfer to a regional centre is encouraged.

or two patients with bleeding varices annually consider sclerotherapy well within their capabilities. However the technique needs experience and the occasional sclerotherapist cannot obtain this. Even more important is the long-term management; the initial sclerotherapy is only one incident in the complete care of the patient. In Western society probably less than 10 per cent of patients admitted with upper gastro-intestinal haemorrhage will be bleeding from oesophageal varices. It is important to recognise this small group of patients as they are liable to have continuing or repeated haemorrhage. If there is a known history of previous variceal bleeding, even though haemorrhage on this occasion may be from another source, the patient should following resuscitation be transferred to a centre with a special interest in portal hypertension (Fig. 1). When an endoscopist finds unexpected varices on endoscopy for upper intestinal haemorrhage, the same principle of referral applies no matter how trivial the episode. With major bleeding balloon tamponade may be required before transfer; in this case a nurse must accompany the patient in the ambulance. In the specialised unit experienced nursing and medical staff should be able to minimise the reported difficulties of tamponade, manage possible renal problems, undertake injection sclerotherapy and proceed if necessary to surgica¹ management of the portal hypertension.

Financial considerations

Patients suffering from cirrhosis of the liver, portal hypertension and bleeding varices are an expensive drain on national medical resources. It has been shown that the cost of admission of a patient with bleeding varices to a medical unit is three times that of an average medical admission [2]. If in addition sclerotherapy or surgery are required, the admission cost is even greater. It has been suggested that the money used for treating individual alcoholic cirrhotics could 'perhaps be better used to find ways of detecting patients at risk from developing cirrhosis' [1]. Certainly more could be done world wide to try and prevent alcoholic liver disease where that is the main problem, to vaccinate against Hepatitis B where it is rife and to eliminate schistosomiasis in endemic areas. However in the meantime we must continue to treat patients with established portal hypertension and bleeding varices. Dykes and Keighley suggest that patients with Child's Grade C liver disease and bleeding varices should either not be resuscitated or efforts should be concentrated on stopping bleeding and saving blood by simple methods such as vasopressin, tamponade and injection but no more [3]. However I believe it would be wrong for clinicians to allow themselves to be pressurised into a 'no treatment' category for all Grade C patients as many are salvaged from the acute bleeding episode, give up alcohol, improve their Child's grading and live for many years. Financial considerations cannot be the sole determinant of therapy.

Timing of interference

The severity of the liver disease is the main determinant in the mortality rate for variceal bleeding in the cirrhotic patient. Most deaths occur in the first two weeks following the onset of bleeding and thus the management in this early period is vital. It is essential to get control of the initial haemorrhage as quickly as possible and then try and prevent recurrent bleeding. It is worth remembering that bleeding stops spontaneously in about one half to two thirds of patients [4]. However about one third will rebleed within the next couple of days and two thirds within one week. Should the patient therefore have urgent endoscopy soon after admission followed by immediate slcerotherapy if varices are found to be the source of bleeding? Theoretically this sounds ideal but injection sclerotherapy in the presence of bleeding can be technically difficult unless one uses general anaesthesia and a rigid oesophagoscope which not only allows one to control the bleeding point with the wide bore instrument, but also permits the use of a large sucker for evacuation of blood. Generally it is more satisfactory to do any definitive procedure in daylight hours with a fully staffed theatre familiar with the techniques. For the patient with major bleeding oesophageal tamponade can be used temporarily for control, sclerotherapy being performed on the next day's list.

Prevention of recurrent bleeding

One would like to be able to say that we can now select the appropriate operation for each individual patient on the basis of scientific data, but unfortunately this is not so. Often the patient's management is determined more by the enthusiasm of the clinician involved and the local expertise available rather than by any other factors. Perhaps the value of this enthusiasm outweighs many other considerations in the depressing field of bleeding oesophageal varices. Back in 1877 Eck, the Russian surgeon, performed the first portacaval shunts on eight dogs [5]. One died within twenty-four hours, six within seven days and the only relatively long-term survivor escaped after two and a half months and was lost to follow up. Although the other seven dogs died from peritonitis or strangulation of the intestine he proceeded to suggest that this would be a perfectly safe operation for humans. It was certainly not on the basis of this scientific data that shunt surgery eventually found popularity from 1945 onwards. For the next quarter of a century some form of shunt surgery was considered the obvious surgical treatment for variceal haemorrhage but the last decade has seen a swing of the pendulum away from shunt surgery because of the high incidence of post-shunt encephalopathy and the failure to improve survival. When the results of four controlled studies of portacaval shunt versus medical therapy were combined there was no significant difference in survival between the shunted and non-shunted groups [6]. Even the selective distal splenorenal shunt with its possible lower encephalopathy rate does not give better survival than a programme of chronic injection sclerotherapy [7]. Therefore on a scientific basis we cannot recommend shunt surgery and yet one has a 'gut feeling' that for selected individuals it still has a role. For example, the young non-alcoholic cirrhotic with good liver function can have the risk of bleeding from varices virtually eliminated while being exposed to a relatively low chance of developing serious clinical encephalopathy. Another situation where the possibility of shunt must be considered is the patient with bleeding gastritis in the presence of portal hypertension, medical therapy having failed. Obviously injection slcerotherapy or direct ligation transection procedures have nothing to offer since they do not lower the portal pressure. The shunt operation is not yet dead and should not be buried. If we reserve shunt surgery for that small select group of patients under fifty years of age with Child's Grade A liver disease, provided they are not actively bleeding or suffering from diabetes or schistosomiasis, the operative mortality is negligible, the risk of rebleeding small and the incidence of clinical encephalopathy low. Obviously such a policy of selection excludes 80 to 90 per cent of patients who will require some other form of treatment, such as chronic injection sclerotherapy or one of the devascularisation-transection procedures. The first recorded use of injection sclerotherapy was for the control of acute bleeding in a patient with portal vein thrombosis [8]. Its efficacy in the control of acute bleeding was adequately demonstrated in the Belfast series of 117 patients with a 93 per cent control rate of acute bleeding [9]. Subsequent review of 25 years' experience of acute injection sclerotherapy in 264 patients during 396 admissions gave a similar control rate of 91.4 per cent [10]. The Cape Town study suggests that changing to a programme of repeated chronic injections does not improve mortality when compared to repeated acute injections for each new haemorrhage [11]. However deliberately waiting for a further bleeding episode before giving repeat injection sclerotherapy is somewhat unsatisfactory both for the patient and the doctor. Innumerable studies have now demonstrated that a programme of chronic injection sclerotherapy eradicates varices in the majority of patients and carries a low morbidity and mortality. Once the varices have been eradicated the risk of rebleeding is low but a lifetime follow up is required. In 1979 we began using a chronic injection sclerotherapy programme for patients considered unfit for surgical intervention. In the next eight years 65 patients entered the programme. Thirteen patients had an episode of bleeding between the first and second injections before being got under control. Twenty other patients had 47 episodes of bleeding during the programme but often the amount of haemorrhage was relatively minor. During the period 1979 to 1986 only three patients in the series died from bleeding. One death occurred very soon after an injection and this was the only death precipitated by injection. Although 16 other patients have died during the follow up period, these deaths were mostly due to liver failure. The success of any chronic injection programme depends on patient compliance to a lifetime follow up regime. This aspect of repeated visits can be a problem in countries where patients are reluctant to attend in the absence of symptoms. Where there is a risk than one may get only 'one bite at the cherry' a more definitive procedure that sclerotherapy may have to be considered. Terblanche has also recently highlighted the problem of the few patients who are not controlled by sclerotherapy and suggests that early on, another option should be considered for them [12].

Direct sub-diaphragmatic devascularisation for variceal haemorrhage by coronary vein ligation was first reported by Walters and colleagues from the Mayo Clinic [13]. Since those early days many modifications and combinations of transection, ligation and devascularisation have been suggested. Undoubtedly the best reported results are for the Sugiura procedure of transthoracic para-oesophageal devascularisation and oesophageal transection combined with an abdominal component of splenectomy, devascularisation of the upper stomach, vagotomy and pyloroplasty. In a series of 671 patients the operative mortality was only 4.9 per cent and the rebleeding rate from all causes only six per cent [14]. Since only 74 per cent of their patients suffered from cirrhosis and only 10 per cent of the cirrhosis was due to alcohol, it might be difficult to reproduce their excellent results in Western patients. The development of the circular stapling gun facilitated subdiaphragmatic oesophageal transection [15, 16]. In the ten year period of 1976 to 1985 we performed 121 oesophageal transections combined with subdiaphragmatic devascularisation. Twenty-six patients in the series had emergency transections with a mortality of 27 per cent compared to a 13.7 per cent mortality for the 95 patients who had a more elective procedure [17]. Although 33 patients in the series had recurrent haemorrhage in the total follow up period, only six patients died as a result of haemorrhage. Recurrent oesophageal varices were shown to be the source of bleeding in just under half of these rebleeders and accounted for two of the deaths. It must be emphasized that although the incidence of recurrent bleeding has been disappointing many of the episodes of bleeding were minor in nature and only six patients in the whole series died as a result of haemorrhage. Endoscopic doppler probe studies have shown that even where some varices persisted following transection no significant blood flow could be detected [18]. Residual or recurrent varices following transection can be treated effectively by secondary injection sclerotherapy; twenty patients in the series have had post-transection injections.

Geographic differences

Hepatic schistosomiasis is the second main cause of portal hypertension world wide after cirrhosis, occurring chiefly in Africa, Asia and South America. The infestation produces chronic inflammatory changes in the liver with fibrosis in the portal tracts but true cirrhosis does not develop and hence the patients do not usually exhibit the stigmata of chronic liver disease. The patients are usually relatively young when compared with the average cirrhotic patient.

Although they do get portal hypertension, massive splenomegaly and bleeding varices, liver function remains good and ascites, jaundice and portal systemic encephalopathy are rare in the absence of surgical intervention. Thus management of these patient with bleeding varices must not include portacaval shunt which carries a prohibitive 60–70 per cent chance of producing encephalopathy. In an excellent prospective randomised study comparing conventional splenorenal shunt, Warren distal splenorenal shunt and oesophago-gastric devascularisation with splenectomy for schistosomiasis Raia found that the incidence of recurrent bleeding was approximately the same in all three groups [19]. However the encephalopathy rate in the conventional splenorenal shunt was 31.2 per cent compared to 13.3 per cent for the Warren shunt; no encephalopathy was encountered in the splenectomy devascularisation group. It would appear that patients with portal hypertension due to schistosomiasis do not tolerate portal systemic shunts and bleeding varices in these patients should probably be managed by either injection sclerotherapy or some form of transection-devascularisation procedure.

Although alcohol is a major cause of cirrhosis in Western society, it accounts for only a small number of the patients with portal hypertension in Africa and Asia. Here, Hepatitis B, nutritional causes, non-cirrhotic portal fibrosis and schistosomiasis are responsible. Thus in Japan only about 10 per cent of the patients presenting with bleeding varices have an alcoholic aetiology. Perhaps about twice as many have ideopathic portal hypertension, which carries a good prognosis. The Japanese have generally abandoned portal systemic shunting procedures with the exception of the Inokuchi shunt, in favour of a direct attack on the varices because of the high post-shunt encephalopathy rate in their patients. Initially they used the Siguira type of operation, but now injection sclerotherapy is increasing in popularity [20]. Similarly in Egypt injection sclerotherapy is tending to replace the Hassab operation [21].

One must be careful about making direct comparisons of results emminating from different countries. For example, where low rebleeding rates are reported it is necessary to know the adequacy of the follow up of the patients and whether or not the initial procedure was done prophylactically prior to any bleeding episode. Thus, if about 20 to 30 per cent of the operations are done prophylactically it is incorrect to talk about 'recurrent bleeding' in these patients [22]. The important point is that a programme of treatment suitable for one society may be inappropriate for another area where the aetiology of the portal hypertension is different, the indications for treatment are different and patient compliance and follow up are often a problem.

Problems of selection

How do we solve the problem of choosing the right procedure for each patient with bleeding oesophageal varices? I suggest the following.
1. All patients with acute bleeding should have injection sclerotherapy within twenty-four to forty-eight hours of admission whether or not bleeding stops spontaneously.
2. As a general principle Grade C patients should not be considered for any form of surgery, but sclerotherapy is well worthwhile.
3. At present chronic injection sclerotherapy seems the 'best buy' for the prevention of recurrent haemorrhage where patient compliance is likely to be good.
4. A transection-devascularisation procedure should be considered for patients likely to fail to re-attend for sclerotherapy or where sclerotherapy fails to control bleeding. In addition this procedure may be the best option for portal hypertension due to schistosomiasis or non-fibrotic cirrhosis.
5. Shunt surgery still has a place for a very small select group of younger patients with good liver function as outlined above and also where serious bleeding gastritis is a problem.
6. We look forward to a day when adequate medical means of reducing portal pressure may become available to prevent recurrent haemorrhage but the initial acute episode will still be with us even if that day arrives.
7. A possible way of preventing bleeding would be the establishment of a prophylactic injection programme but more evidence is needed before embarking on this.
8. Eradication of the preventable causes of portal hypertension would be the most sensible and positive step in the management of the problem.

Management of non-variceal problems in the cirrhotic patient

It has been estimated that 10 per cent of all patients with liver disease undergo operative procedures during the last two years of their lives [23]. Not all of these operations are related directly to the intrahepatic disease. Obviously these patients are liable to the usual surgical problems of the general populus, but in addition they have an increased risk of certain diseases. For example, the risk of gallstones is about twice that of the general population [24, 25]. The incidence of peptic ulceration is higher and in patients with ascites hernias are more common as previously empty hernial sacs become filled with ascitic fluid. The cirrhotic patient with depressed immune response, coagulation problems, disturbances of renal function, abnormalities of pulmonary circulation and possibly cardiomyopathies carries an immensely greater than average operative risk. In a series of 100 consecutive celiotomies for non-shunt surgery 30 per cent died and major complications occurred in another 30 per cent [26]. In that series where the surgical treatment was done on an urgent basis the mortality was 57 per cent compared to 10 per cent where the procedures were done electively. In the last few years there have been a lot of rather worrying publications in relation to the operation of cholecystectomy in the presence of liver cirrhosis and I want to look at this problem in some more detail.

Cholecystectomy in the cirrhotic patient

It is generally accepted that the incidence of cholelithiasis is doubled in patients with liver cirrhosis. In the majority of patients the stones are of the pigment variety secondary to excess haemolysis associated with hypersplenism. Thus the use of drugs aimed at dissolution therapy is contra-indicated on two counts, namely, the non-cholesterol composition of the stones and the presence of a sick liver. Where cholecystectomy has been undertaken, the reported mortality varies from zero [27] to 21 per cent [26]. Perhaps the 10 per cent mortality reported by Bloch and colleagues in 1985 is fairly representative and rather worrying when one compares this with a less than 0.5 per cent mortality in the non-cirrhotic population [28]. The deaths were due to exsanguinating haemorrhage, hepatic failure, renal failure or sepsis culminating in multiple organ failure. Operative haemorrhage occurs because of coagulation abnormalities coupled with the presence of portal hypertension. Abnormalities of coagulation include decreased synthesis of most of the clotting factors, platelet deficiency and increased fibrinolysis. A prothrombin time of 2.5 seconds greater than the control carries a poor prognosis [29]. These deficiencies can be compensated for by providing an adequate supply of the factors required intravenously before, during and after the operation. Portal hypertension however presents a more serious problem. Serious bleeding tends to occur from two sites, namely the gallbladder bed and the free edge of the lesser omentum if common duct exploration is required. Although division of adhesions may give rise to some bleeding, control is usually relatively simple with ligations. Partial cholecystectomy leaving the intrahepatic portion of the gallbladder in place with cauterisation of the mucosa avoids the troublesome hepatic bleeding from the gallbladder bed. Even cholecystostomy with simple removal of gallbladder calculi is acceptable in these patients who do not have a long life expectancy in any case. Kaufman and colleagues demonstrated the value of cholecystostomy in a series of 24 non-cirrhotic high risk patients, the majority of whom had purulent peritonitis [30]. Twenty-two of their patients survived and twenty were symptom-free one to eleven years later.

Objective evidence of choledocholithiasis by ERCP, ultrasound or cystic duct cholangiogram should be present before duct exploration is carried out. As Dr Walt pointed out in a discussion of Arahana's paper, 'All that is jaundiced is not stone' [31]. There is growing body of opinion that routine drainage of the sub-hepatic space is not required after a simple cholecystectomy in the non-cirrhotic patient. In the presence of cirrhosis, I would suggest that routine drainage is contra-indicated if one is to avoid the risk of troublesome ascitic fluid leak post-operatively. Also a drain provides an easy entry route for exogenous infection of an ideal culture medium, namely ascitic fluid. Finally cholecystectomy in the presence of cirrhosis is not a job for a junior surgeon. This is one place where experience is essential and I believe it is unfair and indefensible to leave the task to a trainee.

Herniorrhaphy

Abdominal wall herniae are particularly common in cirrhotic patients with ascites but it is doubtful whether the majority of these should have herniorrhaphy. In most patients the accumulation of ascitic fluid can be controlled medically making herniorrhaphy unnecessary; fortunately strangulation is uncommon in the presence of ascites. Although ulceration, rupture and leakage of ascitic fluid may occur in the case of umbilical herniae, this is a fairly rare occurrence. In a series of 39 patients subjected to umbilical herniorrhaphy, 24 had uncontrolled ascites and in this group the mortality was 8.3 per cent compared with zero mortality in the 15 patients who had functioning peritoneo-venous shunts [32]. The authors suggest that cirrhotic patients with ascites who require an umbilical herniorrhaphy should undergo peritoneo-venous shunting prior to the repair of the hernia. However I would caution that the possible complications of peritoneo-venous shunts are greater than the risk of obstruction, strangulation or rupture if the hernia were left alone. Repair of a hernia merely for cosmetic reasons is unjustifiable in the presence of cirrhosis.

Peptic ulceration

Although peptic ulceration is commoner in cirrhotic patients than in the general population, it is not often that one has to operate solely for the ulcer. Long term maintenance therapy with H2 antagonist drugs has drastically reduced the number of patients who now require surgery because of persisting pain. Perforation is rare in cirrhotic patients but serious haemorrhage from posterior ulcers does occur and requires urgent therapy. Where a patient has concomitant bleeding oesophageal varices and the presence of a peptic ulcer, this may influence the prefered method of therapy. If one does an oesophageal transection-devascularisation procedure this can be easily combined with a vagotomy and drainage procedure at the same time. In our series of 121 oesophageal transections, nine patients had simultaneous truncal vagotomy and gastrojejunostomy for concomitant duodenal ulceration. The gastrotomy for insertion of the circular stapler was made low down on the anterior wall of the stomach and then used for the gastrojejunostomy.

Primary liver cell carcinoma

In many parts of the world Hepatitis B virus plays an aetiological role in both cirrhosis and hepatocellular carcinoma and half to three quarters of patients with primary hepatoma already have cirrhosis [33]. The incidence of primary hepatocellular carcinoma is increasing in countries where Hepatitis B infection is common; China has 150,000 cases annually. In Japan screening programmes in high risk asymptomatic patients using ultrasound, CT scan and alphafetoprotein estimations have resulted in much earlier detection, half of the tumours found being less than five centimetres in diameter [34]. Resectional surgery may be undertaken if the lesion is less than 50 per cent of liver volume and liver function is good. Yukaya and colleagues reported a resectability rate of 64.3 per cent in a series of 205 patients presenting at their hospital in Hiroshima; the operative mortality rate was only 6.8 per cent [35]. In the Japanese patients three year survival of greater than 50 per cent has been achieved where it is considered that a potentially curative procedure has been carried out. In Western society where hepatocellular carcinoma is often discovered late and usually in patients with a major degree of liver impairment due to cirrhosis, the role of surgery is limited. In addition multifocal tumours are rather more common and encapsulation less often a feature. In a fourteen year period Bismuth and colleagues found that resection was applicable in only 35 of a consecutive series of 363 patients with histologically proven hepatocellular carcinoma [36]. There were only five post-operative deaths but a further 17 patients died with recurrence within one to forty months. Professor Okuda feels that liver transplantation should be considered for patients where resection is not possible provided there are no detectable extrahepatic metastases [37]. However there is a high incidence of recurrent disease even after resection of the whole liver and the risks inherent in such major surgery must be balanced against this. For non-resectable tumours and for multicentric lesions non-surgical treatments are under investigation. However an eleven year prospective randomised trial found that hepatic dearterialisation, intrahepatic arterial chemotherapy, portal vein chemotherapy or external radiation gave the same dismal results as symptomatic treatment alone [38]. Perhaps by localising cytotoxic agents to the tumour area using lipiodol incorporation of the drug or by means of degradable starch microspheres one may accomplish better results with less systemic side effects [39, 40].

Sepsis in the cirrhotic patient

Sepsis is a major problem in patients with cirrhosis and it is estimated 10 to 25 per cent of deaths in patients with liver disease are due to bacterial infection [41]. Since the reticuloendothelial system forms a major defence mechanism and since Kuppfer cell numbers are reduced in cirrhosis the host defence mechanism is impaired [42]. Phagocytosis of particulate matter is reduced and the patient is therefore at greater risk from bacteriaemia. The already impaired defence mechanism may be further depressed by both gastro-intestinal bleeding and blood transfusion. Spontaneous bacterial infections of ascitic fluid can develop insidiously and unless there is a high index of suspicion, mortality can be 50 to 100 per cent. Infection leads to endotoxaemia, encephalopathy, renal failure, hepatic and multiple organ failure. There may be remarkably little abdominal tenderness and therefore any patient with ascites who is 'off colour' should have diagnostic aspiration of ascitic fluid for polymorphonuclear leucocyte count and culture; a count of greater than $250/\mu l$ is the best criteria for the diagnosis of spontaneous bacterial peritonitis [43]. Endoscopic injection sclerotherapy undoubtedly precipitates bacteriaemia but this is usually transient and does not result in established sepsis. It is likely that bacteria are introduced at the time of injection and this may occur in up to half of the patients [44]. In our own series of over 600 episodes of injection sclerotherapy, we have had only one patient who developed a distant abscess. Four days after sclerotherapy she developed quite severe neck pain in the absence of clinical or radiological evidence of oesophageal damage. She was subsequently found to have osteomyelitis of the body of the fifth cervical vertebra which required bone grafting after eradication of sepsis. Post-injection cerebral abscess has also been reported in an insulin dependent diabetic; she recovered with drainage and antibiotic therapy [45]. When laparotomy is undertaken for any reason in the cirrhotic patient prophylactic antibiotic therapy should be employed. This applies whether or not the gastro-intestinal tract is being opened. The mortality from established sepsis is very high.

Conclusion

Emergency surgery in the cirrhotic patient carries a significant mortality, but obviously the increased risk is justified in the presence of a life threatening situation. However before embarking on an elective procedure serious consideration must be given to all the 'pros and cons'. One must be careful that the dangers of surgery are not greater than the risks arising from the pathology itself. When interference is deemed necessary time should be spent in patient assessment and preparation pre-operatively. This may mean a period of medical treatment to control ascites, replacement therapy for coagulation defects, the appropriate use of prophylactic antibiotics, etcetera. Above all an experienced team must be responsible for the operation, no matter how trivial it may at first appear.

References

1. Anonymous: Why treat cirrhosis? Leading article Br Med J 283: 338, 1981
2. Burroughs AK, Oadiri M, D'Heygere F, et al.: Hospital costs of upper gastro-intestinal bleeding in cirrhosis. Paper presented to British Society of Gastroenterology, Lancaster, April 1986
3. Dykes PW, Keighley MRB: Gastro-intestinal haemorrhage. Wright 1981, Bristol, London and Boston, 1981, p 455
4. Graham DY, Smith JL: The course of patients after variceal haemorrhage. Gastroenterology 80: 800–809, 1981
5. Eck NV: On the question of ligature of the portal vein. Voen Med J 130: 1 (Translation in Surg Gynaecol Obstet 96: 375, 1953), 1877
6. Conn HO: A plethora of therapies. In: Westaby D, MacDougall BRD, Williams R (eds) Variceal Bleeding. Pitman, Bath, 1982, p 241
7. Warren WD, et al.: Distal splenorenal shunt versus endoscopic sclerotherapy for long-term management of variceal bleeding. Preliminary report of a prospective, randomized trial. Ann Surg 203: 454–462, 1986
8. Crafoord C, Frenckner P: New surgical treatment of varicose veins of the oesophagus. Acta Otolaryngol 27: 422–429, 1939
9. Johnston GW, Rodgers HW: A review of 15 years' experience of sclerotherapy in the control of acute haemorrhage from oesophageal varices. Br J Surg 60: 797–800, 1973
10. Spence RAJ, Anderson JR, Johnston GW: Twenty-five years' of injection sclerotherapy for bleeding varices. Br J Surg 72: 195–198, 1985
11. Terblanche J, Bornman PC, Khan D, et al.: Failure of repeated injection sclerotherapy to improve long-term survival after oesophageal variceal bleeding. A five year prospective controlled clinical trial. Lancet ii: 1328–1332, 1983
12. Bornman PC, Terblanche J, Kahn D, Jonker MAT, Kirsch RE: Limitations of multiple injection sclerotherapy sessions for acute variceal bleeding. SAMJ 70: 33–36, 1986
13. Walters W, Rowntree LG, McIndoe AH: End result of tying the coronary vein for prevention of haemorrhage from oesophageal varices. Proc Staff Mayo clinic 4: 263, 1929
14. Sugiura M, Futagawa S: Esophageal transection with paraoesophagegastric devascularisation (the Sugiura procedure) in the treatment of esophageal varices. World J Surg 8: 673–682, 1984

15. Vankemmel M: Resection-anastomose de l'oesophage sus-cardial pour rupture de varices oesophagiennes. Nouvelle Presse Medicale 5: 1123–1124, 1974
16. Johnston GW: Treatment of bleeding varices by oesophageal transection with the SPTU gun. Annals of Royal College of Surgeons of England 59: 404–408, 1977
17. Johnston GW: Ten years' experience of oesophageal transection for bleeding varices using the circular stapler. Dig Surg 3: 112, 1986
18. Hoskins SW, Johnston AG: What happens to oesophageal varices after transection and devascularisation. Paper presented to Association of Surgeons of Great Britain and Ireland, London, April 1986
19. Raia S, Mies S, Macedo AL: Surgical treatment of portal hypertension in schistosomiasis. World J Surg 8: 738–752, 1984
20. Hasagawa H, Takada T, Yasuda H, et al.: Endoscopic sclerosing therapy for the bleeding oesophageal varices – comparative studies of the treatments. Paper presented to First World Congress of Hepatico-Pancreatico-Biliary Surgery, Lund, Sweden, June, 1986
21. Barsoum MS, Hussein AM, Zakaria S, et al.: Sclerotherapy How and what? Paper presented to First World Congress of Hepatico-Pancreatico-Biliary Surgery, Lund, Sweden, June 1986
22. Inokuchi K: Present status of surgical treatment of oesophageal varices in Japan: a nationwide survey of 3588 patients. World J Surg 9: 171–180, 1985
23. Jackson FC, Christophersen EB, Peternel WW, et al.: Preoperative management of patients with liver disease. Surg Clin North Am 48: 907–930, 1968
24. Bouchier IAD: Postmortem study of the frequency of gall stones in patients with cirrhosis of the liver. GUT 10: 705–710, 1969
25. Nicholas P, Rinaudo PA, Conn HO: Increased incidence of cholelithiasis in Laennec's cirrhosis; a postmortem evaluation of pathogenesis. Gastroenterology 63: 112–121, 1972
26. Garrison RN, Cryer HM, Howard DA, Polk HC: Clarification of risk factors for abdominal operations in patients with hepatic cirrhosis. Ann Surg 199: 648–655, 1984
27. Kogut K, Aragoni T, Ackerman MB: Cholecystectomy in patients with mild cirrhosis. Arch Surg 120: 1310–1311, 1985
28. Bloch RS, Allaben RD, Walt AJ: Cholecystectomy in patients with cirrhosis – a surgical challenge. Arch Surg 120: 669–672, 1985
29. Aranha GV, Sontag SJ, Greenlee HB: Amer J Surg 143: 55–60, 1982
30. Kaufman M, Schwartz I, Weissberg D: Cholecystostomy as a definitive operation. Dig Surg 3: 147, 1986
31. Walt AJ: In discussion of paper – Cholecystectomy in cirrhotic patients: a formidable operation by Aranha GV, Sontag SJ, Greenlee HB. Amer J Surg 143: 55–60, 1982
32. Leonetti JP, Aranha GV, Wilkinson WA, Stanley M, Greenlee HB: Umbilical herniorrhaphy in cirrhotic patients. Arch Surg 119: 442–445, 1984
33. Ying Yue-Ying, Yan Rui-Qi, Xu Bing-Dong, et al.: Relationship of hepatocellular carcinoma, liver cirrhosis and Hepatitis B virus. Chinese Medical Journal 97: 758–764, 1984
34. Halliday C, Henahan J: Congress report – World Congress of Gastroenterology in Practice 2: 6–12, Brazil 1986
35. Yukaya H, Nagasue N, Ogawa Y, Sasaki Y, Chang Y-C: Clinical experience with 132 hepatic resections for hepatocellular carcinoma. Paper presented to First World Congress of Hepatico-Pancreatico-Biliary Surgery, Lund, Sweden, June 1986
36. Bismuth H, Houssin D, Ornowski J, Meriggi F: Liver resections in cirrhotic patients: a western experience. World J Surg 10: 311–317, 1986
37. Okuda K, Obata H, Nakajima Y, Ohtsuki T, Okazaki N, Ohinishi K: Prognosis of primary hepatocellular carcinoma. Hepatology 4: 35–65, 1984
38. Lai ECS, Choi TK, Tong SW, Ong GB, Wong J: Treatment of unresectable hepatocellular carcinoma: Results of a randomized controlled trial. World J Surg 10: 501–509, 1986

39. Kanematsu T, Inokuchi K, Sugimachi K, *et al.*: Selective effects of lipiodolized anti-tumour agents. Journal of Surgical Oncology 25: 218–226, 1984

40. Miura T, Haida K, Haida S: Hepatic arterial administration of 5-FU and mitomycin C with degradable starch microspheres and local hypothermia. Paper presented to First World Congress of Hepatico-Pancreatico-Biliary Surgery, Lund, Sweden, June 1986

41. Wyke RJ: Susceptibility to infection in liver disease. Current Opinion in Gastroenterology 2: 471–477, 1986

42. Rimola A, Soto R, Bory F, Arroyo V, Piera C, Rodes J: Reticuloendothelial system phagocytic activity in cirrhosis and its relation to bacterial infections and prognosis. Hepatology 4: 53–58, 1984

43. Scemama-Clergue J, Doutrellot-Philippon C, Metreau J-M, *et al.*: Ascitic fluid pH in alcoholic cirrhosis: a re-evaluation of its use in the diagnosis of spontaneous bacterial peritonitis. GUT 26: 332–335, 1985

44. Sauerbruch T, Holl J, Ruckdeschel G, Forsti J, Weinzierl M: Bacteriaemia associated with endoscopic sclerotherapy of oesophageal varices. Endoscopy 17: 170–172, 1985

45. Cohen FL, Koerner RS, Taub SJ: Solitary brain abscess following endoscopic injection sclerosis of esophageal varices. Gastrointest Endosc 31: 331–332, 1985

20. Selective and total shunts in portal hypertension: facts and myths

I.S. BENJAMIN

History of portal-systemic shunting

The first clinical portal-systemic diversion procedure is correctly attributed to the French surgeon Vidal, who in 1903 presented a paper to the XVI Congress of French Surgeons on the surgical treatment of ascites, which before this time had been managed by omentopexy [1, 2]. Finding the omentum unavailable in a young alcoholic cirrhotic he carried out an end-to-side portacaval anastomosis, and suggested in his presentation parenthetically but prophetically that bleeding from varices might prove to be an indication for portal-systemic diversion. Vidal observed however that 'all absorption of albuminoides provoked a very severe intoxication. Thus it is to hydrocarbons that one must turn for recourse'. Vidal's patient suffered a recurrent haematemesis at 6 weeks, but ultimately died of sepsis. Thus in one very early report this pioneer clearly described the indications, the technique and the complications of an operation which still forms a part of our practice almost a century later.

Only a very few anecdotal reports appear in the literature from that time until the presentation by Whipple [3] to the American Surgical Association in 1945 ushered in the modern era of portal diversion. In the 1950's, McDermott and Adams [4] and Hubbard [5] reported portal-systemic encephalopathy (PSE) in patients who had required end-to-side portacaval shunt during pancreatico-duodenectomy for tumour. Within a few weeks all patients reported had developed episodic hepatic encephalopathy, along with malnutrition, fatty infiltration of the liver and hypoalbuminaemia. This rediscovery of the risk of PSE was made at a time when the surgical management of bleeding varices by means of portal diversion had become an established part of clinical practice [6]. The term 'portal systemic encephalopathy' was in fact first coined by Sherlock and her colleagues in 1954, when the crucial relationship between the syndrome and impaired hepatocellular function was also recognized [7]. Ten years later the same group [8] reported encephalopathy in 15% of non-cirrhotic patients undergoing portal diversion because of portal vein thrombosis. Thus the major risk of the only truly effective therapy for portal hypertension with bleeding varices had become well established. Prior to this time the concern of the surgeon in this field was with operative mortality and protection from bleeding, and technical improvements including new varieties of shunt such as the side-to-side shunt and central splenorenal shunt followed, but no controlled information was available to demonstrate major advantages for any of these techniques.

The first information from *controlled trials* came from the Boston Inter-Hospital Liver Group between 1969 and 1974. The first report [9] described the results of a controlled study of *prophylactic* portacaval shunting versus conventional medical management in patients with portal hypertension and oesophageal varices without previous bleeding. This study failed to demonstrate improved survival in shunted patients, apparently because the increased incidence of severe liver failure and PSE counterbalanced the beneficial effects of reduced bleeding. One important aspect of this work was the careful definition and standardized prospective recording of neurological changes. This group defined mild PSE as three or less episodes of encephalopathy precipitated by gastrointestinal bleeding, diuretic or depressive drugs or by terminal events, while severe PSE was defined as more than three episodes not induced by these agents, or continuous symptoms, or a need for protein restriction or oral antibiotic therapy. Almost 20% of patients in each group had experienced at least one episode of PSE before inclusion in the trial, but only one patient had suffered severe spontaneous recurrent PSE (in the control group). During a mean follow-up of four years, mild individual episodes of PSE occurred in approximately one-third of each group, but severe and recurrent PSE occurred in some 20% of patients with prophylactic shunts, compared with 2% of the unshunted control patients. It thus appears that although cirrhotic patients without a surgical shunt may develop sporadic PSE, the severe continuous and incapacitating form occurs almost exclusively in patients with shunts. These studies may be said to mark the close of the era of unbridled enthusiasm for shunting in cirrhotic patients. It is interesting that the first report from Warren and his co-workers [10] suggesting the need for an improved form of portal diversion pre-dated these important reports, and at this time Hassab and others [11] were also abandoning the portal diversion procedure in favour of a direct approach to the oesophago-gastric vascular bed.

The 1970's saw a number of reports demonstrating that in a controlled study *therapeutic* portacaval shunt also failed to produce a major improvement in survival, again because of the increased incidence of liver failure and encephalopathy in the surgically treated group. Resnick and his colleagues [12] showed an incidence of severe PSE of only 4% in the medically treated group compared with 13% in the surgical group. Paradoxically, there was apparently a higher rate of chronic PSE in the medically treated patients (35% versus 20%):

however, this apparently higher rate was due to retention within this group of 7 patients who had been randomized to medical treatment but required an emergency end-to-side shunt for recurrent bleeding, 3 of whom developed PSE. Moreover, the randomly selected medically treated patients had a higher frequency of prior PSE at the onset of the study (57% versus 34%). Similar data emerged from other controlled studies. Rueff and his colleagues [13] showed no difference in acute encephalopathy in 89 alcoholic cirrhotics randomized to portacaval shunt or to medical treatment. However, during follow-up there was no incidence of chronic PSE in the control group, while this occurred in 25% after shunting. More recently, Reynolds and his colleagues [14] showed an equal incidence of acute encephalopathy in a randomized controlled study, but the development of spontaneous PSE was again limited to the surgical group, and was considered severe in 22%. The combined incidence of moderate and severe PSE in this group was 35%.

All of these studies indicate that great care must be taken evaluating the results of encephalopathy reported in the literature. Unless PSE is carefully defined important differences in its incidence may fail to be revealed even in prospective studies. The present consensus from these and other controlled trials does suggest that the incidence of spontaneous, and particularly that of severe, PSE is greater following a surgical end-to-side shunt than in a comparable group of medically treated patients. However, since the rate of bleeding is generally higher in medically treated groups, the incidence of *acute* PSE as a result of haemorrhage may counterbalance this if a careful distinction is not made between these two varieties of encephalopathy.

The influence of primary liver disease

It was an early observation that both postoperative mortality and long-term survival were closely related to the quality of liver function in patients with portal hypertension. A group of factors (bilirubin, albumin, nutritional status, ascites and neurological function) was identified by Child in 1964 [15], and these factors have been used for the last 20 years to classify patients into the so-called Child's grades A, B or C. It is remarkable that numerous attempts to improve Child's prognostication have failed to make a marked impact [16], although a modification suggested by Pugh and his colleagues at King's College Hospital [17] which adds the factor of prothrombin time has been adopted more recently. The patients in Child's grade C have both a high perioperative mortality and an unacceptable incidence of encephalopathy following total portal diversion. While it is generaly assumed that patients in Child's grade A sustain the diversion of portal blood well, we have already noted that early work [4, 5] showed that even the previously normal human liver is sensitive to diversion of portal blood. More recent experience attests to the relative safety of portal diversion in patients with normal livers. In particular Starzl and his colleagues have undertaken numerous total portal diversion procedures for patients with metabolic diseases such as glycogen storage disease or familial hypercholesterolaemia. Following such patients for periods of 5 to 20 years these workers have shown only rare and transient encephalopathy [18, 19]. Another relevant group of patients is those with extrahepatic portal venous obstruction. Many of these patients develop a system of hepatopetal collaterals, and when a surgical shunt is constructed this collateral flow to the liver is 'stolen' through the shunt resulting in some diminution of portal flow [20]. Nonetheless, the majority of such patients are without encephalopathy during long term follow-up [21]. Similar results have been reported following shunting in children for portal vein thrombosis [22].

However, there is no doubt that even patients with previously normal liver function do have some impairment as a result of the shunt. In Starzl's series [18, 19] low grade elevations of serum transaminases and alkaline phosphatase are common, and blood ammonia levels were always increased beyond the upper limits of normal. Mikkelsen and his colleagues [23] have observed encephalopathy following portal diversion for extrahepatic portal block, and Warren's group [20] have shown reversal of this encephalopathy following disconnection of the shunt. Voorhees [24] made the important observation that following shunting for extrahepatic portal block in children there was a high incidence of psychological and psychiatric abnormalities, which might possibly represent a variant of PSE. A further interesting exception is schistosomiasis, a disease which produces a largely pre-sinusoidal portal block, and should allow of a good prognosis following shunting. However, this has not been found to be the case and indeed some of the most devastating encephalopathy has been reported following shunts for schistosomiasis [25]. However, it is possible that the effects of schistosomiasis may not be an entirely mechanical pre-sinusoidal block, and other pathological factors may be involved in deterioration of these patients' liver function.

Notwithstanding the above comments on hepatic function, it is apparent that at least in part the outcome of portal diversion procedures depends upon changes in hepatic circulation. It is thus important to examine the role of haemodynamics in shunting, particularly in relation to PSE.

Haemodynamics of portal diversion

Since Warren's observations in 1967 [10] numerous workers have tried to relate hepatic haemodynamics, and in particular the degree of hepatopetal flow before shunting, to the outcome of portal diversion procedures. Much of the older work in this area was technically unreliable, particularly studies attempting to make firm haemodynamic conclusions from angiography [26]. Indeed, numerous attempts to find specific haemodynamic parameters which correlate with the outcome of surgery have been largely fruitless [27, 28]. Attempts to maintain hepatopetal portal flow by means of side-to-side portacaval shunts (of which the splenectomy with central splenorenal shunt is but one variety) have been shown to be futile, and this type of shunt has no obvious clinical advantage over end-to-side portacaval shunt [29–31]. The original report by Drapanas of the mesocaval interposition graft suggested an encephalopathy rate as low as 11% [32]. This has never been substantiated by other workers. Mulcare [33] in a retrospective survey reported a 32% incidence of PSE 'of sufficient gravity to require active medical therapy'. This did not appear to relate to preoperative liver function. Reznick *et al.* [34] reviewed 30 survivors of 47 mesocaval shunts: 10 (33%) had mild PSE and 6 (20%) severe, defined as 'disabling or requiring hospitalization'. There have been two controlled trials of mesocaval shunts against conventional PCS. Malt [26] found no advantage in emergency cases, though the mortality rate was high (73%). Stipa [35] also showed little difference in survival or in overall PSE (43–44%) in electively shunted Child's A and B patients, though the rate of *severe* PSE was unusually low in his series (1 out of 46 patients). Drapanas's original observation that the mesocaval shunt maintained hepatopetal flow has also not been confirmed by other workers, and these results carry an important lesson on the dangers of haemodynamic interpretation of angiographic data. Coeliac or superior mesenteric injections may show filling of the portal vein, but fail to distinguish between hepatopetal and hepatofugal flow – a misinterpretation termed 'portal pseudoperfusion' by Warren's group [36]. Splenic arterial injection may clarify the situation and demonstrate that the shunting of portal blood is total or near total [34].

While the majority of authors have attempted to study changes in *portal* flow following shunting, Burchell and his colleagues [37] made important observations regarding changes in *arterial* flow. These workers demonstrated that following a total PCS there was a variable increment in the volume of hepatic arterial flow to the liver. Moreover, follow-up studies demonstrated that those patients who had an increment of hepatic arterial flow greater than 100 mls per minute had a very low incidence of encephalopathy, while those with a lesser increment in arterial flow suffered a significantly higher incidence [38]. This is important evidence relating the *volume* rather than the *character* of hepatic blood flow to the incidence of encephalopathy. Also based on the hypothesis that maintenance of the total volume of portal flow might be of value, Maillard and his colleagues [39] reported the use of arterialization of the portal venous stump in association with PCS in order to avoid the complication of PSE. While this proved to some extent effective it carried a high rate of com-

plications due to increased sinusoidal pressure, including intrahepatic cholestasis and marked portal venous sclerosis. This procedure does not appear to
be of clinical value.

However difficult it may be to prove the hypothesis that maintenance of hepatic portal perfusion bears a strong relationship to a good outcome following
portal decompression, the concept remains both important and attractive. It
was this concept which led Warren and his colleagues to the development of a
selective shunt, designed to decompress the dangerous oesophago-gastric variceal bed, while leaving intact the residual portal flow to the liver. This concept
is considered in the next section.

The selective (distal splenorenal) shunt

This shunt is illustrated schematically in Fig. 1. The concept of the operation
differs radically from other portal diversion procedures, in which the objective
is to produce a generalized lowering of pressure within the entire portal venous
system, with the beneficial effect of decompressing oesophago-gastric varices,
but the inevitable detrimental effect of reducing the residual portal venous inflow to the diseased liver. The concept of the distal splenorenal shunt (DSRS)
is that blood from the gastro-oesophageal portal bed is shunted by way of the
short gastric veins and the plexus of veins in the splenic hilus, and diverted via
the splenic vein into the left renal vein and hence into the systemic circulation.
The formation of this shunt is complemented by ligation of the venous collaterals in the gastrohepatic and gastrocolic ligaments, thus dividing the coronary, right gastric and right gastroepiploic veins. The objective is to separate
the portal venous beds of the abdomen into two compartments, that from the
major part of the mesenteric and pancreatic bed draining to the liver in a normal manner through the intact portal vein, while that from the oesophagus and
stomach drains into the systemic circulation. There is no attempt to lower the
pressure in the 'right-sided' venous compartment so that portal blood continues to have the maximum opportunity to perfuse the liver selectively, while the
'left-sided' compartment is under low pressure and is safe from bleeding.

In addition to preserving the high pressure of portal perfusion of the liver
there are two other theoretical advantages to this operation. Firstly, much of
the hormone-rich venous effluent from the pancreas is still selectively directed
towards the liver. Experimental work has attempted for more than 50 years to
elucidate the nature of the process which determines hepatocyte mass and controls atrophy and hyperplasia within the liver. Early work by Rous and Larimore [40] suggested that 'hepatotrophic' substances in portal venous blood
were essential to the maintenance of the liver, while subsequent experiments
by Mann [41] suggested the prime role of the quantity of hepatic blood flow.

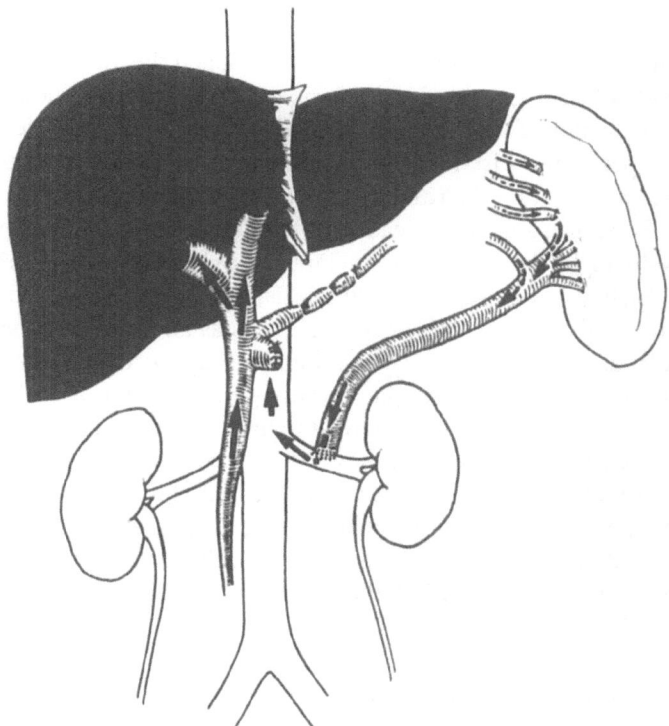

Fig. 1. The distal splenorenal shunt. (Courtesy of Dr W Dean Warren and Year Book Medical Publishers Incorporated, Chicago).

(The reader is referred to the major review of this subject by Starzl and his colleagues [19] for an up-to-date account of the controversy). However, despite difficulties and subtleties in interpretation, it does appear that hormonal substances within the pancreatic contribution to the portal hepatic blood supply do play at least a supportive or permissive role in maintenance of normal liver mass and function. It is thus beneficial to maintain this component of hepatic blood flow. The second marginal benefit of DSRS lies in the preservation of a degree of increased pressure in the veins of the small intestines. It has been shown that a degree of venous hypertension retards intestinal absorption of some of the metabolic products which may be associated with encephalopathy [42, 43].

There is clearly a conceptual and practical problem in attempting to produce artifically a high pressure and a low pressure venous bed side-by-side within the abdomen. Intraoperative and early postoperative studies suggest that this is in fact achieved [44, 45]. Hepatopetal portal perfusion was reported in more than 90% of patients in the early postoperative period. However, when late postoperative studies are performed the percentage of patients with continued antegrade portal flow diminishes to 50% or less [44], indicating a gradual loss of selectivity. Maillard's group [44] indeed abandoned the attempt to achieve disconnection of the right-sided and left-sided portal beds by venous ligation following the results of their early clinical and angiographic experience, and continue to perform a distal splenoral shunt *without* venous disconnection. These workers claim that the results of the two procedures are identical. This group has also shown angiographically that the DSRS carries a high flow which is partially driven by the splenic arterial input. This has the effect of protecting the splenorenal anastomosis from thrombosis, but may also produce a 'steal' effect on the hepatic portal flow because it acts as an arteriovenous fistula. Nonetheless, data from Warren's own group [46] suggest that this conversion from a selective to a total shunt may be very gradual: 9 out of 11 patients in Warren's randomized studies who agreed to have follow-up angiography at a mean of 7.4 years after DSRS were shown to have continued hepatic perfusion following a superior mesenteric injection. The situation may be further complicated by the effect of the primary liver disease on haemodynamics: it has been suggested that alcoholic patients suffer a much greater loss of portal venous inflow to the liver after DSRS than do non-alcoholic patients [47].

Clinical evaluation of the selective shunt

Three questions must be posed in order to establish the true clinical role of the DSRS:
1. Can it be accomplished with an acceptable mortality?
2. Is it as effective in reducing variceal bleeding as the conventional (total) shunt?
3. Does it have any advantage in terms of a reduced rate of post-shunt encephalopathy?
These three questions can only be answered in the light of an increasing breadth of published worldwide experience, and best of all in the performance of carefully controlled randomized clinical trials.

The DSRS has in the past enjoyed the reputation of being an extremely technically demanding procedure, with a high failure rate. While it is certainly more difficult than some of the other conventional shunts, it has now become clear through increasing experience that it can be performed with an acceptable success rate and low mortality rate as long as there is careful attention to detail. The principal area of difficulty is in the dissection of the splenic vein from the pancreas. This does require great care and particularly in patients with fibrosis due to chronic pancreatitis may be a hazardous procedure because of bleeding from small veins in the unyielding pancreatic substance. Mobilization of the left renal vein may also prove difficult. It is the author's practice to request left renal venography in combination with selective angiography whenever possible before performing elective shunt surgery, as a disadvantageous position of the left renal vein can be detected before undertaking the dissection. The left renal vein is retroaortic in less than 5% of patients, but this may pose a particular problem requiring division of the vein with end-to-end splenorenal anastomosis. It may also be necessary in some difficult cases when the splenic vein cannot be mobilized from the pancreas to perform an end-to-side renal vein-splenic vein anastomosis with ligation of the splenic vein in continuity to the right of the anastomosis. The use of a jugular vein interposition graft has also been described [48]. Warren has recently published an excellent, detailed technical description of his own current procedure [49].

Long-term patency of the DSRS has also been questioned. This in fact compares quite favourably with total shunts, and may even be better than the 82% patency documented for the central splenorenal shunt [50]. In the most recent study from Warren's group [51] there was only one shunt occlusion (which was followed by recurrent variceal bleeding) in 35 patients. The incidence of occlusion after DSRS in Warren's much larger collected series of several hundred patients was only 7%, all but 2 of whom were detected immediately after surgery and were due to technical errors: late thrombosis was very rare with only 2 late shunt occlusions during a 10 year follow-up [43]. Maillard's group reported no shunt thrombosis in 44 patients, all subjected to selective angiography [52].

As regards the efficacy of the procedure, 6 controlled investigations have been published comparing the DSRS with other forms of portal decompression surgery [30, 45, 53–56]. All 6 of these trials show comparable operative mortalities and long-term survival figures. The numbers in these trials were necessarily small (ranging from 27 to 89 patients randomized). Warren's [57] rather larger collected experience in fact shows a lower operative mortality for the DSRS (14/348, 4.1%) than for non-selective shunts (22/156, 14.1%). This difference in operative mortality was not found in Warren's controlled studies (11.5% and 10.3% respectively) [58]. There is a clear effect in the non-randomized series of increasing experience with the DSRS, with a mortality rate in patients operated since 1976 of only 3.4% in 322 cases. This is paralleled by a rise in mortality to 15% in 127 non-selective shunts, reflecting also the larger number of poor risk patients and emergency operations in the latter group. However, long term survival in the randomized studies from Warren's group remains the same for selective and non-selective shunts.

Preservation of hepatic function, as measured by biosynthetic processes such as urea synthesis, is better maintained after DSRS. However, in a randomized trial of DSRS versus endoscopic sclerotherapy, Warren's group showed better maintenance of galactose elimination capacity in patients managed by sclerotherapy than in those undergoing selective shunting [51]. This serves to highlight the inevitable deterioration in liver function which follows shunting even when attempts are made to preserve portal flow.

As far as lowering of the rate of PSE is concerned, there is now good evidence from the controlled clinical trials that DSRS is of some value [30, 45, 56]. Langer's results [56] showed that only 3/22 patients surviving a selective shunt procedure had a significant encephalopathy, classified as mild in all cases. In contrast 14 out of 28 patients with end-to-side portacaval shunt had encephalopathy, 9 mild and 5 (18%) severe. Conn and Lieberthal [59] combined the available data from Warren's, Langer's and the Boston/New Haven Liver Group and showed a lower incidence of PSE of all grades (7/50 versus 20/52) and particularly of severe encephalopathy (1/50 versus 12/52). Reichle *et al.* [30] also showed a significantly lower incidence of PSE after DSRS when compared with mesocaval shunt. Adson [31] reviewed the Mayo Clinic experience (uncontrolled) of 71 Warren shunts over 10 years. They described an operative mortality rate of 4%, with a a 76% actual 3 year survival and a 'probable' shunt occlusion rate of 10%. The incidence of PSE was 5.6 or 7%, the latter figure including one patient who 'becomes confused when drunk'! Marni and his colleagues [60] however showed no advantage of selective shunting, although this was a very small and uncontrolled series. Similarly, Mikkelsen [31, discussion] reported no overall difference in PSE between Child's A and 'high B+' patients undergoing DSRS or portacaval shunt. However, in both Marni's and Mikkelsen's study, selection of the lowest risk patients for inclusion may have considerably influenced the outcome.

Selective shunt – facts or myths?

The above discussion has been an attempt to review briefly what is a very complex literature, addressing simultaneously a number of problems relating to technical detail, liver function, variceal bleeding, encephalopathy, and other more subtle issues. It is true that a certain mythology has developed surrounding the Warren shunt, but fortunately the waters now appear to be clearing somewhat and it is possible to make some fairly firm conclusions and begin to de-mythologise this procedure.

1. Liver perfusion and liver function are normal following the operation – *myth*. There is now good evidence to show that both liver perfusion and liver function deteriorate following DSRS. However, this does take place gradually, and it may be that this gradual process allows of either haemodynamic or metabolic adaptations or both. Indeed it is necessary to postulate such an adaptation now in order to explain the difference in encephalopathy rates.
2. The operation produces less encephalopathy than a total shunt – *fact*. If one

restricts definition of PSE to severe, *spontaneous* attacks of encephalopathy, and excludes those associated with recurrent haemorrhage, then
controlled trials now demonstrate conclusively that there is a significant difference in the incidence of PSE. Whatever the mechanism, and this remains
far from clear, the one major advantage for which the operation was designed does appear to be a real one.

3. There is a high shunt thrombosis rate following the Warren shunt – *myth*.
Good studies including angiographic and ultrasonographic follow-up have
demonstrated that DSRS can be achieved with a very low thrombosis rate.
Clearly attention to technical detail is important to achieve this result, but
failure to do so can no longer be regarded as a fundamental criticism of the
operation.

4. The operation is so technically demanding that it should be restricted to use
in specialist centres – *part fact, part myth*. There is no doubt that it is a difficult procedure, and indeed the evidence of a progressive improvement in
operative mortality even in the hands of Warren himself [57] suggests that
the best results will certainly be achieved by those who are performing the
procedure regularly. Nevertheless, the operation can reasonably take its
place alongside more conventional procedures in the management of variceal bleeding.

5. The operation is unsuitable as an emergency procedure – *myth*. The higher
mortality in patients treated as an emergency is merely a reflection of the increased mortality for patients of this type undergoing any form of shunting
[61].

6. The Warren shunt does not improve thrombocytopaenia – *myth*. although
not reviewed in this paper, there is now adequate evidence from most of the
studies cited that both thrombocytopaenia and leukopaenia improve significantly, and are often associated with a significant decrease in spleen size
[60]. This emphasizes that splenectomy is rarely necessary for hypersplenism in patients with portal hypertension.

The one major issue which has not been addressed in this discussion is that of
the relative place of shunting, whether selective or total, since the widespread
availability of endoscopic sclerotherapy for long-term control of variceal
bleeding. This is a much more difficult question, and not part of the remit of
this chapter. However, it is important to note that Warren's group have recently published the results of a prospective randomized controlled trial of DSRS
versus endoscopic sclerotherapy [51]. Their conclusions were that sclerotherapy does produce a significantly improved survival in the management of
variceal bleeding, and also does not suffer from the inevitable deterioration of
liver function which follows the shunting procedure. There was in fact a higher
re-bleeding rate in this trial in patients treated by sclerotherapy compared with
DSRS: however, the structure of the trial was such that patients who were de-

344

fined as having 'failure of sclerotherapy' crossed over into the DSRS group. While Warren and his colleagues commented that DSRS was a valuable and highly successful back-up procedure for uncontrolled re-bleeding, other groups using sclerotherapy as their primary method of management would criticize this early recourse to surgery, favouring further intensive injection sclerotherapy as the method of control for patients with breakthrough bleeding (D. Westaby, personal communication). I think it is necessary to regard the choice of therapy between sclerosis and shunting as a question which is still open, and we must await the results of further controlled trials before we have a definitive answer.

References

1. Vidal ME: Traitment chirurgical des ascites dans les cirrhoses du foie. XVIth Cong Fran de Chir 16: 244, 1903 (See reference 2.)
2. Donovan AJ, Covey PC: Early history of the portacaval shunt in humans. Surg Gynec Obstet 147: 423–430, 1978
3. Whipple AO: Problem of portal hypertension in relation to hepatosplenopathies. Ann Surg 122: 449–475, 1945
4. McDermott Jr WV, Adams RD: Episodic stupor associated with an Eck fistula in the human, with particular reference to the metabolism of ammonia. J Clin Invest 33: 1–9, 1954
5. Hubbard Jr TB: Carcinoma of the head of the pancreas: resection of the portal vein and portacaval shunt. Ann Surg 147: 935–944, 1958
6. Blakemore AH: Portacaval shunting for portal hypertension. Surg Gynecol Obstet 94: 443–454, 1952
7. Sherlock S, Summerskill WHJ, White LP, Phear EA: Portal-systemic encephalopathy: neurological complications of liver disease. Lancet ii: 453–457, 1954
8. Thompson EN, Williams R, Sherlock S: Liver function in extrahepatic portal hypertension. Lancet ii: 1352–1356, 1964
9. Resnick RH, Chalmers TC, Ishihara AM, Garceau AJ, Callon AD, Schimmel EM, O'Hara ET, The Boston Interhospital Liver Group: A controlled study of prophylactic portacaval shunts: A final report. Ann Int Med 70: 675–688, 1969
10. Warren WD, Zeppa R, Fomon JJ: Selective trans-splenic decompression of gastroesophageal varices by distal splenorenal shunt. Ann Surg 166: 437–455, 1967
11. Hassama: Gastroesophageal decongestion and splenectomy in the treatment of oesophageal varices in bilharzial cirrhosis: further studies with a report on 355 operations. Surgery 61: 169–176, 1967
12. Resnick RH, Iber FL, Ishihara AM, Chalmers TC, Zimmerman H, The Boston Interhospital Liver Group: A controlled study of the therapeutic portacaval shunt. Gastroenterology 67: 843–857, 1974
13. Rueff B, Degos F, Degos J-D, Maillard J-N, Prandi D, Sicot J, Sicot C, Fauvert R, Benhamou J-P: Controlled study of therapeutic portacaval shunt in alcoholic cirrhosis. Lancet i: 655–659, 1976
14. Reynolds TB, Donovan AJ, Mikkelsen WP, Redeker AG, Turrill FL, Weiner JM: Results of a 12-year randomized trial of portacaval shunt in patients with alcoholic liver disease and bleeding varices. Gastroenterology 80: 1005–1011, 1981

15. Child CG, Turcotte JG: Surgery and portal hypertension. Major Probl Clin Surg 1: 1–85, 1964
16. Campbell DP, Parker DE, Anagnostopoulos CE: Survival prediction in portocaval shunts: a computerized statistical analysis. Am J Surg 126: 748–751, 1973
17. Pugh RNH, Murray-Lyon IM, Dawson JL, Pietroni MC, Williams R: Transection of the oesophagus for bleeding oesophageal varices. Br J Surg 60: 646–648, 1973
18. Starzl TE, Putnam CW, Porter KA, Halgrimson CG, Corman J, Brown BI, Gotlin RW, Rodgerson DO, Greene HL: Portal diversion for the treatment of glycogen storage disease in humans. Ann Surg 178: 525–539, 1973
19. Starzl TE, Porter KA, Francavilla A: The Eck fistula in animals and humans. Curr Probl Surg 20: 688–745, 1983
20. Warren WD, Millikan WJ, Smith RB III, Rypins EB, Henderson JM, Salam AA, Hersh T, Galambos JT, Faraj BA: Noncirrhotic portal vein thrombosis. Physiology before and after shunts. Ann Surg 192 (3): 341–349
21. Fonkalsrud EW, Myers NA, Robinson MJ: Management of extrahepatic portal hypertension in children. Ann Surg 180: 487–493, 1974
22. Alvarez F, Bernard D, Brunelle F: Portal obstruction in children II. Results of portosystemic shunts. J Pediatr 103: 703–707, 1983
23. Mikkelsen WP, Edmondson HA, Peters RL, Redeker AG, Reynolds TB: Extra- and intrahepatic portal hypertension without cirrhosis (hepatoportal sclerosis). Ann Surg 162: 602–620, 1965
24. Voorhees Jr AB, Chaitman E, Schneider S, Nicholson JF, Kornfeld DS, Price JB: Portasystemic encephalopathy in the noncirrhotic patient. Effect of portal-systemic shunting. Arch Surg 107: 659–663, 1973
25. Nel CJC, Honiball PJ, van Wyk FAK: Portal hypertension in schistosomiasis. S Afr J Surg 12: 233–239, 1974
26. Malt RA: Portasystemic venous shunts (in two parts). New Engl J Med 295: 24–29, and 80–86, 1976
27. McDermott Jr WV: Evaluation of the haemodynamics of portal hypertension in the selection of patients for shunt surgery. Ann Surg 176: 449–456, 1972
28. Reynolds TB: The role of haemodynamic measurements in portosystemic shunt surgery. Arch Surg 108: 276–281, 1974
29. Bismuth H, Franco D, Hepp J: Portal systemic shunt in hepatic cirrhosis: does the type of shunt decisively influence the clinical result? Ann Surg 179: 209–218, 1974
30. Reichle FA, Owen OE: Haemodynamic patterns in human hepatic cirrhosis. A prospective randomized study of the haemodynamic sequelae of distal splenorenal (Warren) and mesocaval shunts. Ann Surg 140: 523–534, 1979
31. Adson MA, van Heerden JA, Illstrup DM: The distal splenorenal shunt. Arch Surg 119: 609–614, 1984
32. Drapanas T: Interposition mesocaval shunt for treatment of portal hypertension. Ann Surg 176: 435–448, 1972
33. Mulcare RJ, Halleran D, Gardine R: Experience with 49 consecutive Dacron interposition mesocaval shunts. A unified approach to portasystemic decompression procedures. Am J Surg 147: 393–399, 1984
34. Reznick RK, Langer B, Taylor BR, Lossing A, Blendis LM, Colapinto RF: Results and hemodynamic changes after interposition mesocaval shunt. Surgery 95: 275–279, 1984
35. Stipa S, Ziparo V, Anza M, Fabrini G, Lupino R: A randomized controlled trial of mesentericocaval shunt with autologous jugular vein. Surg Gynec Obstet 153: 353–356, 1981
36. Fulenwider JT, Nordlinger BM, Millikan WJ, Sones PJ, Warren WD: Portal pseudoperfusion. An angiographic illusion. Ann Surg 189: 257–268, 1979
37. Burchell AR, Moreno AH, Panke WF, Nealon Jr TF: Haemodynamic variables and prognosis following portocaval shunts. Surg Gynec Obstet 138: 359–369, 1974

346

38. Burchell AR, Moreno AH, Panke WF, Nealon Jr TF: Hepatic artery flow improvement after portacaval shunt: a single haemodynamic clinical correlate. Ann Surg 184: 289–302, 1976
39. Maillard JN, Rueff B, Prandi D, Sicot C: Hepatic arterialization and portacaval shunt in hepatic cirrhosis: an assessment. Arch Surg 108: 315–320, 1974
40. Rous P, Larimore LD: Relation of the portal blood to liver maintenance; a demonstration of liver atrophy conditional on compensation. J Exp Med 31: 609–632, 1920
41. Mann FC: The portal circulation and restoration of the liver after partial removal. Surgery 8: 225–238, 1940
42. Price Jr JB, McCullough W, Peterson L, Britton MD, Voorhees Jr AB: Increased intestinal absorption resulting from portal-systemic shunting in the dog and man. Surg Forum 17: 367–368, 1968
43. Warren WD, Millikan Jr WJ, Wisgut L, Kutner M, Smith III RB, Fulenwider JT, Salam AA, Galambos JJ: Ten years portal hypertensive surgery at Emory. Results and new perspectives. Ann Surg 195: 530–534, 1982
44. Maillard JN, Flamant YM, Hay JM, Chandler JG: Selectivity of the distal splenorenal shunt. Surgery 86: 663–671, 1979
45. Rikkers LF, Rudman D, Galambos JT, Fulenwider JT, Millikan WJ, Kutner M, Smith III RB, Salam AA, Jones Jr PJ, Warren WD: A randomized, controlled trial of the distal splenorenal shunt. Ann Surg 188: 271–282, 1978
46. Warren WD: Control of variceal bleeding. Reassessment of rationale. Am J Surg 145: 8–16, 1983
47. Henderson JM, Millikan WJ, Wright-Bacon L, Kutner MH, Warren WD: Hemodynamic differences between alcoholic and nonalcoholic cirrhotics following distal splenorenal shunt – effect on survival? Ann Surg 198: 325–334, 1983
48. Raju S: A modification of the Warren Shunt. World J Surg 6: 450–457, 1982
49. Warren WD, Millikan WJ: Selective transsplenic decompression procedure: changes in technique after 300 cases. Contemp Surg 18: 11–29, 1981
50. Mehigan DG, Zuidema GD, Cameron JL: The incidence of shunt occlusion following portosystemic decompression. Surg Gynec Obstet 150: 661–663, 1980
51. Warren WD, Henderson JM, Millikan WJ, Galambos JT, Brooks WS, Riepe SP, Salam AA, Kutner MH: Distal splenorenal shunt versus endoscopic sclerotherapy for long-term management of variceal bleeding. Preliminary report of a prospective, randomized trial. Ann Surg 203: 454–462, 1986
52. Maillard JN, Lacaine F: The French experience with shunt procedures. In: Westaby D, McDougall BRD, Williams R (eds) Variceal Bleeding. Pitman, London, 1982, pp 113–119
53. Villamil F, Redeker A, Reynolds T, Yellin A: A controlled trial of distal splenorenal and portacaval shunts. Hepatology 1: 557, 1981
54. Fischer JE, Bower RH, Atamian S, Welling R: Comparison of distal and proximal splenorenal shunts: a randomized prospective trial. Ann Surg 194: 531–544, 1981
55. Conn HO, Resnick RH, Grace ND, Atterbury CE, Horst D, Groszmann RJ, Gazmuri P, Gusberg RJ, Phayer B, Berk D, Wright SC, Zollman R, Tilson DM, McDermott WV, Cohen JA, Kerstein M, Toole AL, Maselli JP, Razvi S, Ishihara A, Stern H, Trey C, O'Hara ET, Widrich W, Aisenberg H, Stansell HC, Zinny M: Distal splenorenal shunt versus portal-systemic shunt: current status of a controlled trial. Hepatology 1: 151–160, 1981
56. Langer B, Taylor BR, Mackenzie DR, Gilas T, Stone RM, Blendis L: Further report of a prospective randomized trial comparing distal splenorenal shunt with end-to-side portacaval shunt: an analysis of encephalopathy, survival, and quality of life. Gastroenterology 88: 424–429, 1985
57. Galambos JT, Millikan WJ, Henderson JM, Smith RB, Warren WD: Ten years of shunt surgery: the current status of the selective distal splenorenal shunt. In: Westaby D, McDougall BRD, Williams R (eds) Variceal Bleeding. Pitman, London, 1982, pp 104–112

58. Millikan WJ, Warren WD, Henderson JM, Smith RB III, Salam AA, Galambos JT, Kutner MH, Keen JH: The Emory prospective randomized trial: selective versus nonselective shunt to control variceal bleeding. Ten-year follow-up. Ann Surg 201: 712–722

59. Conn HO, Lieberthal MM: The hepatic coma syndromes and lactulose. Williams and Willkins, Baltimore, 1979

60. Marni A, Trosji C, Belli L: Distal splenorenal shunt. Haemodynamic advantage over total shunt and influence on clinical status, hepatic function and hypersplenism. Am J Surg 142: 372–376, 1981

61. Potts III JR, Henderson JM, Millikan WJ, Warren WD: Emergency distal splenorenal shunts for variceal hemorrhage refractory to nonoperative control. Am J Surg 148: 813–816, 1984

21. Use of BCAA enriched nutritional regimens in hepatic failure and sepsis: facts or fancy

P.B. SOETERS and J.P. VENTE

Introduction

The past two decennia have witnessed a surge of interest in artificial nutrition. The development of nutrients, that could be mixed and administered intravenously without untoward side effects, or that could be administered via small bore catheters into the gut has greatly improved our ability to feed patients that otherwise would have become severely depleted, either because the gut could not resorb nutrients sufficiently, or because the gut was inaccessible via the oral route. At the same time this development has greatly stimulated interest and research in areas like intermediary metabolism, immunology and nutritional assessment, in the laboratory, in healthy controls and in patients. Especially during the last decennium artificial enteral or parenteral feeds have become widely available. In the area of all three basic nutrients a large array of products were develoρed that could be administered safely, had proven to have nutritional value, and that could be tailored to the needs of the individual patient.

New carbohydrates and polyalcohols have been employed as energy source. Lipid emulsions have been proven to be safe and useful as energy source and in addition as a source of essential fatty acids. Furthermore the quality and nutritional value of nitrogen in artificial nutrition was improved. Originally the nitrogen source employed in parenteral nutrition consisted of hydrolysates of different proteins like lactalbumin, casein, etc. The disadvantage of these hydrolysates was that they contained small peptides up to 20% and could potentially cause allergic reactions, and that the AA composition was unpredictable. A first development was that cristalline AA solutions were produced that within limits could be composed according to the views developed in the past years concerning optimal nutritional value, etc. Such solutions contained no peptides, caused fewer allergic reactions, and had a more stable composition than the hydrolysates. A later development consisted of the composition of specific AA mixtures, presumably to tailor the needs of specific disease states.

Especially those disease states are involved in which handling of nitrogen is disturbed in some way like renal failure, hepatic failure, sepsis, severe trauma, etc. For reasons to be described later on in this chapter the addition of extra branched chain amino acids (BCAA) to the AA mixture has received much attention. For theoretical reasons this might be of benefit especially in patients suffering from hepatic failure or in patients suffering from severe sepsis or trauma. Parenteral or eneteral nutrition mixtures containing extra BCAA have been used in several randomized trials both in hepatic failure and sepsis/trauma. In this chapter the rationale for BCAA enrichment of the nutritional regime in specific disease states will be discussed and the results of trials at hand, in which BCAA enrichment was employed, will be evaluated.

Biochemistry of BCAA

BCAA(leucine, isoleucine, valine) are essential AA which characteristically have a branched carbon chain. Because the liver lacks BCAA transaminase which catalyzes the first step in the degradation of BCAA, the BCAA relie for their degradation on peripheral tissues, predominantly muscle and adipose tissue. All other essential AA (phenylalanine, methionine, lysine, threonine and tryptophan) are broken down in the liver. Although twenty different AA are biologically active in man, the three BCAA constitute up to one third of all body protein. Because of the ability of peripheral tissues to degrade the essential BCAA and because of their large share in total body protein the BCAA have been in the center of interest during the last fifteen years.

Rationale for BCAA enrichment

Alternative energy source

BCAA have for several hypothetical reasons during the last decade been considered to furnish fuel in peripheral tissues under circumstances where ordinary fuel like carbohydrate and fat was supposedly lacking. Under circumstances of severe stress, trauma or sepsis glucose intolerance is well documented. Furthermore high insulin levels prevailing under these circumstances due to their antilipolytic effect may limit the utilization of fat as a fuel source. Therefore both carbohydrate and fat may be less available to cover energy requirements. Due to the ability of the peripheral tissues to degrade BCAA these AA might then serve as alternative energy source. Objections can be raised against this hypothesis.
1. Glucose intolerance although well documented during trauma/sepsis only

implies that more insulin is needed to metabolize the same amount of glucose. It does not imply that glucose can not be utilized at all.

2. Although theoretically hyperinsulinaemia may inhibit lipolysis several independent reports in the literature have revealed that fat can be well degraded during severe trauma/sepsis and utilized to cover energy needs [1].

3. It can be calculated that if indeed BCAA serve as alternative fuel source not more than approximately 5% of total energy requirements can be covered by the degradation of BCAA.

4. Other hypotheses have been put forward to explain accelerated peripheral proteolysis in severe disease states. Clowes has suggested that peripheral proteolysis serves to furnish AA that in the liver can be used as building stones for proteins that are operative in the defense against trauma/sepsis/stress [2].

Effects on protein synthesis

In the laboratory it has been repeatedly demonstrated that BCAA and especially leucine stimulates protein synthesis *in vitro* [3]. Furthermore BCKA (branched chain keto acids result after transamination of BCAA: the first step in the degradation of BCAA) have been demonstrated to inhibit BCAA degradation, equally *in vitro*. No convincing experimental evidence has ever been put forward however that net protein gain can be achieved *in vivo* after enrichment of the diet with BCAA in any form or quantity.

Normalization of plasma AA profile

Originally a distorted plasma AA profile (low plasma BCAA; high plasma aromatic AA) present in hepatic failure has been linked with hepatic encephalopathy [4]. All neutral AA share a common transport system into the brain so that a distorted plasma AA profile is reflected in the brain. There the AAA serve as precursors for neurotransmitters so that increased AAA transport into the brain ultimately may result in a distorted neurotransmitter profile and subsequently in encephalopathy. BCAA enrichment of the diet might normalize abnormal plasma AA profiles and improve hepatic encephalopathy [5].

On the other hand it is possible that in severe sepsis/trauma or hepatic failure, metabolic changes induced by these severe disease states also include an amino acid pattern which is less optimal for protein synthesis. Normalization of the plasma AA profile and consequently (hopefully) also normalization of the composition of body AA pools may then theoretically optimize the precursor pattern for protein synthesis and improve nitrogen balance [6].

Effect on ammonia levels

It has been demonstrated that infusion of ammonium salts results in a depression of plasma BCAA levels [7]. Alternatively infusion of BCAA has been suggested to decrease plasma ammonia levels. BCAA might furnish the amino group with which α-ketoglutarate yields glutamic acid which in peripheral tissues (adipose tissue, muscle) can take up ammonia. The resulting glutamine is then released in the circulation where it is relatively non toxic despite its high concentration (500 μmol/L).

Problems in trials to demonstrate the efficacy of BCAA

The difficulty to demonstrate the efficacy of BCAA enrichment in patients either with hepatic failure, or with sepsis/trauma chiefly arises from the fact that nutritional repletion in such patients can at best have only a minor influence on outcome.

Outcome will be chiefly determined by progression of the underlying disease or by the succes of primary treatment modalities such as stabilization of fractures, excision of damaged tissue, relief of sepsis, etc.

Therefore to detect the effect of a secondary treatment modality like BCAA enrichment during nutritional repletion large numbers of patients are required, even more so because such patients vary greatly and generally suffer from complex problems. Another difficulty is what control group should be used. In the trials to be discussed control groups were used that received no nutritional support, or that received isonitrogenous nutritional support of conventional AA composition. Against all these control groups valid criticisms can be raised. To meet these criticisms a four or five armed trial should be undertaken. Due to the secondary nature of BCAA enrichment as treatment modality, the complex nature of the patient material under study and the requirement to include several control groups, such a trial is virtually impossible. To settle the issue of efficacy of BCAA enrichment in liver disease and sepsis/trauma we have therefore to rely on trials which are always too small to furnish a definitive and convincing answer. Studies in liver disease are generally carried out in patients admitted to surgical or medical wards, or to intensive care units, with chronic hepatic failure, temporarily aggravated by superimposed illness, operation, drugs, etc. The result of nutritional support in such patients is very difficult to measure, firstly because the duration of such trials is by necessity very short (approximately one week), and secondly because succesful abolition of the precipitating factor like intercurrent sepsis, diuretics, etc., in itself influences parameters that are used to assess nutritional state (e.g. plasma proteins). Nitrogen balances measured under such circumstances are liable to errors because they have to be corrected for changes in body water, urea accumulation or loss, administration of blood and blood products, insensible losses, etc. Finally for theoretical reasons BCAA enrichment might have a beneficial effect on mental state, more as the consequence of a pharmacological action, than of nutritional repletion [4]. Such a pharmacological effect may become evident after relatively short time periods (1–2 days) and is therefore the more likely beneficial result to be detected in short term trials.

BCAA enrichment in hepatic failure and hepatic encephalopathy

Although some twenty anecdotal or randomized series have been presented as oral presentation, in abstract form or as full publication only five studies, that have employed a randomized set up, have appeared as complete publications in the literature. We will consider only these five studies in this review [8–12].

In these studies chronic liver patients are described suffering from acute deterioration of mental state. By necessity the duration of these studies could never be long (7–10 days). As discussed in the preceding section the aims of nutritional repletion and BCAA enrichment in patients with hepatic failure are threefold:
1. Improvement of liver function, morbidity, mortality.
2. Nutritional repletion.
3. Improvement of hepatic encephalopathy.
In Table 1 the published trials are listed including the form of nutritional support. It will be appreciated that not one study is identical with anyother study, which is also evident from the amounts of protein and calories employed in these studies.

Morbidity and mortality (Table 2)

Morbidity scores are rarely mentioned in the trials under review. Mortality rates are not significantly different between control groups and the groups receiving BCAA enrichment. Only the US multicenter study shows significantly improved survival already during the study in the BCAA enriched group. For reasons mentioned earlier this would suggest that BCAA enrichment is not just a superior method to replete liver patients nutritionally thereby exerting a beneficial modulating effect on the result of primary treatment but may act as pharmacological treatment, waking patients up, thereby reducing complications secondary to the comatose state, or even ameliorating hepatic function. It is a pity however that there is no indication in the paper itself that this is the case, nor is there in the other studies which do not confirm improved survival. Therefore as yet there is no convincing evidence that BCAA enrichment has a

Table 1.

Author	Nutritional treatment groups (BCAA %)	Nutritional regime		
		AA	glucose (calories)	fat (calories)
Rossi Fanelli 1982	1) Lactulose + Dextrose 20%	–	1600/24 hr	–
	2) BCAA + Dextrose 20%	56 g/24 hr	1600/24 hr	–
Fiaccadori 1984	1) Lactulose + Dextrose 30%	–	2500/24 hr	–
	2) AA (BCAA 45%) + Dextrose 30%	0.8–1 g/kg/24 hr	2500/24 hr	–
	3) Lactulose + AA (BCAA 45%) + Dextrose 30%	0.8–1 g/kg/24 hr	2500/24 hr	–
Michel 1985	1) Glucose/fat + Conv. AA (BCAA 20%)	60 g/24 hr	1060/24 hr	540/24 hr
	2) Glucose/fat + AA (BCAA 45%)	60 g/24 hr	1060/24 hr	540/24 hr
Wahren 1983	1) Glucose/fat + Dextrose 5%	–	20 Cal/kg/24 hr	15/kg/24 hr
	2) Glucose/fat + Dextrose 5% BCAA	40 g/24 hr	20 Cal/kg/24 hr	15/kg/24 hr
Cerra 1985	1) Neomycin + Dextrose 25%	–	27 Cal/kg/24 hr	–
	2) AA (BCAA 38%) + Dextrose 25%	1.1 g/kg/day	27 Cal/kg/24 hr	–

beneficial effect on survival in chronic liver patients suffering from acute deterioration of mental state.

Nutritional repletion

Very few data are available concerning the efficacy of nutritional repletion in the trials under review. It is not to be expected however that improvement of nutritional parameters (anthropometric, plasma protein, immunological) can be obtained within 10 days. This may be the reason that they are not mentioned in most studies and that only nitrogen balances are recorded. Only the US multicenter trial records a clear improvement in nitrogen balance in the group receiving extra BCAA (+0.8g N/24hr in BCAA treated group versus −8.6g N/24hr in control group). All other studies either do not mention nitrogen balance [8, 9, 11], or do not show a benefit [10]. It should be noted that only in the study of Michel [10] a control group received isonitrogenous amounts of AA of conventional composition.

Hepatic encephalopathy (Table 2)

It is clear from the trials under review that BCAA enrichment does not further deteriorate hepatic encephalopathy and that arousal was as fast or faster and in a larger proportion of patients than in control groups receiving conventional treatment (generally 20–25% dextrose + neomycin/lactulose). It also appears that BCAA enrichment allows quantities of protein to be administered from 0.6–1.1g AA/kg/24hr. It is bothering however that in only one study a control group received isonitrogenous amounts of a conventional AA mixture. In this study no differences were observed between the two AA mixtures [10]. It should therefore be concluded that parenteral AA mixtures, administered up to 1.1g AA/kg/24hr allow a wake up response which is a favourable or better than with conventional treatment (hypertonic dextrose, neomycin/lactulose).

Table 2. Mortality from hepatic failure and recovery from encephalopathy to grade 0–1.

Author	Mortality (%)		Recovery HE (%)	
	Control	BCAA	Control	BCAA
Rossi Fanelli	29	23	47	70
Fiaccadori	?	?	62	94
Michel	25	30	25	35
Wahren	20	40	48	56
Cerra	55	17	17	53

It is not certain however that this is due to the BCAA content of the AA mixture.

Conclusions

In conclusion it is unlikely and indeed it has not been demonstrated in the studies published that BCAA enrichment improves survival from acute hepatic encephalopathy, and nutritional state in chronic hepatic failure. It is likely that parenteral administration of BCAA enriched glucose (− AA) mixtures improves mental state as well or better than conventional types of treatment. It further allows administration of amounts of AA up to 1.1g/kg/24hr. It is not demonstrated however that this is specifically due to the BCAA content of the mixtures.

BCAA enrichment in sepsis/trauma

Similar as with hepatic failure the aims of BCAA enrichment are threefold:
1. Improvement of morbidity and mortality.
2. Nutritional repletion.
3. Improvement of mental state.
In recent years many studies concerning the efficacy of trauma/stress have been carried out. In this review only prospective randomized trials will be considered (Table 3).

Most studies deal with patients with severe stress and/or sepsis because of polytrauma or after major operations. The number of patients in all studies is relatively small with the exception of the Maastricht study (101 patients). Protein intake varied from 1 to 1.5g/kg/day. Non-protein calories were given glucose only (30–35 Cal/kg/day) or in combination with fat (15–50% of non-protein calories). Freund [13] compared a 5% dextrose solution with different BCAA solutions in 5% dextrose while the other studies compared AA solutions containing different BCAA concentrations (15–100%).

Morbidity and mortality (Table 4)

As discussed earlier it is not to be expected that morbidity and mortality will be influenced within the short time period of the studies mentioned. Indeed in the studies which mention clinical outcome no differences in outcome between treatment groups occurred.

Table 3. Types of nutritional support and BCAA content.

Author		Nutritional support				Nutrition treatment groups, BCAA %
		N/Cal	Protein g/kg/24 hr	Glucose Cal/kg/24 hr	Fat Cal/kg/24 hr	
Freund	1	–	0	6–8	–	0%
1979	2	1:40	1.0	6–8	–	22%
	3	1:40	1.0	6–8	–	35%
	4	1:40	1.0	6–8	–	100%
Cerra	1	1:215	1	35	–	15.5%
1982	2	1:215	1	35	–	50%
Cerra	1	1:190	1.0	30	–	16% (0.15 g/kg)
1983	2	1:150	1.5	30	7	20% (0.30 g/kg)
	3	1:190	1.0	30	–	50% (0.50 g/kg)
	4	1:150	1.5	30	7	50% (0.70 g/kg)
Nuwer	1	1:150	1.5	30	7	24%
1983	2	1:150	1.5	30	7	45%
Cerra	1	1:150	1.5	30	7	24%
1984	2	1:150	1.5	30	7	45%
Bower	1	1:150	1.5	28	9	25%
1986	2	1:150	1.5	28	9	45% Valine ↑
	3	1:150	1.5	28	9	45% Leucine ↑
Lundholm	1	1:240	1	20	20	100%
1986	2	1:240	1	20	20	38% (only EAA)
	3	1:240	1	20	20	15%
Maastricht	1	1:200	1.12	28	5	18% (0.19 g/kg)
1986	2	1:200	1.12	28	5	50% (0.56 g/kg)

Nutritional repletion (Table 4)

It has already been mentioned on page 335 that it is difficult to obtain improvement in nutritional state within 7–10 days. If this would be achieved it is difficult to measure because most established parameters react slowly, but in addition can also be influenced by the disease itself. Recovery from illness achieved by non nutritional means may therefore also result in improvement of parameters generally used for nutritional assessment. Endeavours to establish improvement in nutritional status have for these reasons been limited to measurement of short half life plasma proteins synthesized by the liver, and of nitrogen balance and 3-methylhistidine excretion.

With the exception of Lundholm [14], all studies report an improved nitrogen balance when BCAA containing solutions are used.

Significantly increased nitrogen balances in BCAA enriched solutions are reported by Cerra [15–17], Nuwer [18] and Bower [19]. Lundholm finds no im-

Table 4. Nitrogen balance, plasma proteins, immune status, morbidity and mortality.

Author		BCAA %	N-Balance during treatment	N-Balance compared other groups	N-Balance cumulative	3-Meth. hist. excretion	Plasma proteins	Immune status	Morbidity/mortality
Freund 1979	1	0	↓				↓ (A1b)		no diff.
	2	22	↑	↑↑ (gr 1)			↓ (A1b)		
	3	35	=	↑↑ (gr 1)			↓ (A1b)		
	4	100	↑ (day 6)	↑↑ (gr 1)			↓ (A1b)		
Cerra 1982	1	15.5		↑↑ (gr 1; day 3)	–	no diff.			not studied
	2	50.0			–	no diff.			
Cerra 1981	1	16	↑		–	→			not studied
	2	20	↑	↑↑ (gr 1; day 4)	–	→			
	3	50	↑		–	→			
	4	50	↑	↑↑ (gr 1, 2, 3; day7)	–	→			
Nuwer 1983	1	24			no diff.	no diff.	↑↑ (Ly;C; DHC)		no diff.
	2	45		↑↑ (gr 1)		no diff.			
Cerra 1984	1	24		↑↑ (gr 1)		→	↑↑ (Ly;C; DHC)		not studied
	2	45		↑↑ (gr 1; day 6, 7)	↑↑ (gr1)	→	↑ (transf; PAlb; RBP)		
Bower 1986	1	25				→	=		no diff.
	2	45 (val)		↑↑ (gr 1)	↑ (gr2)	→	↑ (transf; PAlb) ↑↑ RBP		
	3	45 (leu)		↑↑ (gr 2)	↑ (gr 2)				
Lundholm 1986	1	100	} no diff.		} no diff.				not studied
	2	38		↓↓ (gr 2)					
	3	15		↓↓ (gr 2)					
Maastricht 1986	1	18	↑	moderate stress	} no diff.				no diff.
	2	50	↑	severe stress					

provement in N-balance, independent of the BCAA solution used, when the nitrogen intake from blood products was not accounted for. The urinary 3-methylhistidine excretion, which is considered as a parameter for muscle degradation, decreases in most studies. Differences in primary 3-methylhistidine excretion between the various BCAA solutions are not found. This suggests that muscle proteolysis is not influenced. Immune function was investigated by Nuwer [18] and Cerra [17]. Both found a significant increase in absolute lymphocyte count and delayed cutaneous hypersensitivity in the group of patients receiving BCAA enriched nutrition. Bower [19] and Cerra [17] found a significant increase in short half life plasma proteins like transferrin and prealbumin.

In these studies relatively few patients are included and not much information is furnished regarding the clinical characteristics of the population under study. It is therefore impossible to ascertain whether the improvements observed are due to BCAA enrichment or are the result of clinical differences between groups.

Improvements of mental state

Although BCAA enrichment and improvement in mental state have generally been linked with liver disease some reports mention improvement of mental state with BCAA enrichment also in patients with sepsis/trauma, who indeed frequently suffer from metabolic encephalopathy. Such patients often exhibit BCAA/AAA ratio's between 2 and 1.5 but never reach values around 1, encountered in hepatic encephalopathy. Not much systemic work is done in this respect, nor is the pathogenesis of septic encephalopathy clear.

Conclusion

For several theoretical reasons there is a rationale to enrich the AA part of parenteral or enteral nutritional regimens in patients with hepatic failure, or sepsis/trauma. In this chapter only short term (5–10 days) prospective randomized studies are reviewed employing parenteral BCAA enrichment in both patient groups mentioned above. Although a BCAA enriched AA composition in the nutritional regimen may be of higher biological and nutritional value under circumstances of severe disease and liver failure the length of the studies does not allow major changes to become visible. In addition the result of nutritional assessment is strongly influenced by the succes with which the disease itself can be influenced by primary (non nutritional) treatment. This also explains why it is difficult to demonstrate a clinical benefit regarding morbidity and mortality: nutritional repletion as a secondary treatment modality can only have a modulating effect on outcome, and in that instance only after longer time periods. Indeed no clinical benefit has been demonstrated as yet. There is a suggestion in some studies however that in trauma/stress nitrogen balances are improved and synthesis of short half life plasma proteins is stimulated. In liver disease some studies suggest that AA administration up to 1.1 g/kg/24 hr relieves hepatic encephalopathy at least as well or better as conventional treatment (glucose 20–25%, neomycin, lactulose). Due to the nature of the randomized trials it is not certain that this is specifically the result of the BCAA content.

References

1. Carpentier YA, Askanazi J, Elwyn DH, Kinney JL: Effects of hypercaloric glucose infusion on lipid metabolism in injury and sepsis. J Trauma 9: 649, 1979
2. Clowes GHA, George BC, Villee CA, et al.: Muscle proteolysis induced by a circulating peptide in patients with sepsis or trauma. N Engl J Med 308: 545, 1983
3. Buse MG, Reid SS: Leucine, a possible regulator of protein turnover in muscle. J Clin Invest 56: 1250, 1975
4. Fischer JE, Baldessarini RJ: False neurotransmitters and hepatic coma. Lancet 2: 75, 1971
5. Fischer JE, Rosen HM, Ebeid AM, James JH, Keane JM, Soeters PB: The effect of normalization of plasma amino acids on hepatic encephalopathy in man. Surgery 80: 77–91, 1976
6. Soeters PB: Amino acid metabolism in liver disease: nutritional aspects. In: Holm E and Kasper H (eds) Metabolism and Nutrition in Liver Disease. Proceedings of the 41st Falk Symposium, Freiburg im Breisgau, West Germany, June 15–16, 1984, MTP Press Ltd, pp 57–66
7. Leweling H, Holm E, Staedt U, Striebel J-P, Tschepe A: Intra- and extracellular amino acid concentrations in ammonium-infused rats. Evidence that hyperammonemia reduces BCAA levels. In: Kleinberger G, Ferenci P, Riederer P, Thaler H: Advances in Hepatic Encephalopathy and Urea Cycle Diseases. Proceedings 5th International Symposium on Ammonia, Semmering, Austria, May 16–19, 1984, Karger, pp 552–555
8. Rossi-Fanelli F, Riggio O, Cangiano C, et al.: Branched chain amino acids vs lactulose in the treatment of hepatic coma: A controlled study. Dig Dis Sci 27: 929–935, 1982
9. Fiaccadori F, Ghinelli F, Pedretti G, et al.: Branched-chain enriched amino acid solutions in the treatment of hepatic encephalopathy: a controlled trial. Ital J Gastroenterol 17: 5, 1985
10. Michel H, Pomier-Layrargues G, Duhamel O, Lacombe B, Cuilleret G, Bellet H: Intravenous infusion of ordinary and modified amino acid solutions in the management of hepatic encephalopathy. In: Capocaccia L, Fischer JE, Rossi Fanelli F (eds) Hepatic Encephalopathy in Chronic Liver Disease, Plenum Press, 1984, pp 323–333
11. Wahren J, Denis J, Desurmont P, Eriksson LS, et al.: Is intravenous administration of branched chain amino acids effective in the treatment of hepatic encephalopathy? A multicenter study. Hepatology 3: 475–480, 1983
12. Cerra FB, Cheung NK, Fischer JE, et al.: Disease-specific amino acid infusion (FO80) in hepatic encephalopathy: a prospective, randomized, double-blind, controlled trial. JPEN 9: 288–295, 1985
13. Freund H, Hoover Jr HC, Atamian S, Fischer JE: Infusion of the branched chain amino acids in postoperative patients. Ann Surg 190: 18–23, 1979
14. Lundholm K, Bennegard K, Wickström I, Lindmark L: Is it possible to evaluate the efficacy of amino acid solutions after major surgical procedures or accidental injuries? Evaluation in a randomized and prospective study. JPEN 10: 29–33, 1986

15. Cerra FB, Upson D, Angelico R, Wiles Ch III, Lyons J, Faulkenbach L, Paysinger J: Branched chains support postoperative protein synthesis. Surgery 92: 192–198, 1982
16. Cerra FB, Mazaski J, Teasley K, Nuwer N, Lysne J, Shronts E, Konstantinides F: Nitrogen solution in critically ill patients is proportional to the branched chain amino acid load. Crit Care Med 11: 775–778, 1983
17. Cerra FB, Mazaski J, Chute E, Nuwer N, Teasly K, Lysne J, Shronts E, Konstantinides F: Branched chain metabolic support. Ann Surg 199: 286–291, 1984
18. Nuwer N, Cerra FB, Shronts E, Lysne J, Feasley K, Konstantinides F: Does modified amino acid total parenteral nutrition alter immune response in high level surgical stress. JPEN 7: 521–524, 1983
19. Bower R, Muggia-Sullam M, Vallgren S, Hurst J, Kern K, Lafrance R, Fisher J: Branched chain amino acid enriched solutions in the septic patient. Ann Surg 203: 13–20, 1986

22. Pancreas transplantation

G. TYDÉN and C.G. GROTH

Insulin dependent diabetes mellitus ranks as one of the major disease entities in the world. It is widespread in industrialized countries as well as in developing countries. In spite of the considerable improvements in conventional diabetes therapy during the past few years, severe secondary complications still develop in most patients. The National Commission on diabetes in the United States has reported that patients with insulin dependent diabetes are 25 times more prone to blindness, 17 times more prone to kidney disease, five times more often afflicted with gangrene and twice as often afflicted with heart disease than non diabetic individuals. In Sweden diabetes is now the second most common cause of uremia and it is the most common cause of blindness in adults. The life expectancy for the diabetic patient is approximately 1/3 less than that of the general population. Since the metabolic abnormalities that prevail in diabetes mellitus are due to abolished beta-cell function, it would seem logical to treat this disease by the transplantation of normally functioning islets of Langerhans. This operation should correct the metabolic abnormalities and presumably prevent or delay the severe secondary complications. There are two ways of transplanting the endocrine pancreas, either by means of a vascularized graft or by providing free, isolated islets. Unfortunately it has not been possible, so far, to correct diabetes in humans with islet transplantation. However, during the last years there has been substantial progress in the field of vascularized pancreatic transplantation and the results are now beginning to approach those obtained with other organs such as the kidney, heart and liver.

Patient selection

Since the purpose of pancreatic transplantation is to prevent the secondary complications of diabetes, the procedure should ideally be undertaken before renal and other organ damage has occurred. Earlier, some centers, including ours, did in fact carry out transplantations in non-uremic diabetics [1–3]. However, because of the hazards of the immunosuppressive treatment, most groups have offered pancreatic transplantation only to uremic diabetic patients who require a renal transplantation as well. These patients must be given immunosuppressive therapy for the renal graft in any case and the renal and pancreatic transplantations can be performed simultaneously. The use of such a combined procedure does not seem to increase the hazards for the patient. In a recent Stockholm series (1981–1985) the patient survival rate and the renal graft success rate was no different from that obtained in diabetic patients undergoing renal transplantation only [4]. Alternatively, diabetic patients carrying well functioning renal grafts have been given subsequent pancreatic grafts. However, with the improved results now seen and the safer immunosuppressive protocols now available, the indications have again been expanded. Thus, the Minneapolis group has recently begun to treat mostly non-uremic patients [5] and several other groups have included some such cases in their series. Many of the patients have been selected because they were suffering from rapidly progressing diabetic nephropathy (massive proteinuria, declining glomerular filtration). These patients would be candidates for renal transplantation within a year or two. By performing pancreatic transplantation at the pre-uraemic stage instead the gains for the patient are much greater, while the risks are similar, with a successful transplantation diabetes will be cured and hopefully the kidneys will be protected from further deterioration. Other pre-uraemic diabetic patients who are candidates for pancreatic transplantation are those with severe management problems, for instance patients with hyperlabile diabetes.

The surgical procedure

Pancreatic grafts are most frequently obtained from ABO – blood group – compatible cadaveric donors. However, since it is enough to transplant a segment of the pancreas, it is also possible to use relatives as graft donors (Fig. 1). This approach has been pioneered by the Minneapolis group and they have have now performed some 50 segmental pancreatic transplantations with grafts obtained from parents or siblings.

At removal from the donor the pancreatic graft is cooled by intra-arterial perfusion with an electrolyte solution and it is then stored in the cold (5°C). The cold ischemia time, i.e. the time from the initiation of the cold perfusion to the revascularization of the graft in the recipient, should be as short as possible; preferably below 6 hours.

Originally when only cadaveric grafts were employed pancreatico duodenal grafts were chosen [6]. When it was found, however, that the duodenum could

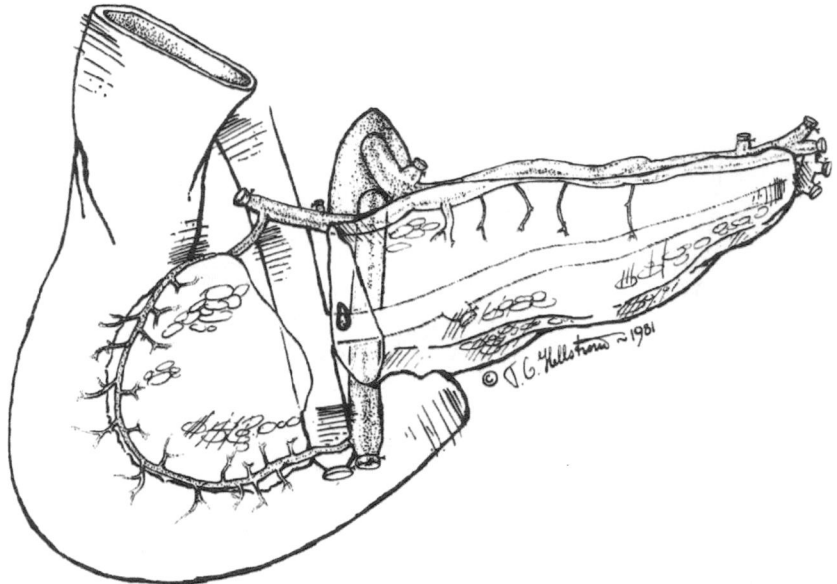

Fig. 1. Since it is enough to transplant a segment of the pancreas the donor pancreas is usually transected above the portal vein and the graft then consists of the body and tail of the pancreas. Blood supply to the graft is through the splenic artery and vein. Med. ill.: Tommy Hellström, Stockholm, Sweden.

cause complications segmental grafts consisting of the body and tail of the pancreas became popular (Fig. 1). Recently, however, several groups have started again to use the whole pancreas with or without part of the duodenum [7–10]. This has the advantage of increasing the islet mass and also making possible the use of a physiological outlet for exocrine secretion by including a duodenal patch or segment. However, regarding islet mass, so far no difference in the glucose tolerance has been reported between patients with functioning segmental grafts and those with whole organ grafts. It should also be noted that in the living donor situation, and in the case when the cadaveric liver as well as pancreas is to be retrieved, only segmental grafts can be obtained.

The handling of the exocrine secretion in pancreatic transplantation has been a subject of controversy. Thus in the 10 centers most active in the field of pancreatic transplantation, no less than 5 different techniques are presently used to handle the exocrine secretion of the pancreatic graft. Dubernard introduced an ingenious method, namely injection of a polymer into the ductal system, a measure that ablates not only the escape of the exocrine juice but its actual formation [11]. This method has been used in the majority of cases over the past few years. However, the ductal filling causes fibrosis and atrophy of

366

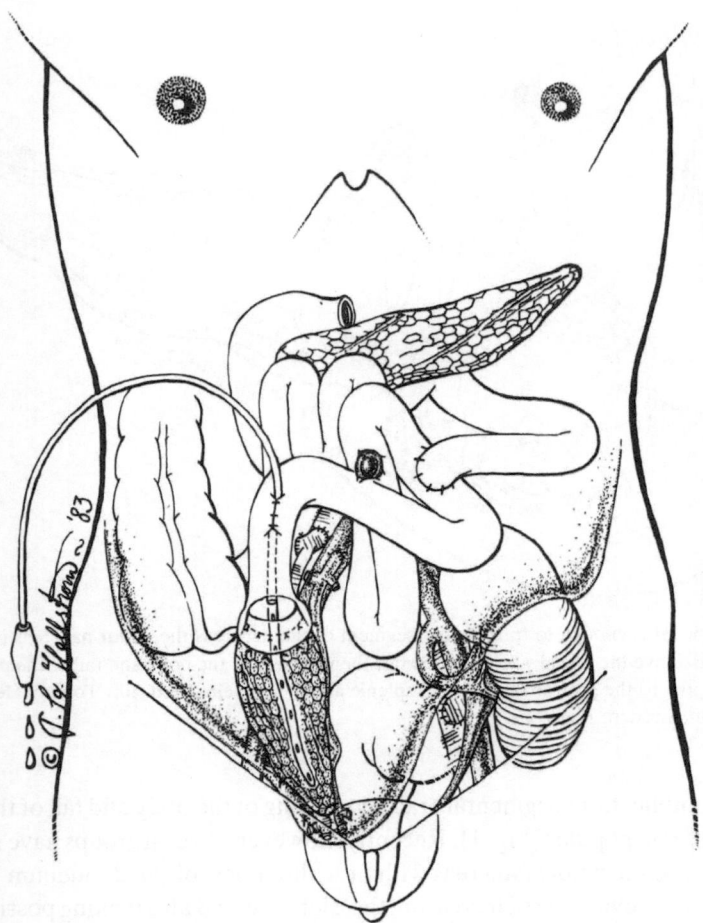

Fig. 2. The technique used for intraperitoneal segmental pancreatic transplantation with pancreatico-enterostomy to a jejunal Roux loop with temporary pancreatic duct tube drainage to the exterior. The concomitantly transplanted kidney is placed extraperitoneally on the contralateral side. Med. ill.: Tommy Hellström, Stockholm, Sweden.

the exocrine pancreas and this may eventually lead to impairment of endocrine function. Furthermore, measures of the exocrine activity may be of aid in the diagnosis of rejection episodes [10–12], a possibility which is lost if the exocrine part has been destroyed by ductal obliteration.

A more physiological approach to handling the exocrine pancreatic secretion is by diversion to the recipients bowel. In Stockholm pancreatico-enterostomy was first used in 1974 but initially there was a high incidence of anastomotic leakage which usually led to loss of the graft [13]. Following modifications in the technique (Fig. 2) with intra instead of extraperitoneal placement of the graft and temporary diversion of the exocrine secretion by pancreatic duct tube drainage [14] the incidence of this technical complication has been reduced to a very low figure. We have found a very high amylase activity in the peri-pancreatic fluid during the first postoperative days proving that the graft initially sweats a fluid rich in pancreatic enzymes. This finding emphasizes the importance of intra-, as opposed to extraperitoneal placement of pancreas grafts, thereby taking advantage of the absorbant capacity of the peritoneum. Also, during the first postoperative days, the amylase activity and lipase concentration in the juice has been found to be extremely high, probably due to an ischemic graft injury. By diverting the exocrine juice to the exterior for the first postoperative days, the pancreatico-enteric anastomosis is protected from this highly concentrated juice [15]. Indeed, improved pancreatic duct catheter patency has probably contributed to recent improvements in results in the Stockholm series by reducing the incidence of anastomotic leaks.

Early findings that many patients with enteric diversion developed a contaminated pancreatic fistula, led to the search for alternative sites for the diversion [16, 17]. By diverting the exocrine secretion to the recipient stomach the risk of enteric contamination is reduced. Previously, pancreatico-gastric anastomosis has been used with satisfactory results in the Whipple procedure [18]. If the graft is telescoped into the stomach, endoscopic biopsies are made possible, at least early after transplantation. In one of our patients so operated upon, a biopsy was indeed obtained 2 months after transplantation [19]. Later on mucosa covered the end of the graft. We abandoned this method in spite of its potential advantages, because of severe complications seen in the case of graft pancreatitis. Good results with gastric exocrine diversion have, however, been obtained using a ducto-gastric anastomosis with the graft placed in a paratopic position above the native pancreas [20]. In this series pancreatitis has not constituted a problem. Another possible site for exocrine diversion is the urinary tract. This approach was pioneered by Gliedman [3] who performed a ducto-ureteric anastomosis, the exocrine secretion from the graft could then be monitored by measuring urinary amylase. More recently, urinary tract diversion by means of an anastomosis between the pancreas and the recipients urinary bladder has gained popularity [10].

Irrespective of surgical technique early graft pancreatitis may occur. This dangerous complication is characterized by high serumamylase levels and local tenderness over the graft. The pancreatitis is probably due to an ischemic injury consequent to an excessive ischemic time. There is reason to believe that pancreatitis predisposes for graft thrombosis and exocrine leakage. At our institution, when cold ischemia was limited to no more than six hours, the incidence of this serious complications was much reduced [21]. This finding is in agreement with the data from the International Pancreas Registry where an analysis showed better early function and survival rate for grafts preserved for less than 6 hours compared to those stored for more than 6 hours [22].

The incidence of graft vascular thrombosis in most series of pancreatic transplantations has been about 20%. The reason for this complication at least in segmental grafts is believed to be due to the abnormal hemodynamic situation created by the removal of the spleen. The large splenic artery is then left to drain via the small pancreatic branches and this low outflow may promote thrombosis. Attempts have been made to alleviate this complication by the use of anticoagulants [9, 23, 24], the creation of a distal arterio-venous fistula between the splenic artery and vein [20], by interposing the splenic artery into the internal iliac vascular bed [25], and, more recently, by the inclusion of the spleen in the graft [7, 9, 10]. The latter approach is of course the most physiological but because of the occurrence of graft versus host disease, the spleen is now usually removed after the completion of the vascular anastomoses. The use of anticoagulants seems to be effective in reducing the incidence of vascular thrombosis. Thus, in the first part of the recent Stockholm series several grafts were lost due to arterial or venous thrombosis. However, following the adoption of aggressive anticoagulant therapy in the second part, no more grafts were lost because of thrombosis. The price paid is, however, an increased risk of bleeding. In several of our patients transient intestinal bleeding necessitating transfusions occurred. In three patients bleeding was massive and one graft had to be removed because of this complication. Similar complications due to anticoagulant therapy in pancreatic transplantation have been reported by other groups [24]. The creation of a distal arteriovenous fistula between the splenic artery and vein has so far not proven to significantly reduce the incidence of graft thrombosis [20].

Graft rejection

Ever since the early days of pancreatic transplantations, it has been speculated whether or not the pancreas is more or less prone to rejection than other organ grafts. In 1971 Lillehei reported a patient who had been subjected to combined renal and pancreatico-duodenal transplantation and lost the renal graft in acute rejection while the pancreas was retained [6]. Based on this finding, Lillehei suggested that the pancreas may be less antigenic than the kidney. Similar observations have been made by us [26] and by others [27, 28]. It may be that the pancreas is less prone to rejection than the kidney, but it could also be that the laboratory methods used for diagnosing rejection in the kidney are more sensitive than those used for the pancreas. Thus it is well known that 90–95% of the islet mass must be destroyed before the fasting blood glucose rises. A further possibility is that rejection manifests itself earlier in the renal graft. If this is the case, the anti-rejection therapy then given would mask or prevent pancreatic

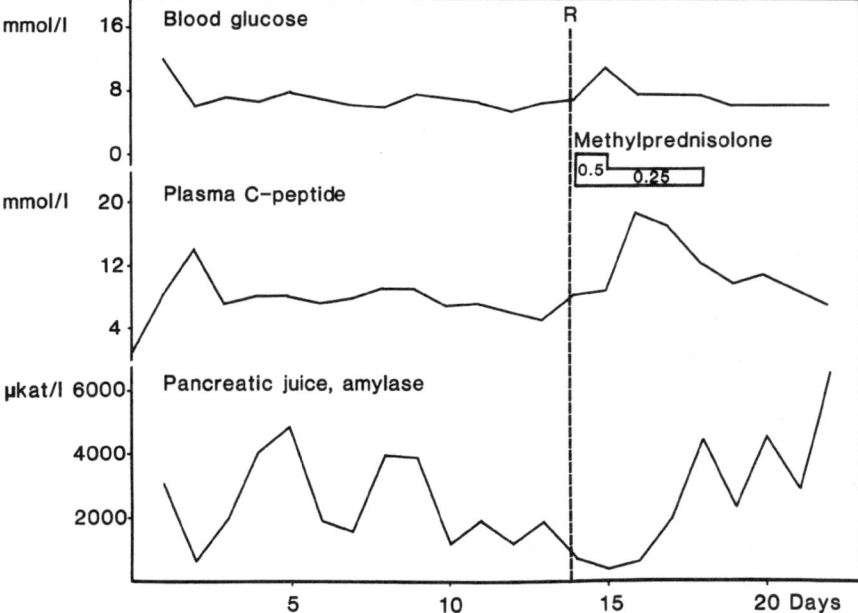

Blood glucose, C–peptide and pancreatic juice amylase in a patient with a suspected rejection episode of the pancreatic graft. The renal graft was not functioning because of posttransplant ATN

Fig. 3. Fasting blood glucose, fasting plasma C-peptide and pancreatic juice amylase in a patient in whom pancreatic graft rejection was diagnosed by a drop in the amylase activity in the pancreatic juice. Following rejection treatment with methylprednisolone the activity recovered. Note the increase in C-peptide output during steroid treatment indicating intact endocrine function in spite of impaired exocrine function of the graft.

graft rejection. Be that as it may, it is clear that the kidney serves as an excellent marker for immunological events in the recipients of combined grafts [29]. With pancreatic transplantation alone, the diagnosis of rejection must obviously be based on measures of pancreatic function. As for the endocrine portion of the graft, increase in the postprandial blood glucose is sometimes an early sign of graft rejection [30]. Also declining C-peptide or insulin levels should occur with islet injury [31]. In grafts where the exocrine part has not been destroyed by ductal occlusion, the earliest signs of graft rejection might, however, be from the exocrine tissue. Thus, Sollinger has reported that the urinary amylase output decreased before the blood glucose rose during rejection in patients carrying grafts with exocrine diversion to the bladder [10]. Similar findings were recorded in one of our patients in whom the exocrine secretion was studied by means of a pancreatic duct catheter (Fig. 3). Also, it was noted several years ago by us and by Largiadér that changes in blood glucose were often preceeded by a transient, small elevation in the serum amylase level [32, 33]. Recent studies in the dog have confirmed that rejection may firstly afflict the exocrine, and then the endocrine portion of the graft [12].

Aid in the differential diagnosis between rejection and other conditions causing pancreatic graft malfunction can be obtained by angiography. With rejection, the graft vasculature shows characteristic destructive changes [34]. The final option is open biopsy, a method often applied by the Minnesota group [35].

Metabolic control

Usually, an excellent metabolic control can be achieved by pancreas transplantation as exemplified in Figs. 4 and 5. Following revascularization of pancreatic grafts with exocrine diversion, exogeneous insulin can usually be discontinued promptly and the recipient becomes normoglycemic within a few hours [36]. In recipients of duct obliterated grafts, supplemental exogeneous insulin may be required for one or several weeks [37, 24]. However, following this delay in onset of function, it seems that all the recipients of technically successful grafts maintain normal fasting and postprandial glucose levels and normal glucosylated hemoglobin levels. Also 24 h metabolic profiles have been found to be normal for as long as 5 years after transplantation [5]. In animal experiments, ductal obstruction has been found to lead eventually to impairment of the endocrine function of the graft. To what extent such a chain of events takes place in man is unclear. The Minnesota group and Calne have reported that some of their duct occluded grafts ceased to function after several months or years and that this might have been due to fibrosis. Rejection could, however, not be excluded as an alternative cause in many of the cases. In patients with functioning duct obliterated pancreatic grafts, there seems, however, to be no deterioration in metabolic control with time [38, 39].

Oral glucose tolerance tests and intravenous glucose tolerance tests have been reported to be normal in 50–80% of the patients with functioning pancreatic grafts. Several factors may explain the impaired glucose tolerance observed in some patients, such as insufficient islet mass, denervation of the graft, systemic hormone delivery, impaired renal function and the immunosuppressive treatment. The diabetogenic effect of steroids is well known. Also, evidence is mounting that cyclosporin impairs the glucose tolerance. Thus, we reported in 1981 that when intravenous glucose tolerance tests were performed in pancreatic transplant recipients during azathioprine treatment and again after a switch to a high dose cyclosporin, a significant decrease in the K-value was found: On the other hand, when the cyclosporin dose was

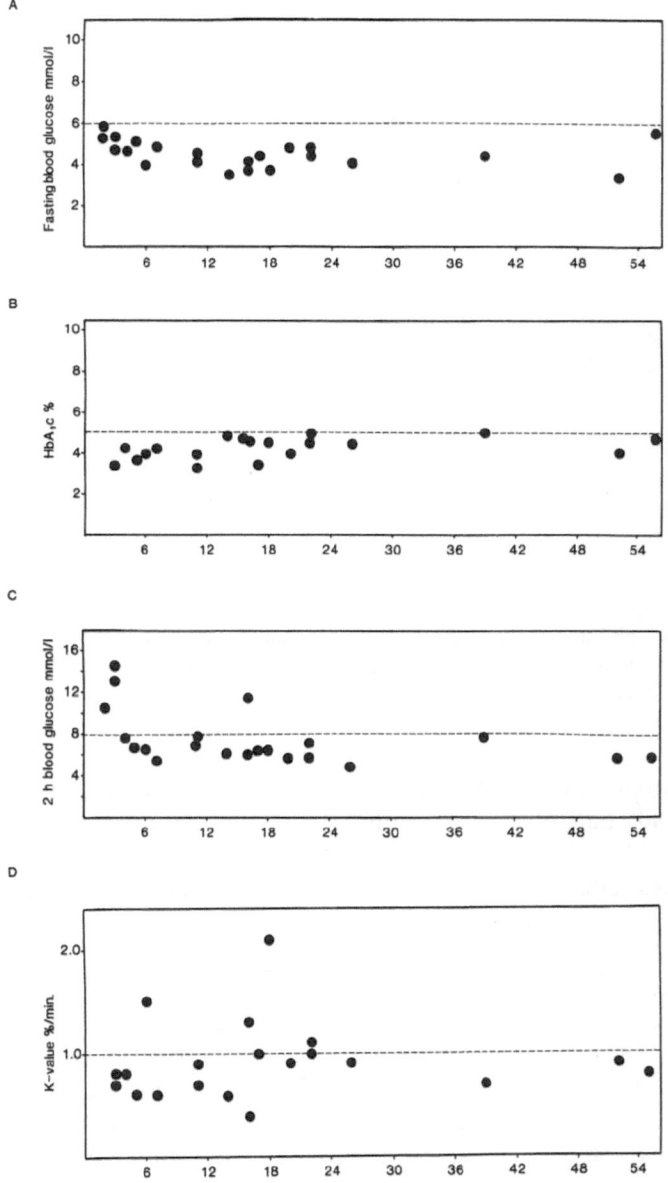

Fig. 4. Fasting blood glucose, glucosylated hemoglobin, 2 hour blood glucose of the oral glucose tolerance test and K-value of the intravenous glucose tolerance test in patients with functioning pancreatic grafts. Dotted lines indicate reference value.

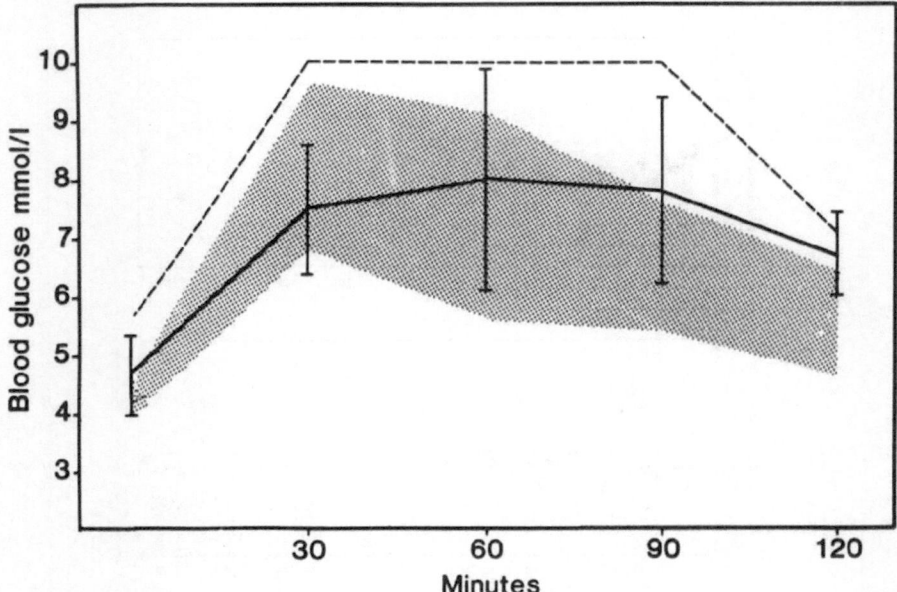

Fig. 5. Oral glucose tolerance tests performed in 17 patients with functioning pancreas grafts at 4 months to 4 years following transplantation. Vertical lines indicate the standard deviations. The shaded area indicates the range (2 standard deviations from the mean) of values in 39 oral glucose tolerance tests carried out in non-diabetic controls.

reduced from high to maintenance levels, there was a significant increase in the K-value [40]. Later these observations were confirmed and extended by us and others [41, 42]. The diabetogenic effect of cyclosporin can be explained by a B-cell toxic effect, or possibly that a steroid mediated peripheral insulin blockade may be induced.

Normally, the insulin delivery is achieved via the portal system. However, for technical reasons the venous anastomosis has, in the vast majority of pancreatic graft recipients been to the iliac vein, thus, the insulin delivery has been via the systemic circulation. It is possible, however, to accomplish portal delivery either to the mesenteric vein as was done in a few cases by us [19], or to the splenic vein as advocated by Calne [20]. However, systemic insulin delivery seems to carry no metabolic disadvantages though the peripheral insulin levels are almost double those seen in normal subjects. In fact, there is data to indicate that the oral glucose tolerance is actually better in patients with systemic rather than portal insulin delivery [20, 43]. It has also been shown that hepatic glucose regulation is entirely normal in recipients of pancreatic grafts with systemic insulin delivery [44].

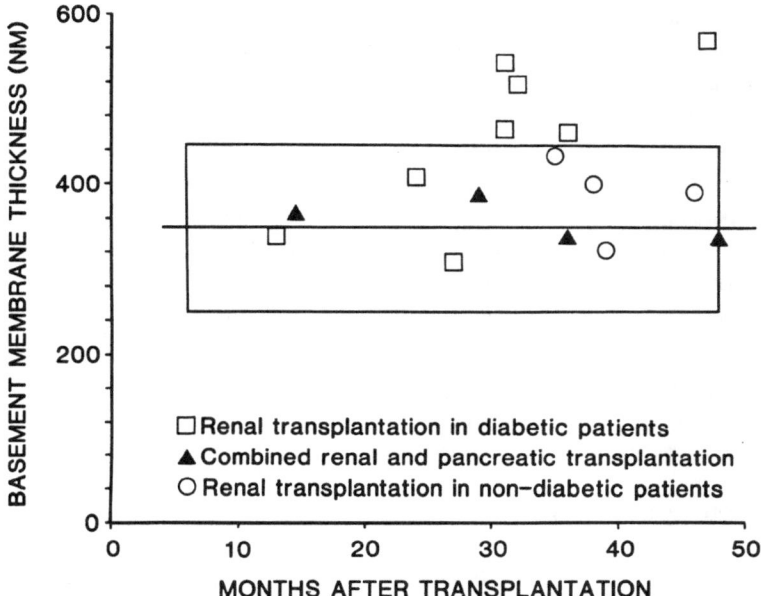

Fig. 6. Glomerular basement membrane thickness in renal graft biopsies performed in diabetic patients subjected to kidney transplantation only or combined kidney and pancreas transplantation and in non-diabetic patients subjected to kidney transplantation. Rectangular area indicates the range (2 standard deviations from the mean) of values in non-diabetic controls [48].

Effect on secondary lesions

A most remarkable effect of successful pancreatic transplantation is the improvement in the patients quality of life. The fact that insulin injections are no longer required creates a sense of freedom and this feeling is further enhanced by the abolition of all dietary restrictions.

The ultimate benefit of pancreatic transplantations lies, however, in the prevention or reversal of the secondary complications of the disease. So far, however, the results have in this respect been eqivocal. In many patients an improvement in neuropathy has been observed both subjectively and objectively [36, 38, 39], but a recent carefully controlled study has shown that the improvement in nerve conduction velocity is only moderate and no greater than the improvement occuring after renal transplantation only [45]. Several reports have indicated that visual acuity is stabilized after pancreatic transplantation [5, 16, 38, 39]. However, in a recent study from Minnesota it was found that the evolution of retinopathy was no different in patients with well functioning pancreatic grafts when compared to patients who had lost their graft early in the course (R.C. Ramsay, personal communication). An explanation for these negative findings could of course be that the secondary lesions in the diabetic patients with end-stage renal disease were so severe that reversal was impossible.

The use of combined kidney and pancreas transplantation in diabetic patients creates a unique opportunity to assess whether pancreas transplantation can prevent the development of diabetic kidney lesions. In our patients renal graft biopsies obtained 1–4 years after transplantation have failed to show a thickening of the glomerular basement membranes [46], a finding which would be indicative of recurrence of diabetic nephropathy (Fig. 6). Already after two years, such a thickening has been found in diabetic patients subjected to renal transplantation alone. Another encouraging observation is that the glomerular mesangium in a renal graft may diminish when the patient is provided with a subsequent pancreatic graft [5].

Overall activity and results

In the late 1970s, fewer than 20 pancreatic transplantations were performed per year in the world. Since then, there has been a rapid expansion, and over 200 such transplantations were carried out in 1985. The overall results have improved each year. The 1-year patient survival rates for the periods before 1977, 1978 – 1982 and 1983 – 1986 were 40%, 72% and 79% and the corresponding 1-year graft success rates were 3%, 20% and 42% respectively [47]. However, individual groups have obtained figures that are better than these. Thus, in the most recent Stockholm series, the 1-year graft success rate survival was 72% (Fig. 7) and similar figures have been obtained in Pittsburgh and Iowa City (62% and 57% respectively) using a whole organ graft with a duodenal patch as devised by Starzl [7, 9]. With the paratopic technique used by Calne [20], the recent 1-year graft success rate is 60% and with exocrine drainage to the urinary bladder, as employed in Madison, the 1-year graft survival is now 74% [10]. Also, with duct obliterated grafts, recent improvements in graft survival have been obtained and the 1-year graft survival in the Munich series is now 54%, in Lyon 40% and in Oslo 60% [23, 24, 37]. In Minneapolis, where the largest experience with pancreas transplantation exists (130 cases since 1966), the overall pancreas graft success rates (related and cadaveric donors and uremic and non-uremic recipients) have improved from 27% before 1983 to 43% in 1984–1985 [5]. However, the functional survival rate of related donor grafts has greatly exceeded that of cadaveric donor grafts, this being most evident when only technical successful allografts were analyzed. In this subgroup, 76% of grafts from HLA-identical siblings were functioning at 1 year compared to 30% from cadaveric donors [5].

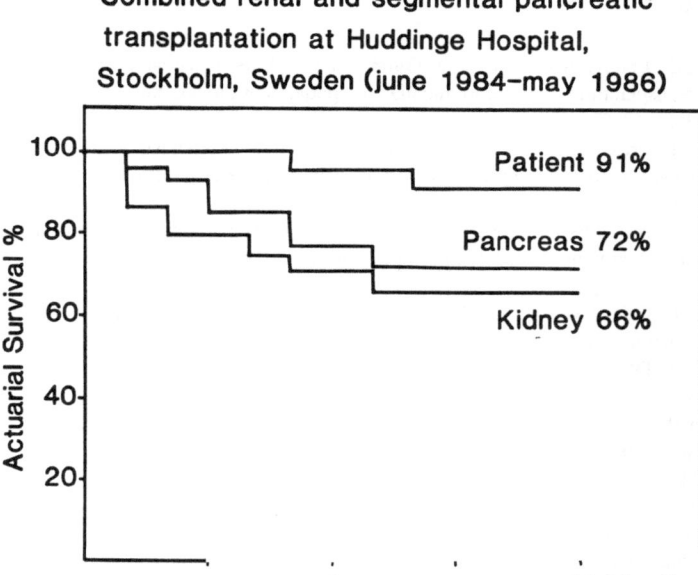

Fig. 7. Actuarial patient, renal graft and pancreatic graft survival in 28 recipients of combined renal and pancreatic grafts at Huddinge Hospital, Stockholm, Sweden. (June 1984 – May 1986).

Summary

In the last few years there has been a considerable improvement in results with pancreatic transplantation. Several centers now report a 1-year graft survival rate of 50–70%. Patients with well functioning grafts become insulin independent and have normal or near normal fasting and postprandial glucose levels and normal glycosylated hemoglobin values. The glucose tolerance, as measured by oral and intravenous glucose tolerance tests, is normal in 50–80% of the patients but subnormal in the others. One important reason for subnormal glucose tolerance is the medication with cyclosporin and prednisolone. In most cases an improvement in neuropathy is found and retinopathy seems to be stabilized. Preliminary data indicate that the provision of a pancreatic graft prevents the occurrence of diabetic nephropathy in a simultaneously or previously transplanted kidney.

376

References

1. Groth CG, Lundgren G, Östman J, Gunnarsson R: Experience with nine segmental pancreatic transplantations in preuremic diabetic patients in Stockholm. Transplantation Proceedings 12: 68–72, 1980
2. Sutherland DER, Goetz FC, Carpenter AM, Najarian JS, Lillehei RC: Pancreaticoduodenal grafts: Clinical and pathological observations in uremic versus nonuremic recipients. Transplantation and Clinical Immunology 10: 190–195, 1978
3. Gliedman ML, Tellis VA, Soberman R, Rifkin H, Veith FJ: Long-term effects of pancreatic transplant function in patients with advanced juvenile-onset diabetes. Diabetes Care 1: 1–9, 1978
4. Wilczek H, Gunnarsson R, Lundgren G, Öst L: Improved results of renal transplantation in diabetic nephropathy. Transplantation Proceedings 16: 623–625, 1984
5. Sutherland DER, Goetz FC, Kendall DM, Najarian JS: One Institution's experience with pancreas transplantation. The Western Journal of Medicine 14: 838–844, 1985
6. Lillehei RC, Simmons RL, Najarian JS, Kjellstrand CM, Goetz FC: Current state of pancreatic allotransplantation. Transplantation Proceedings 3: 318–324, 1971
7. Starzl TE, Iwatsuki S, Shaw BW, et al.: Pancreaticoduodenal transplantation in humans. Surgery Gynecology & Obstetrics 159: 265–272, 1984
8. McMaster P, Michael J, Adu D, Vlassis T, Gibby O: Combined kidney and pancreas transplantation in man: Experience at the University of Birmingham. Diabetic Nephropathy 4: 135–139, 1985
9. Corry RJ, Nghiem DD, Schulak JA, Beutel WD, Gonwa TA: Surgical treatment of diabetic nephropathy with simultaneous pancreatic duodenal and renal transplantation. Surgery Gynecology & Obstetrics 162: 547–555, 1986
10. Sollinger HW, Kalayoglu M, Hoffman RM, Belzer FO: Results of segmental and pancreaticosplenic transplantation with pancreaticocystostomy. Transplantation Proceedings 17: 360–362, 1985
11. Dubernard JM, Traeger J, Neyra P, Touraine JL, Tranchant D, Blanc-Brunat N: A new method of preparation of segmental pancreatic grafts for transplantation: Trials in dogs and in man. Surgery 84: 633–639, 1978
12. Schulak JA, Drevyanko TF: Experimental pancreas allograft rejection: Correlation between histologic and functional rejection and the efficacy of antirejection therapy. Surgery 98: 330–336, 1984
13. Groth CG, Lundgren H, Wilczek H, et al.: Segmental pancreatic transplantation with duct ligature or enteric diversion: Technical aspects. Transplantation Proceedings 16: 724–728, 1984
14. Groth CG, Collste H, Lundgren G, et al.: Successful outcome of segmental human pancreatic transplantation with enteric exocrine diversion after modifications in technique. Lancet ii: 522–524, 1982
15. Tydén G, Brattström C, Häggmark A, Groth CG: Studies on the exocrine secretion of human segmental pancreatic grafts. Surgery Gynecology & Obstetrics 164: 404–407, 1987
16. Groth CG, Lundgren G, Gunnarsson R, Hårdstedt C, Östman J: Segmental pancreatic transplantation with special reference to the use of ileal exocrine diversion and to the hemodynamics of the graft. Transplantation Proceedings 12: 62–67, 1980
17. Groth CG, Collste H, Lundgren G, et al.: Surgical techniques for pancreatic transplantation. A critical appraisal of methods used and a suggested new modification. Hormonal and Metabolic Research (Suppl 13): 37–46, 1983
18. Telford GL, Mason RG: Pancreaticogastrostomy: Clinical experience with a direct pancreatic-ductto-gastric-mucosa anastomosis. American Journal of Surgery 147: 832–837, 1984
19. Tydén G, Lundgren G, Östman J, Gunnarsson R, Groth CG: Grafted pancreas with portal venous drainage. Lancet i: 964–965, 1984

20. Calne RY, Brons IGM: Observations on paratopic segmental pancreas grafting with splenic venous drainage. Transplantation Proceedings 17: 340–342, 1985
21. Tydén G, Brattström C, Lundgren G, et al.: Improved results in pancreatic transplantation by avoiding non-immunological graft failures. Transplantation 43: 674–676, 1987
22. Sutherland DER, Kendall D, Goetz FC, Najarian JS. In: Pancreas transplantation in man. The Diabetes Annual. Elsevier Science Publishers, 1985, pp 198–216
23. Brekke IB, Dyrbekk D, Jakobsen A, Jervell J, Sodal G, Flatmark A: Improved pancreas graft survival in combined pancreatic and renal transplantation. Transplantation Proceedings 18: 63–64, 1986
24. Land W, Landgraf R, Illner W-D, et al.: Improved results in combined segmental pancreatic and renal transplantation in diabetic patients under cyclosporine therapy. Transplantation Proceedings 17: 317–324, 1985
25. Kocandrle V, Vanek I, Bartos V, Pavel P: Splenic artery interposition in animal and human segmental pancreatic transplantation. Transplantation Proceedings 16: 1283–1284, 1984
26. Tydén G, Lundgren G, Öst L, Gunnarsson R, Östman J, Groth CG: Are pancreatic grafts prone to reject. Transplantation Proceedings 18: 27–29, 1986
27. Baumgartner D, Largiader F, Uhlschmid G, Binswanger U: Rejection episodes in recipients of simultaneous pancreas and kidney transplantation. Transplantation Proceedings 15: 1330–1331, 1983
28. Dubernard JM, Traeger J, Touraine JL, Betuel H, Malik MC: Rejection of human pancreatic allografts. Transplantation Proceedings 12: 103–106, 1980
29. Florack G, Sutherland DER, Sibley RK, Najarian JS, Squifflet JP: Combined kidney and segmental pancreas allotransplantation in dogs. Transplantation Proceedings 17: 374–377, 1985
30. Groth CG, Lundgren G, Arner P, et al.: Rejection of isolated pancreatic allografts in patients with diabetes. Surgery, Gynecology & Obstetrics 143: 933–940, 1976
31. Östman J, Arner P, Groth CG, Gunnarsson R, Heding L, Lundgren G: Plasma C-peptide and serum insulin antibodies in diabetic patients receiving pancreatic transplants. Diabetologia 19: 25–30, 1980
32. Groth CG, Lundgren G, Gunnarsson R, Arner P, Berg B, Östman J: Segmental pancreatic transplantation with duct ligation or drainage to a jejunal Roux-en-Y loop in nonuremic diabetic patients. Diabetes 29: 3–9, 1980
33. Largiader F, Uhlschmid G, Binswanger U, Zaruba K: Pancreas rejection in combined pancreaticoduodenal and renal allotransplantation in kidney. Transplantation 19: 185–187, 1975
34. Svahn T, Lewander R, Hårdstedt C, Lundgren G, Sundelin P, Groth CG: Angiography and scintigraphy of human pancreatic allografts. Acta Radiologica Diagnosis 19: 297–304, 1977
35. Sutherland DER, Goetz FC, Najarian JS: One hundred pancreas transplants at a single institution. Annals of Surgery 200: 414–440, 1984
36. Tydén G, Wilczek H, Lundgren G, et al.: Experience with 21 intraperitoneal segmental pancreatic transplants with enteric or gastric exocrine diversion in humans. Transplantation Proceedings 17: 331–335, 1985
37. Dubernard JM, Traeger J, Piatti PM, et al.: Report of 54 human segmental pancreatic allografts prepared by duct obstruction with neoprene. Transplantation Proceedings 17: 312–314, 1985
38. Landgraf R, Landgraf-Leurs MMC, Burg D, et al.: Long-term follow-up of segmental pancreas transplantation in type I diabetes. Transplantation Proceedings 18: 1118–1124, 1986
39. Traeger J, Dubernard JM, Monti LD, et al.: Studies in patients with a segmental pancreatic graft functioning more than 1 year. Transplantation Proceedings 18: 1139–1140, 1986
40. Gunnarsson R, Klintmalm G, Lundgren G, et al.: Deterioration in glucose metabolism in pancreatic transplant recipients after conversion from azathioprine to cyclosporine. Transplantation Proceedings 16: 709–712, 1984

378

41. Engfeldt P, Tydén G, Gunnarsson R, Östman J, Groth CG: Impaired glucose tolerance with cyclosporin. Transplantation Proceedings 18: 65–66, 1986
42. Pozza G, Traeger J, Dubernard JM, *et al.*: Endocrine responses of type 1 (insulin-dependent) diabetic patients following successful pancreas transplantation. Diabetologia 24: 244–248, 1983
43. Gil-Vernet JM, Fernandez-Cruz L, Andreu J, Figuerola D, Caralps A: Clinical experience with pancreaticopyelostomy for exocrine pancreatic drainage and portal venous drainage in pancreas transplantation. Transplantation Proceedings 17: 342–345, 1985
44. Wilczek H, Gunnarsson R, Felig P, Wahren J, Groth CG: Normalization of hepatic glucose regulation following heterotopic pancreatic transplantation in humans. Transplantation Proceedings 17: 315–316, 1985
45. Wilczek H, Solders G, Gunnarsson R, Tydén G, Persson A: Effects of successful combined pancreatic and renal transplantation on advance diabetic neuropathy: A one-year follow up study. Transplantation Proceedings 19: 2327–2328, 1987
46. Bohman S-O, Tydén G, Wilczek H, *et al.*: Prevention of kidney graft diabetic nephropathy by pancreas transplantation in man. Diabetes 34: 306–308, 1985
47. Sutherland, DER: Clinical pancreas and islet transplantation. Transplantation Proceedings 18: 1739–1746, 1986
48. Mauer SM, Steffes MW, Ellis EN, *et al.*: Structural-functional relationship in diabetic nephropathy. Journal of Clinical Investigation 74: 1143–1155, 1984

23. Transplantation of hepatic segments

C.E. BROELSCH and J.C. EMOND

Introduction

Wide-spread application of orthotopic liver transplantation (OLT) has evolved since the NIH Consensus meeting on Liver Transplantation in 1983 [1]. Almost exclusively, orthotopic liver transplantation is performed with full sized liver grafts, whereas, heterotopic liver grafting has only received scattered application. With the growing demand for transplants, the development of approaches to increase the pool of donor organs has taken on increasing importance. In pediatric recipients, where size-matched organs are rarely available in a timely fashion, particularly in patients with acute liver failure, the organ supply has not kept pace with the increase in the number of potential recipients despite an overall increase in organ availability in recent years in the United States. At the present time, more than 800 patients in the U.S. are awaiting a liver transplant of whom some 20% are children [2]. An estimated 30 to 40% of pediatric recipients died awaiting a liver in 1986.

An appropriate size match between donor and recipient is a principal requirement in liver transplantation due to the problems of space and circulation of the transplanted organ [3]. It becomes a predominant problem in pediatric transplantation but also in adults if a heterotopic position is chosen [4]. The heterotopic position appears favorable in avoiding the obstacles of the recipient hepatectomy, cross clamping, splanchnic congestion and acute tubular necrosis. Furthermore, in cases of potentially reversible acute liver failure, a heterotopic graft provides a substitute for the host liver with a chance of removal of the transplant if no longer needed. However, these theoretical advantages have not been realized in practice. With increasing success, the treatment of acute liver failure has become orthotopic transplantation with removal of the diseased organ whereas, alternative heterotopic approaches have been abandoned. In the orthotopic position, circulation of the transplant appears to be adequately provided by portal venous and arterial hepatic blood. The hepatic venous outflow condition is hemodynamically more favorable because of the low pressure system in the suprahepatic vena cava. Consequently, the only successful long-term results have been obtained with orthotopic grafting, with few exceptions.

The controversy between the heterotopic and orthotopic position is not yet settled. The actual space limitations in the abdomen for using liver grafts heterotopically has led to employment of reduced size grafts, i.e., hepatic lobes for transplantation in animals [5]. More recently, with the growing importance of pediatric liver transplantation and the limited availability of size matched donor organs, reduced size liver grafting has received a renewed attention and may eventually receive broader clinical application. Consequently, the available technology of reduced size liver grafting could change the perception of heterotopic transplantation since less space and different hemodynamic conditions are required. Detailed studies of the liver anatomy by Couinaud [6] have defined the principles of anatomic liver resections which have received broad application. These studies provide the basis for transplantation of size reduced but functionally intact organs with preservation of physiologic vascular and biliary connections. In experimental models of liver grafting, the reduced size liver graft has been used for nearly 13 years, although with limited clinical application. In this chapter, we present a review of the experimental developments and present clinical experience with reduced size liver grafts in the orthotopic and heterotopic position.

Heterotopic transplantation

In the years following the initial report by Welch, in 1955 [7], heterotopic liver transplantation (HLT) was thought to represent the only practical solution to avoid the overwhelming technical difficulties of total hepatectomy and OLT. The evolution of the approaches to HLT closely followed increased understanding of the physiologic requirements for successful liver grafting in both positions.

The role of portal blood

Early observations of liver atrophy following portal vein ligation by Schalm [8] and Eck Fistula by Hahn [9] and Fischler [10] led to a variety of experimental models involving heterotopic auto- and homografting of the liver to assess the importance of portal blood in maintaining liver function and supporting regeneration.

Marchioro *et al.* [11] demonstrated atrophy of the heterotopic liver graft without portal blood and later [12] demonstrated liver atrophy in hemi-livers perfused with systemic venous blood in a series of portal caval transposition experiments (split portal caval transposition model).

Price *et al.* [5] made similar observations in a heterotopic auto transplantation model. Quantitation of blood flow to the graft receiving systemic blood into the portal vein in the Welch model of HLT indicated that liver atrophy occurred despite adequate blood flow (Daloze 1969) [13].

The trophic effects of portal blood were also observed in the rat liver transplant model by Lee *et al.* [14, 15]. Further quantitation of these observations were provided by Broelsch *et al.* [16], indicating that the regenerative response in partially resected heterotopic isografts was dependent upon portal blood.

Inter liver competition in heterotopic liver grafting

Despite the observations of the beneficial effects of portal blood, considerable interest remains in the possibility of successful HLTX without the technical constraints of providing portal blood to the graft. In a model providing systemic arterial blood as the only inflow to heterotopic liver grafts, Van der Heyde, in 1966 [17] demonstrated successful grafting, provided the host liver was impaired by bile duct ligation and end-to-side portal caval shunting as suggested by Schalm 1956 [5]. His experiment suggested that the fate of the graft was related to its access to unknown trophic factors and that the graft competed with the host liver for its support. Sigel [18, 19], using heterotopic autografts without portal blood also demonstrated that these grafts received systemic stimulation of the regenerative response probably by recirculation of trophic factors. However, only hepatic segments maintained adequate viability at least with reduced blood flow. Chandler *et al.* [14] found a similar effect of competition in dogs and rats if portal blood to the recipient liver was diverted into the systemic circulation exposing the graft and host liver equally to the beneficial effects of portal blood via arterial circulation.

Successful heterotopic grafting, despite the absence of direct portal blood supply to the graft, was further explored by Mito [20], Van der Heyde [21], Wexler *et al.* [22] and Slapak [23], all utilizing models in which the host liver was impaired by bile duct ligation or deprivation of portal blood by a side-to-side portal caval shunt.

Slapak and associates later demonstrated that HLT using the left renal vein to supply the portal vein of the partial autograft could sustain life even after total removal of the host liver [24, 25]. Looking carefully, however, at the mortality rate of these procedures, it became apparent that they are associated with an unacceptably high complication rate.

Hepatic venous outflow

The importance of hepatic venous outflow in liver grafting was addressed by

382

Juxtarenal

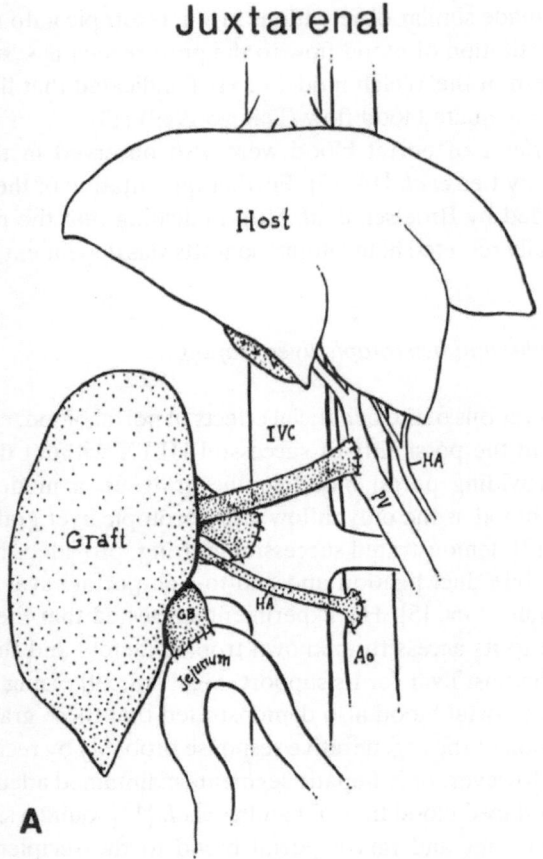

Fig. 1A. Segmental heterograft of the liver in Juxtarenal position in the dog. Hepatic venous outflow at the level of the right renal vein. Portal venous blood is shared with the host liver after removal of the caudate lobe.

Starzl in 1960 in the orthotopic liver transplant model in the dog [26]. Detailed physiologic studies of the consequences of outflow block in the perfused liver were carried out in a variety of species by Eiseman *et al.* [27] in 1963. These observations were later applied to the heterotopic transplant model by Hess *et al.* [28], who demonstrated the importance of proximity to the diaphragm of the vena caval drainage in avoiding the deleterious effects of outflow obstruction. Jerusalem *et al.* [29] in 1972, argued that unfavorable outflow conditions could lead to late failure of heterotopic liver grafts. However, the outflow block described in the dog liver is essentially a different mechanism compared to outflow obstruction due to increased inferior vena cava pressure. The existence of sphincter muscles in the dog liver at the postsinusoidal hepatic veins is mainly responsible for the uncontrollable outflow block frequently

Suprarenal

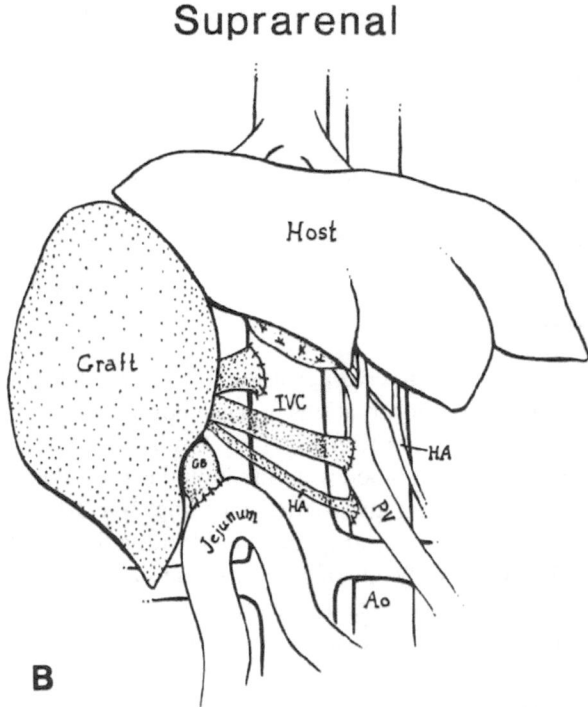

Fig. 1B. Segmental heterograft of the liver in Suprarenal position in the dog. Hepatic venous outflow into the IVC, above the renal vein junction. Portal venous blood is shared with the host liver after removal of the caudate lobe to allow a subdiaphragmatic inplantation of the segmental graft.

Table 1A. Results of auxiliary segmental liver transplants in dogs.

Postop time	Heterotopic, Juxtarenal position, n = 12		
	Complications		Survival
24–48 hrs.	Outflow bloc	n = 3	
	P-V-Thrombosis	n = 1	n = 6
	Tx-Congestion	n = 2	
3–5 d.	Intussusception	n = 1	
	Tx-Congestion	n = 2	n = 4
>5 d.	Rejection	n = 1	n = 2
	None	n = 2	m = 22 d.
			range 16–28 d.)

384

Table 1B. Results of auxiliary segmental liver transplantation in subdiaphragmatic position (N = 6).

Perioperative 24–48 hrs.	3–5 days	>5 days
Cerebral hypoxia + vital graft n = 1	Outflow bloc graft congestion n = 2 (day 3,5)	Intusseption + vital graft n = 2 (day 11,15) Vital graft (day 21) (sacrificed)

occurring after manipulation, cold perfusion and recirculation of a graft [27].

We have pursued these observations in our laboratory in a series of studies using auxiliary partial liver grafts in dogs [30]. Left lobe segmental transplants receiving portal and arterial blood were implanted using either the juxtarenal of the subdiaphragmatic vena cava for drainage [Fig. 1-A, 1-B]. The results are presented in Table 2. Six of 12 transplants failed within the first 48 hours using juxtarenal outflow while only one of 6 grafts in the subdiaphragmatic position failed acutely. These experiments further emphasized the importance of optimal outflow conditions for successful heterotopic liver transplant.

Newer approaches to heterotopic segmental liver graftings

Despite all the reports of successful grafting using non-physiologic implantation of the graft, recent experimental models have attempted to provide portal blood and optimal outflow conditions. Reuvers and Terpstra, *et al.* have recently reported successful auxiliary segmental liver transplants in dogs and pigs [31, 32]. The model uses optimal physiologic conditions for the transplant, providing portal blood from the recipient mesenteric venous system and arterial supply with implantation of the hepatic venous drainage just below the diaphragm. End-to-side portal caval shunt diverts portal blood from the recipient liver. Life sustaining hepatic function of these grafts was demonstrated by Reuvers *et al.* [33] in experiments in which the hepatic arterial circulation of the recipient liver was occluded, producing fatal hepatic necrosis in controlled animals. With an operative technique described in 1968 and 1970, Van der Heyde [17, 22] reported successful heterotopically transplanted livers if the venous anastomosis is placed between the liver and the renal veins [17, 22]. However, only some of the experimental dogs could survive pointing again to the importance of providing favorable hemodynamic outflow conditions.

Table 2. Results of Hopital Paul Brousse. Transplantation of reduced-size adult liver grafts in children: Intra and post operative events.

Patient No	Date of transplantation	Type of hepatectomy	Duration of ischemic time	Volume of intraoperative transfusion (l)	Postoperative transaminase level (ALAT/ASAT)	Complications	Outcome
14	11/25/81	Extended right hepatectomy	4 h	1.5	1000/840	Chronic rejection retransplanted	Alive
55	01/03/86	Right hepatectomy	5 h 30	1.8	600/460	Hepatic artery thrombosis and biliary leakage	Alive
59	02/10/86	Right hepatectomy	5 h	1.2	940/670	–	Alive
62	03/05/86	Right hepatectomy	5 h	1.1	193/352	Portal vein thrombosis rejection Retransplanted in emergency	Died (3 m)
65	04/04/86	Right hepatectomy	6 h	1.8	2208/1242	–	Alive

Clinical applications and heterotopic liver grafting

Despite the theoretical advantages of heterotopic liver transplantation and wide experimental application, only a few successful cases have been reported in the world experience of over 40 cases by Starzl [34], Fortner [35] and Houssin [36]. The problem of space is an important limitation and led to the use of partial heterotopic liver grafts initially reported in 1979 by Galperin and Schumakow in two patients [37]. The successful auxiliary graft in an adult cirrhotic reported by Houssin [36] was in fact a pediatric full sized organ. In the experience of Hopital Paul Brousse [38], 4 other auxiliary heterotopic reduced liver grafts were unsuccessful in a series of decompensated adult cirrhotics, who were transplanted in emergency conditions.

Using the principles developed in their experimental work, Terpstra and others have embarked on a clinical program, based on auxiliary segment liver transplantation in the treatment of urgent indications for liver transplantation. One patient has recently received an auxiliary segmental liver graft (Terpstra, personal communication, January 1987).

Orthotopic transplantation of hepatic segments

OLT provides the optimal physiologic and hemodynamic position for the liver graft. Total recipient hepatectomy represents the major technical obstacle in this procedure. Following the earlier descriptions by Starzl *et al.* [26], eventually achieving a high success rate in dogs and pigs, (Stuart *et al.* 1967 [39], Dent *et al.* 1971 [40]) OLT became the standard clinical procedure for liver grafting by 1982, due to the technical and clinical innovations principally contributed by Starzl [41], Calne [42] and Pichlmayr [43]. Since the introduction of cyclosporine A and improved immunosuppressive therapy, technical improvements, including venous decompression bypass, and the more frequent performance of retransplantation in cases of transplant failure, OLT is now established as effective therapy of end-stage liver disease with an acceptable mortality rate. In this context, the role of segmental liver transplantation is primarily to increase the donor pool and solving the problem of space and non-size matched recipients such as pediatric patients.

Segmental liver grafts in the orthotopic position

Experimental approaches

The use of reduced liver grafts in the orthotopic position has received theoretical consideration in 1969 by Smith [44] and less experimental interest than the great variety of heterotopic models. Mizumoto *et al.* reported a series of dogs receiving orthotopic segmental transplantations in 1974, and demonstrated the feasibility of the technique [45]. The first successful series of orthotopic non-auxiliary segmental liver transplants in dogs was reported by Bax *et al.* in 1982 [46], although a 50% mortality was still observed in recipient animals receiving a 40% reduced donor graft. Beagle dogs were used to avoid the potential loss of animals due to rejection of the graft. We have recently demonstrated a 20% mortality in pigs receiving a 40 and 60% reduced graft in the orthotopic position [47].

Segmental liver grafts in orthotopic position, clinical application

In 1983, Bismuth [48], in 1984, Broelsch [40], reported successful implantation of part of adult donor livers into pediatric recipients following total recipient hepatectomy. These procedures were based on anatomic reduction of the donor liver, using a segmental approach via hepatic resection as described by Bismuth [51]. Since these initial reports, Bismuth has had excellent results in a series of 5 children receiving orthotopic segmental liver grafts with 4 of 5 patients alive [38]. These patients are presented in Table 2. Equally encouraging results have been obtained in the series with 9 of 12 small children alive following orthotopic segmental transplantation (personal communication, Otte, Lambotte 1986). Our experience with segmental liver grafting in the orthotopic position has been confined to a series of 8 children with emergent indications for transplantation. Indications and clinical courses are outlined in Table 3. Three of 8 patients are alive, one later received a size matched re-transplant. Two others with technically successful grafts died of CMV infections, 3 and 6 months after transplantation, while one died from intracranial bleeding with a functioning transplant.

Alternative approaches to orthotopic segmental liver transplantation

An alternative approach to segmental liver transplantation, which preserves the hemodynamic advantages of OLT without requiring total recipient hepatectomy is orthotopic segmental liver transplantation (OSLT). Partial recipient hepatectomy is performed with implantation of the segmental liver graft in the position of the resected organ, the most favorable being the left lobe position (Fig. 2). This approach was initially suggested by Smith in 1969, who proposed the technique and explored its application in dogs and monkeys as a method for ultimately using living donors [44]. Lortat-Jacob [50] in studies of autotrans-plantation of partial liver grafts, had also suggested the use of living donors in men, exploiting the safety of a left lateral segmentectomy (Couinaud segments 2–3) as did Bücherl in a theoretical consideration and dagradi. We

Table 3. Orthotopic segmental liver transplantation in children, Hannover (FRG)/University of Chicago experience.

Indication	Recipient Age/weight	Donor Age/weight	Lobe	Survival
Art. Thromb. Retx	3 y/11 kg	16 y/47 kg	Right	*Alive*
Biliary Atresia	2 y/ 8 kg	42 y/65 kg	Left-Lateral	3 months CMV-Sepsis
Biliary Atresia	11 m/ 9 kg	12 y/33 kg	Left	12 d. Intracran. Bleed
Acute Hepatitis	15 y/61 kg	37 y/90 kg	Left	5 d. Non-viable graft
Art. Thromb. Retx	15 m/10 kg	22 y/64 kg	Left	Intra op. death
Acute Hepatitis	4 y/16 kg	45 y/70 kg	Left-Lateral	6 months CMV-sepsis
Art. Thromb. Retx	6 m/ 7 kg	2 y/13 kg	Right	*Alive* (Retx)
Biliary Atresia	4 m/ 6 kg	7 m/11 kg	Right	*Alive*

Orthotopic

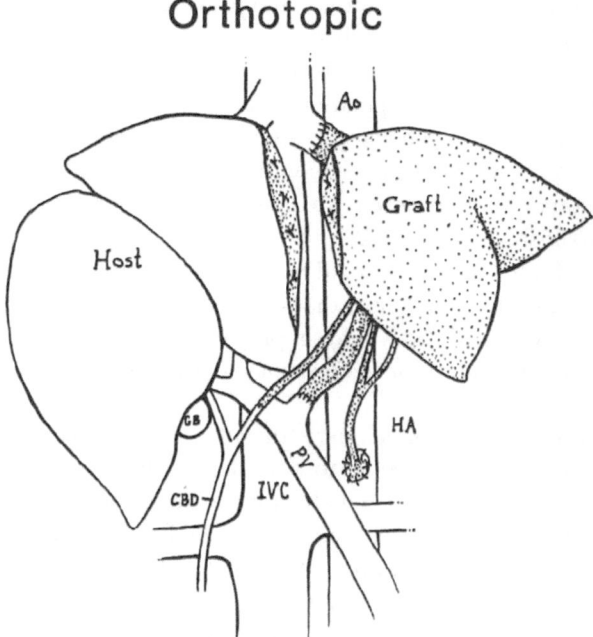

Fig. 2. Segmental heterograft of the liver in orthotopic position after removal of the left hepatic lobe in the dog. Hepatic venous outflow is at the site of the left hepatic vein. Portal venous blood is shared with the host liver.

have explored this technique in the laboratory, using dogs performing allotrans-plantations of a partial graft comprising the left and median lobes into a recipient having undergone partial left hepatectomy [51]. The hepatic vein of the graft is implanted end-to-end and the cut recipient vein with the lateral anastomoses of the graft, portal branch on the intact portal vein of the recipient. Arterial supply is brought directly from the aorta. Ten of 11 dogs survived greater than 5 days with viable grafts. Further exploration of the competition of the graft with the recipient liver on the shared portal vein is necessary.

The technique has been performed in a human patient by Bismuth [38]. The initially functioning graft was lost to rejection on day 13, resulting in death of the critically ill recipient with end-stage cirrhosis.

Conclusions and future avenues of research:

At the present time, transplantation of hepatic segments provides an avenue for increasing the pool of potential donors for pediatric recipients. Auxiliary transplantation of partial liver grafts could provide hepatic support in patients with acute hepatic failure whose liver might eventually recover or in patients with metabolic disorders who simply need correction of enzyme deficiency or support of liver produced coagulation factors.

Both orthotopic and heterotopic approaches to auxiliary hepatic transplantation can be pursued in this context. Predominantly, auxiliary transplantation could be considered for a temporary support of patients with end-stage cirrhosis and acute decompensation to improve the recipients condition until a definite transplant could be performed safely. This concept is still pursued by Galperin who claims that extraperitoneal transplantation of left liver lobes into the iliac fossa would simplify the operation and diminish risk of infection in case of failure or necrosis of the graft (personal communication 1986).

Reservations of the use of auxiliary transplantation can still be posed due to the disappointing clinical results to date despite theoretical advantages. In fulminant liver failure, total hepatectomy with orthotopic OLT has been successful in 4 of 5 recent cases (our unpublished observations) with the only death occurring in a morbidly obese patient. Total hepatectomy and OLT was accomplished with a mean blood loss of 7 units in these patients. Shaw and Wood have recently reported excellent results in a series of patients transplanted in stage 4 hepatic coma [52]. Removal of the diseased liver may be a necessary part of therapy in these acutely ill patients because of the continuous release of toxins and cell detritus.

Orthotopic transplantation of hepatic segments following total hepatectomy in pediatric patients is probably the most promising clinical application of reduced liver grafting. Encouraging results from several centers indicate the feasibility of this approach and justify its continued application. Avenues for continued investigation include more reliable assessment of size requirements in planning the partial hepatectomy in the donor organ. The use of the hepatic veins as vena cava substitutes when transplanting a small left lateral segment from a larger donor into a small child, needs to be explored in a primate model which closely approximates human hepatic vein anatomy. Recent investigations of regeneration and function as well as morphological adaptation of the reduced liver graft can provide a unique investigation into the regulation of regeneration and its relation to functional demands.

The occurrence of fatal cytomegalovirus (CMV) in pediatric recipients receiving a liver from adult donors must stimulate further study into prevention and management of this disease since CMV is common in the adult population. Apparently, there is no protection against recurrent or newly acquired CMV or other viral infections despite previous antibody formation. Antiviral therapy, therefore, becomes an important aspect in the transplantation of adult hepatic segments.

Further studies need to be undertaken to explore the possibility of splitting one liver graft for two recipients with preservation of the vascular supply to the individual lobes. It potentially could lead the way to a living related donation if that becomes necessary due to inefficient supply with donor organs.

This review has been an attempt to integrate past and present experimental approaches utilizing reduced liver grafting with efforts to develop fruitful clinical applications of this technology. It represents an excerpt from the panel conducted on the First World Congress on Hepatobiliary and Pancreatic Surgery in Lund, Sweden and integrates present opinion of all panelists who are further pursuing the application of hepatic segments in preclinical large animal models as well as in selected indications on patients.

Acknowledgements

With cooperation from: Dr. John Guggenheim, Paris, Prof. E. Galperin, Moscow, Dr. Maarten Slooff, Groningen, Prof. Nils Van der Heyde, Amsterdam and, Dr. Reuvers, Rotterdam

References

1. NIH Consensus Development Conference Statement: Liver transplantation, June 20–23, 1983. Hepatology 4: 107S–109S, 1984
2. South Eastern Organ Procurement Foundation, Richmond, VA. Communication, Feb. 1987
3. Starzl TE: The recipient operation man: In: Experiences in Hepatic Transplantation, W.B. Saunders Co., 1969, p 133
4. Starzl TE: Clinical auxiliary Tx. In: Experiences in Hepatic Transplantation, W.B. Saunders Co., 1969, p 492
5. Price JB, Voorhees AB, Britton RC: Partial hepatic autotransplantation with complete revascularization in the dog Arch Surg 95: 59, 1967
6. Couinaud C: Le foie: Etudes Anatomigues et chirurgicales. Masson: Paris, 1957
7. Welch CS: A note on transplantation of the whole liver in dogs. Transplant Bulletin 2: 54, 1955
8. Schalm L, Bax HR, Mansens BJ: Atrophy of the liver after occlusion of the bile ducts of portal vein and compensatory hypertrophy of the unoccluded portion and its clinical importance. Gastroenterology 31: 131–155, 1956
9. Hahn M, Massen O, Nencki M, Pavlov J: Die Eck'sche Fistel Zwischen der Unteren Hohlvene und der Pfortader und ihre Folgen für den Organismus. Archiv f Exp Pathol u Pharmakol XXX11 Bd: 161–210, 1893
10. Fischler F: Physiologie und pathologie der Leber. Verlag-Springer, Berlin, 1925
11. Marchioro TL, Porter KA, Dickinson TC, Faris P, Starzl TE: Physiological requirement of heterotopic auxiliary liver transplants. Surg Gynec Obstet 121: 17, 1965
12. Marchioro TL, Porter KA, Brown BI, Otte JB, Starzl TE: The effect of partial portocaval transposition in the canine liver. Surg 61: 723, 1967
13. Daloze PM, Huguet C, Groth C, Stoll F: Blood flow in auxiliary partial hepatic autografts. Surgery 62 (1): 195–103, 1967

14. Chandler JG, Krubel R, Lee S, Rosen H, Nakaji NT, Orloff MJ: The inter-liver competition and portal blood in regeneration of auxiliary liver transplants. Surg Forum 22: 341, 1971
15. Lee S, Edgington T: Heterotopic liver transplantation utilizing inbred rat strains. Am J Path 52: 649, 1968
16. Broelsch CE, Lee S, Charters A, et al.: Regeneration of liver isografts transplanted in continuity with splanchnic organs. Surg Forum 25: 394, 1974
17. Van der Heyde MN: The role of functional competition in auxiliary liver transplantation. Transplantation 5: 78, 1966
18. Sigel B, Acevedo FJ: Methods and results of partial liver autotransplantation. SG & O 114: 731, 1962
19. Sigel B, Baldia LB, Dunn MR, Menduke H: Humoral control of liver regeneration. SG & O 124: 1023, 1967
20. Mito M, Achroyd FW, Covelli VH, Eyskens E, Katayama I, McDermott WV: Partial heterotopic liver homograft in dogs utilizing portal arterialization. Ann Surg 165: 20, 1967
21. Van der Heyde MN, Schalm L: Auxiliary liver graft without portal blood. Experimental autotransplantation of left liver lobes. Brit J Surg 55 (2): 114, 1968
22. Wexler MJ, Farkouh EF, Farrer P, Slapak M, MacLean L: The renal vein: A satisfactory alternate to the portal vein for temporary auxiliary liver Tx. Surg Forum XXI, 1970
23. Slapak M, Chir M, Beaudoin JG, Lee HM, Hume DM: Auxiliary liver homotransplantation. A new technique and an evaluation of current techniques. Arch Surg 100: 31, 1970
24. Maki T, Blackburn GL, Slapak M, McDermott Jr WV: A life supporting heterotopic autotransplant of the canine liver without portal blood. SG & O 136: 951–57, 6/1973
25. Maki T, Slapak M: Can a heterotopically placed segmental liver graft be life-supporting? An affirmative finding. Br J Surg 61: 33–39, 1974
26. Starzl TE, Knapp HA, Buck DR, Lazarus RE, Johnson RV: Reconstructive problems with canine liver homotransplantation with special reference to the postoperative role of hepatic venous flow. SG & O 110: 733, 1960
27. Eiseman B, Knipe P, Hoh Y, Normell L, Spencer FC: Factors affecting hepatic vascular resistance in the perfused liver. Ann Surg 157: 532, 1963
28. Hess J, Jerusalem C, van der Heyde MN: Advantage of Auxiliary Liver Homotransplantation in Rats. Arch Surg 104: 76, 1972
29. Jerusalem C, van der Heyde MN, Schmidt WJ, Tjebbes FA: Heterotopic liver transplantation. Unfavorable Outflow Conditions as a Possible Cause for Late Graft Failure. Eur Surg Res 4: 186, 1972
30. Broelsch C, Then P, Thistlethwaite JR, Emond J: Heterotoper Oder Orthotoper Leberersatz Durch Lebersegmente? German j Gastroenterology 25, 1987 (in print)
31. Reuvers CB, Terpstra OT, Ten Kate FWJ, Kooy PPM, Molenaar JC, Jeekel J: Long-term survival of auxiliary partial liver grafts in DLA-identical littermate beagles. Transplantation 39 (2): 113, 1985
32. Reuvers CB, Terpstra DT, Tenkate FJ, Kooy PP, Provoost AP, Molenar JC, Jeekel J: Rejection and survival of auxiliary partial liver grafts in non-tissue typed pigs. Eur Surg Res 18: 86–95, 1986
33. Reuvers CB, Terpstra OT, Boks AL, deGroot GH, Terkel J, tenKate FW, Kooy PO, Schalm S: Auxiliary transplantation of part of the liver improves survival and provies metabolic support in pigs with acute liver failure. Surgery 98: 914, 1985
34. Starzl TE, Marchioro TL, Faris TD, McCardle RJ, Iwaski Y: Avenues of future research in homotransplantation of the liver: With Particular Reference to Hepatic Supportive Procedures, Antilymphocyte Serum and Tissue Typing. Am J Surg 112: 391, 1966
35. Fortner JG, Yeh SDJ, Kim DK, Shiu MH, Kinne DW: The case for and technique of heterotopic liver grafting. Transpl Proc 11: 269, 1979

36. Houssin D, Berthelot P, Franco D, Bismuth H: Heterotopic liver transplantation in endstage HBsAg-positive cirrhosis. Lancet May 10: 990, 1980
37. Shumakov VI, Galperin EI: Transplantation of the left liver lobe. Transplant Proc XI: 1489, 1979
38. Guggenheim J, Bismuth H: Personal Communication – Nov. 1986
39. Stuart FP, Torres E, Hester WJ, Dammin GJ, Moore FD: Orthotopic autotransplantation and allotransplantation of the liver: Functional and Structural Patterns in Dog. Ann Surg 165 (3): 325–39, 1967
40. Dent DM, Hickman R, Uys CJ, Saunders S, Terblanche J: The natural history of liver allo- and autotransplantation in the pig. Br J Surg 58: 407, 1971
41. Starzl TE, Iwatsuki S, VanThiel TH, et al.: Evolution of liver transplantation. Hepatology 2: 614–636, 1982
42. Rolles K, Williams R, Neuberger J, Calne R: The Cambridge and King's college hospital experience of liver transplantation. 1968–1983. Hepatology 4: 50S, 1984
43. Pichlmayr R, Broelsch C, Wonigeit K, Neuhaus P, et al.: Experiences with liver trans- plantation in Hannover. Hepatology 4 (1): 56S–60S, 7/1984
44. Smith B: Segmental liver transplant from a living donor. J Ped Surg 4: 126, 1969
45. Mizumoto R, Yokota T, Kohno A, Ohtoshi E, Yasugi H, Ichikawa K, Honjo I: Orthotopic partial hepatic transplantation in dogs. Jap J Surg 4 (2): 121, 1974
46. Bax NMA, Vermeire BMJ, Dubois N, Madern G, Meradji M, Molenaar JC: Orthotopic non-auxiliary homotransplantation of part of the liver in dogs. J Ped Surg 17: 906, 1982
47. Broelsch CE, Then PK: Orthotopic transplantation of hepatic segments in pigs. German j. Gastroenterology 23: 293/4, 1985
48. Bismuth H, Houssin D: Reduced-sized orthotopic liver graft in hepatic transplantation in children. Surg 95 (3): 367, 1984
49. Bismuth H: Surgical anatomy and anatomical surgery of the liver. World J Surg 6: 3, 1982
50. Lortat, Jacob JL: Tentatives experimentales d'auto-transplantation de lobes de foic en position heterotopique. Rev Int Hepat 15: 1491, 1965
51. Broelsch CE, Lygidakis N: Experimental segmental auxilliary orthotopic liver transplanta- tion. Davis & Geck Film Library, 1987
52. Shaw BN, Wood RP: Prospective scoring of relative risk in patients undergoing hepatic transplantation. Hepatology 6: 1227, 1986

24. Pancreatic islet transplantation

I.D.A. JOHNSTON

Introduction

The concept of pancreatic islet cell transplantation to treat diabetic patients dying of ketoacidosis was first enunciated towards the end of the last century and nearly 30 years before the isolation of insulin by Banting and Best.

In December 1893 Dr P Watson Williams and his surgical colleague Mr Harsant [1] at the Bristol Royal Infirmary implanted 3 pieces of freshly killed sheep pancreas into the subcutaneous tissues of a 15 year old boy with diabetes. The experiment was unsuccessful and the boy died in coma 3 days later when it was found that the graft had been destroyed.

A few years later, Ssobolew (1902) [2] and Allan (1903) [3] recommended pancreatic transplantation in diabetic patients suggesting that 'a bigger supply of the sugar destroying substance might result from this procedure'.

Hope did not die after these early failures and Pybus in 1922 [4] reported 2 patients who received subcutaneous grafts of sliced human pancreas obtained from a fresh human cadaver. A transient reduction in glycosuria was recorded in one patient giving a glimmer of hope for the future but the grafts were destroyed rapidly in the recipient and the patients died. Pybus, in his discussion felt that further graft operations were not justified until the 'chemical causes of tissue rejection were understood'.

This was not the end of the story as the prospect of fresh xenografts was pursued by Luisada [5] who in 1927 transplanted portions of duct ligated baboon pancreas beneath the tunica vaginalis of two young diabetic boys. There was no discernable effect.

The rapid and successful introduction of insulin in the management of diabetes bought to an end these early imaginative and futuristic approaches to solve a serious clinical problem. The hopes of these early pioneers remain as valid and as elusive today as 60 years ago.

It took many years, however, to realise that insulin therapy did not prevent the complication of diabetes and while clinical success with islet grafting has yet to be recorded, the large amount of experimental data in small and large animals suggests that the objectives of the early pioneers may still be achieved but long after major whole organ transplantation of heart, liver and kidney has become a routine part of clinical practice.

Once it was realised that insulin treatment did not prevent the serious complications of diabetes, interest in pancreatic transplantation was rekindled. A number of approaches have been used including the transplantation of the pancreas as a vascularised organ with or without destruction of exocrine tissues [6]. The vascularised graft has been used clinically in many centres but will not be considered in any detail in this review.

The transplantation of isolated pure islets of Langerhans has been the most attractive objective from a number of points of view including the availability of adult donor cadavers and the simple and safe transplantation technique of injecting islet suspensions into selected sites as and when required. If storage was effective then repeated transplants when required would be a further advantage.

The possibility of xenogenic grafts while attractive in some respects was abandoned due mainly to the considerable immunological problems associated with this approach.

The prospect of successful islet grafting was brought forward significantly by the successful isolation and transplantation of pancreatic islets in rodents, particularly when it was found that the complications of diabetes in these small animals could be prevented by a successful islet graft. There was a great flurry of laboratory activity following these early reports yet 15 years has elapsed and the clinical objective seems as elusive as ever. The time is therefore opportune to reflect on the achievements of the laboratory and identify the problems that remain before successful islet grafting can become a reality for some diabetic patients.

Rodent experiments

The present era of islet research began in the 1960's when it was shown that both hand microdissection or collagenase digestion could produce viable islets.

Lacy and his colleagues [7] showed that collagenase separated the islets from the surrounding exocrine tissue and suspensions of large numbers of almost pure islets could be made available for experimental use.

The proven method of isolation based on the Ballinger-Lacy technique has been used in many laboratories with success. A combination of collagenase digestion, mechanical chopping and Ficoll layering produces an islet suspension, the purity of which is over 90%. However, the yield from the pancreas remains low and is not much greater than 5% of the total rodent islet population. There have been many attempts to increase the yield with modest success. The problem of yield remains a major difficulty of islet isolation in all species including man. The advantages of various modifications of isolation methods have not been dramatic and the Ballinger-Lacy method [7] is widely used by laboratories engaged in rodent studies.

Ballinger and Lacy [7], however, using their harvesting methods were able to explore the effect of transplantation in experimental diabetes. The first task was to demonstrate that the metabolic consequences of experimental diabetes could be corrected and this was soon demonstrated convincingly in a number of laboratories. The first evidence being the maintenance of normal blood glucose after transplantation in diabetic animals [8, 9].

The method of inducing the diabetic state was irrelevent. Diabetes brought about by pancreatectomy, alloxan streptozotocin or naturally ocurring inbred disease was always abolished in blood glucose terms by successful grafts. Glycosuria was also abolished, plasma glucose and insulin levels became normal. The polydypsia and polyuria of the diabetic state was reversed and normal intravenous glucose tolerance tests were obtained. In the long-term, elevated lipid levels in the metabolic state were lowered subsequently to normal [10].

These encouraging results were a considerable impetus towards the ultimate human goal but the advantage over regular insulin injection was not obvious in these rodent experiments of the 60's and the immunological barriers had not been breached.

The late complications of experimental diabetes are not dissimilar from those encountered in man. Diabetic glomerular pathology, neuropathy and cataract can all be produced experimentally in rodents and the next important challenge was to examine the effect of islet transplantation on these complications.

The renal lesions in experimental diabetes include enlargement of the mesangial space, thickening of the capillary wall, deposition of immunoglobulin and vacuolisation of tubular epithelial cells.

Intraportal islet transplantation resulting in normal blood glucose levels either prevents these lesions from developing or reverses early changes. Advanced renal changes are not reversable but further progression is halted [11, 12].

Site for transplantation

It was soon established that islets placed in the peritoneal cavity of the rat would function to a certain extent. The complete reversal of the diabetic state, however, was only achieved when the islets were either injected into the portal system or placed in a portal venous drainage site and after many studies from different laboratories, it is clear that in the rat, the most effective response requires a well vascularised site in the portal venous system [13].

Graft protection

As part of the efforts to protect the transplanted islets in their new location, an immuno-isolation technique was developed in which the islets were enclosed within a semi-permeable membrane to protect them from a cellular attack. Yet allow them to be bathed in extracellular fluid and thus receive oxygen and nutrients.

A number of separate immuno-isolation devices have been developed including extra, intravascular ultrafiltration or diffusion chambers or micro-encapsulation [14]. Each method is associated with disadvantages such as clotting and anticoagulation difficulties, fibroblast infiltration with poor graft oxygenation, protein deposition and the long-term stability of membranes. No device has been developed to overcome sufficient of these difficulties to allow it to be introduced into clinical trials [15]. In the experimental situation immunological manipulation of the graft appears to be more promising than the isolation approach. Interest in immuno-isolation is not completely finished because it may be a useful temporary measure to protect xenografts in a human situation pending the provision of sufficient human donor islets to complete a transplant procedure. The biotechnological challenge of membrane structure and function remains and if progress is made it may have other applications.

Cryopreservation

If clinical islet transplantation is to be successful it may be necessary to postpone the islet implant until a kidney transplant has been accepted immunologically. It may also be an advantage to store islet tissue for subsequent replacement grafting if graft exhaustion was to occur.

The tightly packed cellular configuration of the islets is a distinct advantage from a cryopreservation point of view.

Cooling and thawing rates which were effective in the rodent were not applicable for large animal tissue and different techniques were required.

It has now been shown that recipients of cryopreserved isografts in diabetic dogs produced prolonged normo-glycaemia and other metabolic benefits similar to those obtained with fresh autografts. The main problem with cryopreservation is the loss of viable islets due to irrepairable damage in the freezing process and as much as 40% of viable islets may be lost during cryopreservation [16].

Sufficient background work has been done to indicate that cryopreservation of human islets will be feasible and that associated cryodamage of remaining exocrine tissue may even be an advantage [17].

Foetal allografts

It has been shown that the rodent foetal pancreas can survive in vitro and selective growth of endocrine cells can occur in tissue culture. Interest in foetal tissue as a source of islets with immunological advantages has been explored in a number of centres [18].

Organ culture was found to produce quite large numbers of islets and, in fact, growth in appropriate media led to functional maturation of foetal cells. Culture conditions could be modified to eliminate passenger leucocytes from the potential graft and it was found that these grafts of cultured foetal islets could be transplanted across histocompatibility barriers without the need for recipient immunosuppression.

Some early studies with human islets showed that they shared some of the properties of rat tissue but the harvesting of the human cells poses serious problems.

Other workers demonstrated that the foetal rat pancreas, when placed under the kidney capsule continued to grow, develop and function sufficiently to reverse streptozotocin induced diabetes. Removal of the foetal pancreas before the critical period of exocrine development and function is possible with the atrophy of the exocrine cells and the survival of the endocrine pancreas in its new site [18].

The possibility of overcoming immunological attack by the use of foetal tissue has been pursued in man. Groth *et al.* in Stockholm infused foetal islets into the portal system but euglycaemia was not achieved [19]. Other workers placed extracts of foetal pancreas intramuscularly but careful monitoring revealed minimal function up to one year.

Islet resistance to immunosuppression

There has been great difficulty in maintaining the function of islet allografts in large animals for long periods of time. It was thought initially that the number of islets used in the allografts was perhaps insufficient but yield alone did not seem to be the main problem.

Steroids are of course potent diabetogenic agents and there is evidence that cyclosporin may interfere with insulin synthesis and release from islets with subsequent degeneration of the islet tissue.

The St Louis group have addressed this vital problem of the ability of islet tissue to function during immunosuppressive therapy and used an autograft model of canine intrasplenic islet implants to test the toxicity of various immunosuppressive regimens.

The control groups maintained normoglycaemia throughout the study. All groups given steroids suffered graft failure within one week. It is clear that the islets were unable to meet the increased demands for insulin when steroids were being given. The relationship between steroid dosage and insulin production by the graft is a delicate one which might, however, be capable of some manipulation [20].

Cyclosporin on the other hand, did not produce the early failure associated with steroids. Cyclosporin treated animals remained normoglycaemic for at least four weeks but thereafter graft failure was observed [20].

There is some evidence from human studies in whole organ vascularised pancreatic grafts that cyclosporin causes an altered tissue sensitivity to insulin. The exact response of islets to long-term cyclosporin administration is uncertain and this has serious implications for clinical islet grafting.

Large animal functional studies

It soon became apparent that the technique of islet cell isolation which worked well in the rodent was not applicable to the large animals. Large animal studies were also limited by the lack of inbred species. The need to use total pancreatecomised animals with subsequent islet autografts was again, not an ideal model. The problem of harvesting enough islets to provide satisfactory grafts without using multiple donors was another major problem.

The lack of numbers and the difficulties of establishing allograft models has made the interpretation of many large animal experiments difficult.

It was clearly necessary to show in the large animal that an islet graft was superior in metabolic terms at least to the regular injection of insulin in a standard diabetic model of a totally pancreatectomised animal.

The Newcastle group addressed themselves to this problem and found that blood sugar levels were not the most precise method of monitoring the metabolic abnormalities of diabetes. Levels of lactate, pyruvate, alanine, glycerol and free fatty acids can all be abnormal in euglycaemic diabetic subjects or animals [21].

Insulin and glucagon levels and the responses to intravenous glucose tolerance tests were found to be identical in diabetic patients and the diabetic dog model created by total pancreatectomy. Subcutaneous insulin in man and the dog produced the similar modifications of the full metabolic and hormonal profile. Successful islet cell transplantation produced a picture which was closer to normal. Glucose tolerance, however, was not restored totally to normal and plasma lipids remained elevated. This failure to completely overcome the metabolic abnormality is a cause of some disappointment.

However, it is clear that the reliance on blood glucose alone as an indicator of islet function is inadequate. The observation that free grafts can undergo a functional improvement after 2 to 3 months is of considerable importance indicating the reintroduction of possible localised neuropeptide control in the graft site with the passage of time [21].

These observations represent an important difference with vascularised grafts which tend to show reduced function as times passes.

The superiority of islet grafts over insulin in restoring full metabolic normality and the evidence of improving function as time passed gives considerable encouragement that the goal of preventing diabetic complications by islet transplantation was achievable.

The difficulties associated with the isolation and transplantation of purified islets in large animals has limited the number of experiments using islet allografts.

Success with fragments of unpurified slices of pancreatic tissue placed in the spleen of dogs as an autograft led to a number of attempts to use what was a relatively simple technique.

Success was limited to the prolongation of euglycaemia in 30% of the animals studied. There were many reports of failure of allografts prepared in this way in large animals. The most interesting report was of successful allografts of unpurified pancreatic fragments beneath the kidney capsule. Long-term normoglycaemia with no immuno-suppression was reported in these studies in which a renal allograft had been introduced initially [22].

One of the possible advantages of free islet transplantation over vascularised grafts is the prospect of obtaining multiple recipient grafts from a single donor pancreas.

Alderson confirmed that there was no simple relationship between the mass of a pancreatic allograft and insulin secretion in dogs with experimentally induced diabetes. These findings indicate that it is realistic to think that one may eventually obtain multiple grafts from a single donor organ [23].

The allograft challenge

The hypothesis that islet cells were less immunogeneic than other tissues in that an immunologically privileged site could be identified were soon dispelled. Islets placed in the portal circulation were usually destroyed within a few days.

Most of the commonly used immunosuppressive agents were ineffective in preventing rejection of pancreatic allografts until antilymphocyte serum was proven to be partially effective but all in all the islet cells were more vulnerable to rejection than other tissues [24] and the same disappointment followed the introduction of cyclosporin which protects most experimental allografts across major autocompatibility barriers [25].

In view of these disappointments attempts were made to alter the immunogenecity of the islets. A tissue culture technique which has shown some promise with thyroid cells was tried.

It was suggested that tissue culture methods could help to remove the passenger leucocytes in the islets which were thought to be mainly responsible for the rapid rejection. Other attempts to clean up the miscellaneous dendritic and other cells around the islet tissue by using monoclonal antibodies were partially effective [26].

While it is accepted that a critical mass is necessary to restore glucose homeostasis, the fact that metabolic abnormalities to persist in spite of the critical mass of functioning cells in the transplant is a source of concern.

It may be that the denervation of the graft or its heterotopic site may be responsible. Many of the dog studies depend on an intrasplenic graft and the spleen may be a very hostile environment for long-term function.

Further studies are required in which the functional integrity of the islets is related to insulin output and the final metabolic result.

Ultraviolet light which is a powerful blocker of dendritic cells was shown to have an effect in preventing rejection.

The Oxford workers made a significant contribution by developing a technique of transplant-induced tolerance in the rat which has potential clinical applications [27].

Vascular organs such as the kidney can be transplanted successfully across major histocompatibility barriers using a variety of immuno-suppressive treatments. Immunotherapy can be withdrawn and a powerful state of donor specific unresponsiveness can remain. This tolerance can provide an immunological umbrella under which islet tissues from the same donor can be transplanted with complete success and without the need of further immunotherapy.

The possibility, therefore, exists of harvesting and storing islets from the same donor for insertion after the transplantation and acceptance of a kidney in patients with diabetic renal failure. This approach requires initially the development of a technique of harvesting and storing sufficient numbers of viable islets and maintaining their viability for variable periods of time.

These aims have been achieved in rat experiments in which islet cryopreserved islets were preserved for six months before being transplanted and found to function effectively.

Rat models have been valuable in allowing immunological manipulation and storage techniques to be studied but some of the results in the large number of rodent experiments can not be applied directly to either the large animal situation or the problem in the human.

Isolation of islets from the human pancreas

The application of the early techniques of isolation used in the rodent experiments were largely unsuccessful. When the islets were transplanted, the yield was less than 50% of the total islet population and cell damage was a problem with subsequent failure to function even in an autograft situation. The trend in mammalian experiments to move away from purity of the islet preparation was somewhat hastily introduced into human studies. Some workers used mechanical chopping with or without collagenase digestion, while others used a period of tissue culture prior to transplantation. Simple sieving was used to separate out large fragments. All these methods were relatively crude so that the purity, viability, and even quantity of actual islets was in considerable doubt in each study reported.

Some attempts were made to use tissue obtained when pancreatectomy was being performed for chronic pancreatitis but the use of diseased pancreas created new complexities and added to the confusion and even attempts to isolate foetal pancreatic islets were unsuccessful.

The main requirement in any isolation technique in man is the provision of an adequate islet volume. The exact numbers of islets required to maintain glucose homeostasis in man is not known. It would appear from large animal studies that at least 10% of the population in the original pancreas is required which represents over 100,000 human islets.

Four groups of workers have made significant progress recently in the isolation and harvesting of human pancreatic islets.

The Oxford group used collagenase digestion and filtration followed by the use of a Ficol gradient. This led to the yield of 1,000 islets per gram of pancreas with an overall purity of less than 30%. Detailed in vitro studies established satisfactory viability and function of the isolated islets [28].

Kneteman and Pafilto added hand teasing of pancreatic tissue after ductal distension with collagenase purification being achieved on a cascade of filters. The yield was about 90,000 islets with a purity of between 20 and 40%. This group explored the effect of cryopreservation of the islet population which had been isolated and achieved some success. The insulin response to glucose perfusion of the isolated islets being used to establish function [29].

Kuhn and colleagues made a valuable contribution again using collagenase digestion after distension of the duct followed by the use of a Velcro adhesive technique to purify the yield which was in the region of 50,000 islets from one gland.

The St Louis workers have added further refinements in the last year with good results. This group emphasised the importance of using highly purified collagenase with high potency in contrast to other groups. This purified collagenase was not contaminated with potentially damaging trypsin. The temperature of the reaction was also very carefully monitored. Ficol purification was again carefully controlled by two-layer separation. Alderson et al carried out 15 successful isolations out of 17 attempts. The yields were $138,000 \pm 22,000$ representing a recovery of $80 \pm 7.6\%$ with about 50% of the final preparation being pure islets [31].

The quality and number of islets obtained by the St Louis team were close to the theoretical requirements needed for successful human transplantation.

There is no doubt now that some significant steps have been taken towards the production of an adequate viable islet preparation for human transplantation.

There are still many problems to be solved in harvesting and the observations by Sharp that perhaps the zero gravity conditions in space lab might be an appropriate environment to complete separation is an interesting twist in the quest for the efficient harvesting of undamaged islet cells.

Human autotransplantation of islets

Islet autotransplantation has been attempted to prevent diabetes when total or near total pancreatectomy has been necessary. The only indication for the procedure is likely to be chronic pancreatitis when near or total pancreatectomy is performed in the management of intractable pain. The number of such patients will always be few and it must be remembered that only about 10% of the total islet mass is needed to prevent the development of diabetes. By 1980, 58 cases of islet transplantation in patients undergoing pancreatectomy had been reported to the World Transplant Registry [32]. The transplant site was the liver following portal vein injection in most patients. The fact that the islets had to be harvested from glands damaged by pancreatitis suggested that the chance of success would be low. Nevertheless, 25 of these patients were reported to be insulin independent but the evidence that a total pancreatectomy had been performed initially was lacking in most cases. Estimation of c. peptide or insulin levels in portal and hepatic vein blood provided some evidence, however, of viability of islets in the various transplantation sites [32].

Cameron and his colleagues however, were disappointed to find that the islets ceased to function within their new location after 6 to 8 months [33]. Islet autotransplantation in man has been associated with serious complications. Some patients have died following the procedure and portal hypertension was recorded, while portal vein occlusion and disseminated intravascular coagulation have been other serious consequences of autografting.

Caution is required, therefore, in advising intraportal injection of islets in man as an autograft and thought should be given to alternative sites such as under the kidney capsule, even though this is not in a portal drainage area.

Between 1981 and 1984 only a further 8 cases were reported to the registry and the contribution of islet autografts to the maintenance of glucose homeostasis in the majority of these patients is difficult to determine.

References

1. Williams PW: Notes on diabetes treated with extract and by grafts of sheep's pancreas. Br Med J 2: 1303, 1984
2. Ssobolew LW: Zur normalen und pathologischen morphologie der inneren secretion der bauchspeicheldruse. Virch Arch Pathol Anat Physiol 168: 91, 1902
3. Allan JW: Transplantation of pancreas in diabetes and of suprarenal gland in Addison's disease. Br Med J 1: 253, 1903
4. Pybus FC: Notes on suprarenal and pancreatic grafting. Lancet 2: 550, 1927
5. Luisada: Cited by Fichera. Implanti omoplastici feto-umani nei cancro e nel diabete. Tumori 14: 434, 1927 (1928)
6. Sutherland DER: Pancreas and Islet Transplant Registry Data. World J Surg 8: 270, 1984
7. Ballinger F, Lacy PE: Transplantation of intact pancreas in rats. Surgery 72: 175, 1972
8. Boyles RR, Seltzer HS: Reversal of Alloxan diabetes in non inbred (allogeneic) rats. Horm Metab Res 7: 210, 1975
9. Gray BN, Watkins E: Isolated islet transplantation in experimental diabetes. Aust J Exp Biol Med Sci 54: 57, 1976
10. Ziegler MM, Rechard CR, Barker CF: Long term metabolism of pancreatic islets. J Surg Res 16: 575, 1974
11. Mauer SM, Steffes MW, Sutherland DER, Najarian JS, Michael AF, Brown DM: Studies of the rate of regression of the glomerular lesions in diabetic rats treated with pancreatic islet transplantation. Diabetes 24: 280, 1975
12. Schmidt RE, Plurad SB, Olack BT, Sharp DW: The effect of pancreatic islet transplantation on experimental diabetic neuropathy. Diabetes 32: 532, 1983
13. Kemp CB, Knight MJ, Sharp DW, Ballinger WF, Lacy PE: The effect of transplantation site on the results of pancreatic islet isographs in diabetic rats. Diabetologia 9: 486, 1973
14. Sun AM, Parisias W, Healey GM: The use in diabetic rats of artificial capilliary units containing cultured islets. Diabetes 26: 1136, 1977
15. O'Shea GM, Grosen MF, Sein AR: Prolonged survival of transplanted islets encapsulated in a biocompatible membrane. Biochem Biophys Acta 804: 133, 1984
16. Rajotte RV, Warnock GL, Bruch LC, Procyshyn AW: Transplantation of fresh and cryopreserved rat islets and canine pancreatic fragments. Cryobiology 20: 169, 1983
17. Rajotte RV, Warnock GL, Kneteman NN: Cryopreservation of insulin producing tissues in rat and dog. World J Surg 8: 179, 1984
18. Brown J, Danilovs JA, Clark WR, Mellen YS: Foetal pancreas as a donor organ. World J Surg 8: 152, 1984
19. Groth CG, Anderson A, Biorken C, Gunnarsson R, Hellerstrom C, Lundgren G, Peterson B, Givenne I: Attempts at transplantation of foetal pancreas to diabetic recipients. Transplantation Proceedings 13 (4): 708, 1980

20. Alderson D, Kneteman NN, Sharp DW: The effect of immunosuppression on islet transplant function in the dog. 1987 (in press)
21. Alderson D, Farndon JR, Alberti KGMM, Johnston IDA: Islet autotransplantation in the pancreatectomised dog. Effect of time on graft function. J Surg 8: 590, 1984
22. Toledo-Pereyra LH, Banalian KU, Gordon DA, Mackenzie GH, Reyman TA: Renal sub-capsular islet transplantation. Diabetes 33: 910, 1984
23. Alderson D, Farndon JR: The effect of transplant mass on insulin release by collagenase dispersed pancreatic fragments in the diabetic dog. World J Surg 8: 598, 1984
24. Kretschmer CJ, Sutherland DE, Matas AJ, Najarian JS: Preliminary experiments with al-lotransplantation of pancreatic fragments to the spleen of pancreatectomised dogs. Transplant Proceedings 11: 537, 1979
25. DuToit DF, Reece-Smith H, McShane P, Denton T, Morris PJ: The effect of Cyclosporin A on allotransplanted pancreatic fragments to the spleen of pancreatectomised dogs. Transplantation 33: 302, 1982
26. Lacy PE: Experimental immunoalteration. World J Surg 8: 198, 1984
27. Reece Smith N, DuToit DF, McShane P, Morris PJ: Prolonged survival of pancreatic allografts beneath the renal capsule. Transplantation 31: 305, 1981
28. Gray DWR, McShane P, Grant A, Morris PJ: A method of isolation of islets of Langerhans from the human pancreas. Diabetes 33: 1055, 1984
29. Kneteman NM, Rajotte RV: Isolation and cryopreservation of human pancreatic islets. Transplantation Proceedings 18: 182–185, 1986
30. Kuhn F, Schulz HJ, Lorenz D, et al.: Morphological investigations in human islets of Langerhans isolated by the Velcro-technic. Biomed Biochm Acta 44: 149–153, 1985
31. Scharp DW, Lacy PE: Human islet isolation and transplantation (Abstract). Diabetes, 3+ (Suppl 1), 5A, 1985
32. Sutherland DER, Najarian JS: In: Brooks JR (ed) Pancreas and islet transplantation in surgery of the pancreas. Philadelphia. WB Saunders & Co, 34, 1983
33. Cameron JL, Mehigan DG, Harrington DP, Zuidema GD: Metabolic studies following intrahepatic autotransplantation of pancreatic islet grafts. Surgery 87: 397, 1980

25. Hepatic dearterialization in hepatic tumours

B. JEPPSSON and S. BENGMARK

The rationale for treating liver tumours by arterial obstruction is based on the derivation of the nutrition of liver tumours from the hepatic artery. Segall showed already in 1923 that hepatic metastases in humans obtain most of the blood supply from the hepatic artery [1]. Later studies by Breedis and Young [2] showed that 80–100% of the human liver tumour circulation is derived from the hepatic artery by studying autopsy specimens of patients with various dye techniques. Similar findings have been described in experimental liver tumours [3–4]. The predominant arterial supply has been verified but around the periphery of tumours a zone of tissue with portal supply could be found. It has also been described that smaller tumours (<30mg) are fed by both the hepatic artery and portal vein while larger tumours have a predominant arterial blood supply. Similar findings have been recently reported on postmortem examination in man [5].

These findings form the basis for treatment of irresectable liver tumours by different devascularization procedures. It was suggested already in 1949 that ligation of the hepatic artery would result in necrosis of liver tumours [6]. In 1966 we first reported the use of hepatic artery ligation in the treatment of human liver tumours [7]. In this study tumour regression following ligation allowed subsequent resection of a previously inexstripable tumour. This favourable result has not been borne out in subsequent clinical trials. We have today, however, a better understanding of the mechanisms of the tumouricidal cytotoxic effects of obstructing the blood supply to liver tumours. This knowledge will hopefully allow us to improve the therapeutic principle.

Pathophysiology of liver ischemia

The reduced arterial blood flow to the liver after hepatic artery ligation or dearterialization leads to a shortage of oxygen and substrates which in turn results in impairment of important liver functions. The ischemia will severely influence the capacity of the reticulo-endothelial system, the hepatic energy storage and the synthesis of lipoproteins and proteins. Recovery of normal liver function has been observed within hours after release of temporary occlusion of the hepatic artery or a few days to one week after permanent occlusion. The recovery after permanent occlusion is considered to be due to the fast revascularization via arterial collaterals [8]. Anoxia – hypoxia following interruption of arterial blood supply is thought to play a significant role for the development of cell necrosis in neoplastic tissues. Hypoxia is known to reduce tumour growth but lack of oxygen is probably not the only etiological factor. In fact, it is known that liver tumours may have cell clones which are dependent on anaerobic metabolism and thereby not influenceable by ischemia. Lack of nutritional factors and accumulation of catabolites have also been suggested to be responsible for cell necrosis after liver ischemia [9].

More recent suggestions have been made on the generation of oxygen-free radicals in liver ischemia and their role in cell damage. It is well known that the production of oxygen-derived free radicals is stimulated by hypoxia or especially by reperfusion following hypoxia [10]. Experimental work by our group has been conducted to investigate the role of free radicals in liver dearterialization. In both a rat and a pig model, we have measured the activity of an enzyme, adenosine diphosphate ribosyl transferase (ADPRT), in the outflow blood from the temporarily dearterialized liver. This enzyme is concerned with repair of DNA strand breaks caused by oxygen free radicals [11]. In this model the enzyme is not activated upon reperfusion of the liver with oxygenetic blood, but within minutes of the arterial occlusion and there is then a steady adaptation as the enzyme activity returns to normal [12]. From these results it seems likely that the small supply of oxygen in the portal blood permits a steady production of cytotoxic oxygen free radicals. The observation that a maximal effect of hepatic arterial occlusion seems to occur very soon has led us to investigate short periods of pulse occlusion instead of long ischemic periods.

Hepatic dearterialization

Hepatic dearterialization can be performed surgically in different ways.
1. Hepatic artery ligation.
    The hepatic artery is ligated as close as possible to the liver.
2. Hepatic dearterialization.
    All connections to the lesser omentum and all structures except the common bile duct and the portal vein in the hepato-duodenal ligament are ligated and divided.

    We perform this procedure via a transrectal incision which with the help of a Rissler retractor gives good access to all parts of the liver. The falciform ligament is first divided. The left triangular ligament is thereafter cut, the left liver lobe is dissected free from the diaphragm until the entrance of the left hepatic vein in the inferior vena cava. Tributaries from the phrenic artery in this area must be ligated. The lesser omentum is thereafter dissected

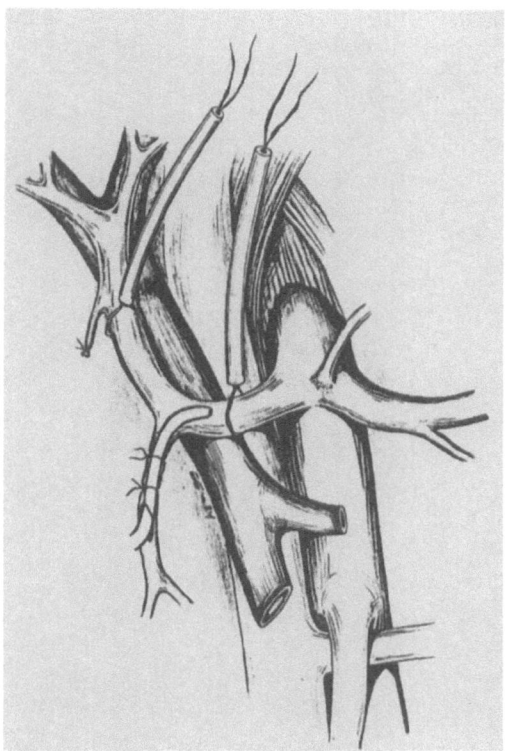

Fig. 1. Model for transient dearterialization. Two occluding slings are applied around the hepatic artery, and a catheter is introduced through the gastroduodenal artery. By pulling the slings occlusion of the hepatic artery is achieved. This technique was used in the early studies of transient dearterialization with a length of occlusion of 16h [21, 25].

and here a big branch from the left gastric artery is usually found and divided. The right liver lobe is thereafter prepared free from all attachments. The peritoneum over the lower dorsal margin of the lobe is incised and with blunt and sharp dissection the attachment to the diaphragm (the right triangular and coronary ligament) can be divided. The dissection is carried out up to the hepatic veins. By first mobilizing the left liver lobe, the whole liver can now be rotated to the left, the right liver lobe lifted up and thereby make possible a good exposure of the posterior liver surface.

The peritoneum on the ventral aspect of the hepatoduodenal ligament is incised and the proper hepatic artery distal to the gastroduodenal artery is dissected. The common bile duct is also isolated and the small lymphatics and blood vessel surrounding the common bile duct and the hepatic artery are divided. The portal vein is isolated dorsal to these structures. The hepatic artery can now be ligated and cut.

410

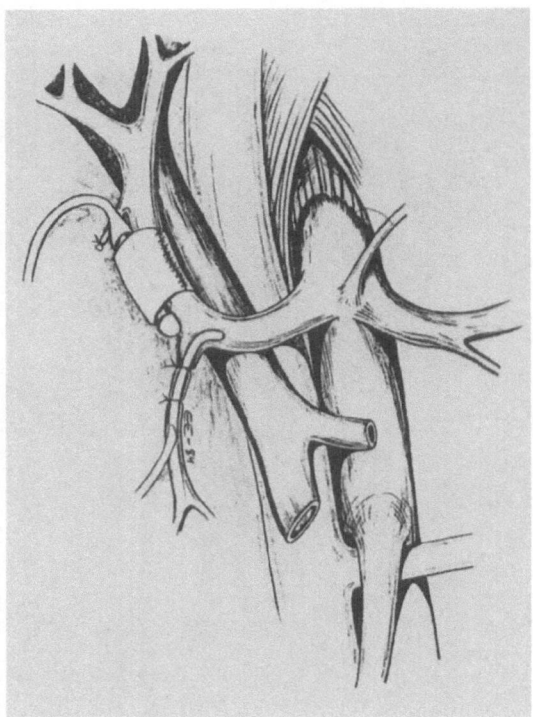

Fig. 2. Recent model for transient dearterialization. The balloon is connected to the plexiglass chamber with a silicon rubber, which is placed subcutaneously in the right hypochondrium. The artery is compressed within the cuff when the balloon is inflated.

3. Repeated transient hepatic dearterialization.

Dearterialization of the liver is carried out as described above. The hepatic artery is either surrounded by occluding slings (Fig. 1) or a vascular occluder (Fig. 2) which allow occlusion of the hepatic artery postoperatively. The vascular occluder consists of a silicon balloon which is attached to sleeves. The sleeves are sewn around the hepatic artery and the balloon is connected via a small catheter to a subcutaneous injection port. By injecting a few ml of saline the balloon is inflated and the artery compressed within the ring.

Clinical results

The prognosis for untreated liver tumours varies in different series and depends on type of tumour and extent of tumour involvement. It is important to recognize the natural history of untreated liver tumours, to use for comparison between results of different therapies. This is especially important since very few randomized trails with untreated controls have been performed regarding dearterialization. The mean survival from time of diagnosis for untreated primary liver cancer is only a few months [13] and for colorectal liver metastases upto six months [14, 15].

Dearterialization in primary liver cancer

Hepatic dearterialization has been performed in the palliative treatment of primary liver cancer since the beginning of 1970. There are only two randomized studies published where dearterialization in combination with cytotoxic drug infusion has been compared with untreated controls (Table 1). In the first study [16] dearterialization was compared with hepatic artery ligation with in-

Table 1. Dearterialization procedures – randomized trials.

Author	Patients	Occlusion	Drug	Survival (mo)	Compl/Mort
Bengmark et al., 1971	39 PLC	–	–	1 (mean)	–
Wood et al., 1976	113 met. colorectal	–	–	6.6 (mean)	
Bengtsson et al., 1981	25 met. colorectal	–	–	4.5 (mean)	
Ong et al., 1975	16 PLC	Deart	–	4.2 (mean)	† 44% at 1 mo
	14 PLC	HAL	5-FU i.p. 15 mg/kg	5.2 (mean)	† 36% at 1 mo
	16 PLC	–	5-FU i.a. 15 mg/kg	5.9 (mean)	† 44% at 1 mo
	12 PLC	–	–	5.2 (mean)	† 42% at 1 mo
Lai et al., 1986	37 PLC	–	–	1.9 (median)	† 27% at 1 mo
	33 PLC	Deart	–	1.1 (median)	† 44% at 1 mo
	30 PLC	HAL	5-FU, i.a. adriamycin	1.1 (median)	† 42% at 1 mo
	29 PLC	HAL	5-FU, i.p. adriamycin	2.7 (median)	† 32% at 1 mo
	37 PLC	Radiation	–	2.2 (median)	† 15% at 1 mo
Taylor et al., 1978	6 met. colorectal	–	–	3.1 (mean)	† 17%
	6 met.	HAL	5-FU, i.a.	3.0 (mean)	† 17%
	7 met.	HAL	5-FU, i.p. + i.a.	9.8 (mean)	† 14%
	5 met.	–	5-FU, i.p.	4.1 (mean)	† 20%

PLC= Primary liver cancer; HAL= Hepatic artery ligation; i.p. = intraportal; i.a. = intraarterial traportal or intraarterial 5-FU infusion and one group without treatment served as control. The length of survival was almost identical in the different groups, averaging 17–21 weeks. Some palliative effect with reduction of tumour size and relief of pain was noted, more often after hepatic dearterialization and hepatic artery ligation. In a more recent study [17] dearterialization was compared to hepatic artery ligation with infusion of 5-FU and adriamycin, irradiation and one group of untreated controls. In this study there was no statistically significant difference in the survival between the different groups. On the other hand, patients who underwent hepatic artery ligation followed by portal vein infusion chemotherapy lived significantly longer than those patients who received infusion by the hepatic artery or those who underwent hepatic artery dearterialization alone. The tumour burden in the different groups was not defined and this makes the evaluation difficult.

Our own experience with dearterialization in primary liver cancer has shown similar results with a mean survival of 4.5 or medium survival of eight months in the two materials published [18, 19] (Table 2).

From these series it can also be seen that dearterialization has a high rate of postoperative complications and it is obvious that it is a difficult technique and applied alone it is of limited value. Combined treatment with cytotoxic drugs has therefore been recommended. This might improve the results but the use of 5-FU in most studies is hard to understand, since this drug has not shown any effect on primary liver cancer. It is therefore today impossible to say if dearterialization and regional chemotherapy has any beneficial effect in the treatment of primary liver cancer.

Table 2. Dearterialization procedures – own results.

Author	Patients	Occlusion	Drug	Survival (mo)	Compl/Mort
Bengmark et al., 1971	39 PLC	–	–	1 (mean)	–
Bengtsson	25 met.	–	–	4,5 (mean)	–
Almersjö et al., 1972	5 PLC 22 met. various	Deart	–	4,5 (mean)	† 37%
Almersjö et al., 1976	10 PLC 30 met. various	26 HAL 14 deart	5-FU i.p. 15 mg/kg (19/40)	8 (median)	† 17,5%
Dahl et al., 1981	20 met. various	Trans. deart.	5-FU i.a. 10 mg/kg	17 (mean)	† 20%

PLC = Primary liver cancer; HAL = Hepatic artery ligation; i.p. = intraportal; i.a. = intraarterial.

Dearterialization in secondary liver cancer

For many tumour types the prognosis of the primary tumour is so poor that the appearance of liver metastases is of no importance. Therefore most studies concerning dearterialization in liver metastases have dealt with metastases from colo-rectal cancers, mammary cancers and some sarcomas. Many studies have been published proposing a beneficial effect of hepatic artery ligation or dearterialization in liver metastases when compared to historic controls. There has to our knowledge only been performed one randomized controled clinical trial of patients with synchronous colo-rectal liver metastases comparing hepatic artery ligation with intraportal cytotoxic drug infusion or portal vein infusion of 5-FU alone [20] (Table 1). The different therapies did not improve symptom-free survival when compared to the untreated controls but the group of patients undergoing both hepatic artery ligation and portal vein infusion had a statistically significant increased survival. The number of patients in the different groups was however small. Our own experience gives some indication of prolonged survival although only compared to historic controls (Table 2). This is especially true when dearterialization is performed as one transient dearterialization [21]. In this material 5-FU was infused in the hepatic artery for a period of at least three weeks following one transient dearterialization for 16 h. In patients with tumour only localized to the liver the medium survival was 24 months and for patients with extrahepatic tumour growth it was 10 months. There was an objected tumour response in 50% of the patients estimated angiographically. The complication rate was however high. Although the overall survival after transient dearterialization was longer in this selected group of patients compared to historic controls, there was no advantage compared to patients treated with regional infusion alone [22].

Dearterialization in metastatic carcinoid tumours

The five year survival of patients with metastatic carcinoid disease and carcinoid syndrome is about 20–30% [23]. Hepatic artery ligation and hepatic dearterialization have shown good results with relief of symptoms in about 50% of patients treated [24]. The operations were however followed by a significant mortality rate. We have used the temporary dearterialization as described above with occluding slings in a series of sixteen patients with carcinoid syndrome without any mortality [25]. In this series there was a clear improvement in the symptoms of the carcinoid patients in fifteen patients after six months and in twelve patients after twelve months. Four patients who preoperatively suffered from carcinoid syndrome were after the temporary dearterialization free of symptoms for 24–62 months and simultaneously there were decreases of serotonin concentrations in blood [26]. One year after the operation a clear

414

therapeutic effect on the tumour volume was still demonstrable in eleven patients.

Repeated short-term transient hepatic dearterialization

The high rate of postoperative complications after dearterialization, as well as the rapid development of arterial collaterals have lead us to develop methods for repeated short-term transient hepatic dearterialization. The advantages of transient repeated dearterialization may be manifold. Development of arterial collaterals does not seem to occur after repeated short-lasting dearterializations [27]. The operative trauma and the trauma of the hepatic ischemia do not coincide which may reduce the complication rate. The development of an implantable occluding device has introduced a great flexibility, especially when combined with a subcutaneous injection port [28] (Fig. 2). This system allows repeated short-lasting episodes of occlusion and administration of cytotoxic drugs via a separate catheter in the hepatic artery or the peritoneal cavity.

In a first pilot study we have now treated three patients with colo-rectal liver metastases with one or two daily occlusions of the hepatic artery lasting for one hour and intraperitoneal infusion of 5-FU 500 mg per day for five days, every third week. The results are encouraging.

Conclusions

There is a wide range of therapeutic manipulations available for the palliative treatment of patients with liver malignancies. The use of the dearterialization principle is today wide spread. The availability of new techniques with implantable equipment for repeated short-lasting ischemia at regular intervals for weeks and months stimulates to further studies.

References

1. Segall MN: An experimental anatomical investigation of the blood and bile channels of the liver. Surg Gynecol & Obstet 37: 152–178, 1923
2. Breedis C, Young G: The blood supply of neoplasms in the liver. Am J Pathol 30: 569–986, 1954
3. Nilsson LAV, Zettergren L: The blood supply and vascular pattern of induced primary hepatic carcinoma in rats. Acta Pathol Microbiol Scand 71: 179–185, 1967
4. Ackerman NV: The blood supply of experimental liver metastases. IV. Changes in vascularity with increasing tumour growth. Surgery 75: 589–596, 1974
5. Lin G, Lunderquist A, Hägerstrand I, Boijsen E: Post-mortem examination of the blood supply and vascular pattern of small liver metastases in man. Surgery 96: 517–519, 1984

6. Markowitz J, Rappaport A, Scott AC: Prevention of liver necrosis following ligation of hepatic artery. Proc Soc Exp Biol Med 70: 305–315, 1949

7. Almersjö O, Bengmark S, Engevik L, Hafström LO, Nilsson LAV: Hepatic artery ligation as pretreatment for liver resection of metastatic cancer. Rev Surg 22: 377–384, 1966

8. Bengmark S, Rosengren K: Angiographic study of the collateral circulation to the liver after ligation of the hepatic artery in man. Am J Surg 119: 620–630, 1970

9. Carlsson G, Hafström LO: Influence of hepatic artery ligation on survival. An experimental study in rats. Am J Surg 147: 688–691, 1984

10. Im MJ, Mansson PN, Bukley GB, Hoopes JE: Effects of superoxide dismutase and allopurinol on the survival of acute island skin flaps. Ann Surg 201: 357–359, 1984

11. Benjamin RC, Gill RM: Poly-CADP-ribosed synthesis in vitro programmed by damaged DNA. J Biol Chem 25: 10502–10508, 1980

12. Puntis MCA, Persson B, Jonsson G, Jeppsson B, Pero RW, Bengmark S: Free radical production in the ischemia rat liver. Surg Res Comm 1: 17–20, 1987

13. Bengmark S, Börjesson B, Hafström LO: The natural history of primary carcinoma of the liver. Scand J of Gastroenterol 6: 351–355, 1971

14. Wood CB, Gillis CR, Blumgart LH: A retrospective study of the natural history of patients with liver metastases from colorectal cancer. Clin Oncol 2: 285–288, 1976

15. Bengtsson G, Carlsson G, Hafström LO, Jöhsson PE: Natural history of patients with untreated liver metastases from colorectal cancer. Am J Surg 141: 586–589, 1981

16. Ong GB, Chan PKW, Alagaratnan TT: Clinical trials of inoperative primary carcinoma of the liver. Bull Soc Int Chir 5: 391–397, 1975

17. Lai ECS, Choi TK, Tong SW, Ong GB, Wong J: Treatment of unresectable hepatocellular carcinoma: results of a randomized controlled trial. World J Surg 10: 501–509, 1986

18. Almersjö O, Bengmark S, Rudenstam CM, Hafström LO, Nilsson LAV: Evaluation of hepatic dearterialization in primary and secondary cancer of the liver. Am J Surg 124: 5–9, 1972

19. Almersjö O, Bengmark S, Hafström LO, Leissner KH: Results of liver dearterialization combined with regional infusion of 5-Fluorouracil for liver cancer. Acta Chir Scand 142: 131–138, 1976

20. Taylor I: Cytotoxic perfusion for colorectal liver metastases. Br J Surg 65: 109–114, 1978

21. Dahl EP, Fredlund PE, Tylén U, Bengmark S: Transient hepatic dearterialization followed by regional intra-arterial 5-Fluorouracil infusion as treatment for liver tumours. Ann Surg 153: 82–88, 1981

22. Ekberg H, Tranberg K-G, Lundstedt C, Hanff G, Ranstam J, Jeppsson B, Bengmark S: Determinants of survival after intraarterial infusion of 5-Fluorouracil for liver metastases from colorectal cancer – a multivariate analysis. J Surg Oncol 31: 246–254, 1986

23. Tilson MD: Carcinoid syndrome. Surg Clin N America 54: 409–425, 1974

24. Farndon JR: The carcinoid syndromes: methods of treatment and recent experience with hepatic artery ligation and infusion. Clin Oncol 3: 365–372, 1972

25. Bengmark S, Ericsson M, Lunderquist A, Mårtensson H, Nobin A, Sano M: Temporary liver dearterialization in patients with metastatic carcinoid disease. World J Surg 6: 46–57, 1982

26. Nobin A, Axelsson S, Frick B, Ingemansson S, Lunderquist A, Mårtensson H, Reichardt W: Selective mesenteric vein catheterization in patients with carcinoid syndrome. World J Surg 7: 223–230, 1983

27. Persson B, Andersson L, Jeppsson B, Ekelund L, Strand SE, Bengmark S: Development of collateral circulation after repeated transient occlusion of the hepatic artery in pigs. World J Surg 1987, in press

28. Persson B, Jeppsson B, Ekelund L, Bengmark S: A new device for temporary occlusion of the hepatic artery. J Exp Clin Cancer Res 3: 155–160, 1984

26. Developments in HPB nursing

K. ULANDER

Purpose of the chapter

The purpose of this chapter is to present the current nursing care being given to patients with disorders in the hepato-pancreatico-biliary tract. The chapter covers the nursing care of the cholecystectomy patient, the patient with pancreatic cancer and the patient with liver disorders. It is not possible naturally to cover every aspect of nursing care in one chapter. The reader will have to turn to other works to get more details. Given and Simmons' 'Gastroenterology in clinical nursing' [1] for example. The intention, is rather to higlight certain aspects being discussed in recent literature.

To start it was necessary to find out what has been written about HPB-nursing care during the last 10 years. A literature search gave 50 titles, which of 12 were in Japanese or Chinese. Half of the articles were published during the 80's. A few of them are written by physicians and contain only medical facts about the etiology and treatment of different HPB-diseases. The great majority of the articles are written by RNs on different levels and contain both information about the medical care and the nursing care. A couple of authors are nursing students presenting case studies.

This chapter is based on the literature and on the knowledge of the nursing profession at the Department of Surgery in Lund.

General dimensions of nursing care

The goal of nursing is to maintain the optimal wellness of patients and, if this state changes, to provide the amount and quality of nursing care the situation demands to direct patients back to wellness or to adjust maximally to their circumstances. Nurses have the knowledge base and the observational skills to assist patients in preventing or recovering from HPB problems. When interviewing these patients, nurses must seek information to allow the patients to adopt the behaviors and acquire the knowledge and skills needed to carry out the prescribed therapeutic regimen.

Knowledge of the disease, medication, diet and other life-style changes are essential components of the therapeutic regimen. The information may need to be repeated throughout the course of treatment.

The nurse can do much to provide support by being aware of the physician's plans for the patient. Being with the physician when these plans are discussed with the patient makes the nurse able to clarify any information that the patient does not understand or has not heard correctly. By being familiar with the patient, the nurse can recognize how the individual is accepting the treatment plan and can encourage the patient to verbalize fears, feelings and misunderstandings.

Therefore it is necessary to organize the nursing care in such a way that these plans may be implemented. The nurse cannot be responsible for the direct care of more patients than she can care for herself. In the general wards at the Department of Surgery in Lund, the RN's are primary nurses for 3–4 patients and assistant/secondary nurses for 2–3 patients.

Nursing care of the cholecystectomy patient

The incidence of gallstones is changing with sex, age, different countries, parts of countries and time. Women have always had a higher frequency of gallstones than men. Approximately 40.000 cholecystectomies per year are performed in Sweden (8 milj inhabitants).

Several experiments have been carried out for the purpose of dissolving gallstones. These means have not seemed to be as effective as the surgical removal of the stones and bladder. Although the nonoperative procedure which involves the use of endoscopic retrograde cholangiopancreatography (ERCP) is useful, it cannot be used to remove stones from the gallbladder itself. Surgery is usually performed when the patient's condition warrants it and after correction of any deficiency.

Preoperative care

Often it seems that little is done to provide individualized care for the preoperative patient beyond the immediate physical needs. Individualized teaching and psychological preparation of the patient may be overlooked if their significance is not realized by those who work with patients daily. The nurse should understand that to each patient surgery is the most important aspect of life at that time. Because surgery carries with it some risk as well as discomfort, emotional stress and a disruption of normal life patterns, the nurse owes the patient an individualized approach that meets his or her specific needs.

When caring for a patient with gallbladder disease, the nurse should be alert to the onset of jaundice. Presence of jaundice may necessitate vitamin K replacement. The nurse must observe closely for signs of bleeding from the gums, nose or injection site. Pain relief and vital signs are other aspects of nursing care that need to be considered during the acute stage. If a chole-dochotomy will be performed the nurse must include teaching regarding the presence and function of the T-tube to be used after surgery. The material covered in each teaching session should be recorded, to make the job easier for the team, and give the patient confidence that the staff are interested in him/her, because they are aware of what has been taught previously.

Postoperative care

If only a cholecystectomy is performed, the patient will be closely observed only until fully awakened from the anesthetic and thereafter return to the general ward. In Lund we mobilize the patient out of bed in the evening the day of surgery and also let the patient have free fluids if tolerated. This early ambulation helps relieve distension and flatulence. A low-fat diet is usually tolerated by the first postoperative day. The patient is then prepared for discharge on the 2nd or 3rd day.

If a T-tube is inserted care should be taken to keep the dressings dry because bile is very irritating to the skin. Special care must be taken to see that no pull is present on the tube and that it does not catch on bed clothing. Output from the tube should be observed, measured and recorded every shift. After the x-ray has showed a clear common bile duct the T-tube will be removed, while the other drain is being removed half a day later.

If complications should occur, making it necessary to keep the T-tube at home, the care of the tube must be fully reviewed with the patient. A record of the teaching must be kept to make sure the patient and family are well informed about how to handle the tube.

Only one case study of a patient undergoing cholecystectomy seem to have been presented in the literature from the nursing field [2]. The patient, 82 yrs old, got the common bile duct explored and got a T-tube inserted. From 18.00 h on the operation day, the patient took sips of water occasionally and tolerated them. On the 10th postoperative day after the acute surgery the patient was discharged to her son's home.

It is difficult to judge from just one case, but it seems that the postoperative phase was quite long. Although it was an old lady going through an acute operation it might have been possible to have prepared her for home earlier.

At our department a patient of the same type would have been discharged after 6–7 days. A patient having undergone elective surgery with a T-tube, would have been at home after 5 days.

Preparation for home

We are just conducting a study trying to cut length of stay further through better preoperative information and education of the patient. The preliminary findings show that the need for better preparation before discharge seem to be of a greater importance than thought before [3].

Nursing care of the patient with pancreatic cancer

Cancer of the pancreas accounts for approximately 15% of the malignant tumors of the digestive tract. Pancreaticoduodenal resection (Whipple's procedure) is the operation of choice for potentially curable cancer of the head of the pancreas.

Nursing care is mostly supportive and symptomatic, depending on the extent of the carcinoma. The aim of care is to provide nutritional support, relief of pain, emotional support, and replacement of pancreatic enzymes, bile salts and vitamin K. Three case studies of patients undergoing Whipple's pancreatico duodenectomy, one article on the equipment in the operating room and one general on the postoperative care have been reported in the nursing literature. The case studies are presenting the medical treatment as well as the nursing care.

Preoperative care

The preoperative preparation follows the guidelines for major gastrointestinal surgery. Osborne [4] comments specifically on the need to explain the significance of that the pancreas will be partially removed. Since many patients don't know the function of the organ, they are not aware of the need for enzyme supplements or the need for insulin. She also stresses the need for correct information about the necessary diet, so that both the patient and the family are informed and can follow the advice for the patient.

Postoperative care

The postoperative care is intensive during the first two days. Whiteford [5] describes the postoperative care in detail. The patient is placed in a pre-heated bed in a semi-recumbent position to obtain a clear airway. The drains and operative site are inspected and the drainage bottles are placed carefully into holders and secured properly. The drainage bottles are emptied at least once per day, the dressing only changed when needed, to prevent introducing infection. Vital signs are observed every half-hour.

Total mouth care is done hourly the first postoperative day. Then from day two these actions are carried out every two hrs. The nurses test and record the urine daily. The colour of stools is noted and as the patient's condition improves the stools became more and more their normal colour.

Maintaining fluid and electrolyte balance is of great importance, but it would take too long to go into all details here. The nurse's role is to assess the amount of drainage and other losses and check the patient for signs of imbalance. On the third day the patient can be allowed his first fluid by mouth – 15 ml of water hourly.

Pain medication ought to be given every four to eight hour as prescribed. It is also important for the nurse to determine if the patient's pain is the typical surgical pain, or if it might be related to another complication like pancreatitis.

The patient must be assisted to breath, cough and to do foot and leg exercises. Whiteford describes how the patient gets a full bed-bath and clean clothes the day after surgery, plus the prevention of pressure sores, using a sheep-skin rug, bootees and massage. The patient can have his family visiting for short periods, as he often is tired postoperatively.

Whiteford advices that the patient's nasogastric (NG) tube is aspirated hourly the first postoperative day. Levine [6] adds that NG suction is continued for several days after the return of peristalsis. This is done in an attempt to reduce the gastric phase of pancreatic stimulation which occurs when the fundus of the stomach is distended.

Hemorrhage is a major common complication following surgery. Prevention of increased pressure on the suture lines is done by maintaining the patency of the nasogastric tube and sump drains. During the immediate postoperative period, the drainage from the naso-gastric tube tends to be grossly bloody. However the physician needs to be notified if the drainage is greater than 75 ml per hour or if it stays grossly bloody for longer than four hours.

Maintain patency of sump drains and fistulas in order to prevent these secretions from disrupting other sites of anastomosis is important. If fistulas should develop, the nurse needs to protect the skin exposed to digestive enzymes of the drainage, by using stoma bags and skin barrier or aluminum paste on any skin that remains exposed around the bag opening. Providing a diet high in calories, protein and vitamins will promote healing. The nurse needs to assess for signs of small bowel obstruction which may result from a chemical peritonitis.

Preparation for home

Before being discharged, all patients who are diabetic will require teaching related to this disease. Patient and family education is essential during this period.

The patient who develops stenosis of the pancreatico-jejunostomy will develop malnutrition and is usually helped by a diet low in fat and by eating six small meals a day. The patient's respons to enzymatic replacement tablets may vary and he needs to know about effects and possible sideeffects.

Nursing care of the patient with liver disorders

The patient with portal hypertension

During pathological circumstances the pressure in the portal vein can rise for many reasons. Mostly the resistence is in the liverparenchym and the damage comes from the use of alcohol. 1/3 of patients with portal hypertension bleed gastro-intestinally. Several different types of shunts have been tried to get decompression. Altshuller and Hilden [7] writes how nurses may take part in informing the patient with portal hypertension about how to prevent and manage bleeding episodes. Many bleeding episodes seem to develop during an upper respiratory infection. Nevertheless, both children and adults need to maintain normal social contacts, but they need to think about avoidance of exposure to persons known to be ill. If a respiratory infection does develop, the early use of cough suppressants may prevent trauma to delicate oesophageal varices.

Some dietary measures are also advocated. Food products that are spicey, rough or of sharp quality may irritate existing varices.

Constipation is a problem to be avoided when possible, as straining increases the possibility for bleeding. Individuals and family need to be able to recognize subtle indications of blood loss, such as melaena, fatigue and pallor. And if a nurse has previously explored with a family the steps needed to reach emergency medical services, should a major bleeding episode occur, the chances are increased for a positive outcome.

Surgical management and nursing care

Some general comments on the care will be discussed here. A prerequisite for good nursing care of the patient with portal hypertension is a clear understanding of the goals of medical and/or surgical management. Without this knowledge it is difficult to give supportive emotional care to the patient and family or to determine realistic objectives for the patient.

It is also important for the medical and nursing staff to have a dialogue about the moral and ethical factors that are involved in patient selection.

Another area to consider is the responsibility, of the nurse to ensure that the patient's rights are being protected. Often the patient is very ill and can not contribute. Then the family needs to have a clear understanding of the possible outcomes of therapy. When information concerning the availability of support systems for follow-up care is not sought from the patient and family, successful surgical intervention may be useless to protect the individual from further liver damage and bleeding episodes.

Pre- and postoperative care

The care will vary according to the condition of the patient. A history of alcohol abuse has significant implications for the nursing observations. Men with moderate to advanced hepatic disease often report physical and libidinal changes. Information on sexual patterns is useful, according to King, for helping the patient adjust psychologically to both his illness and his surgery [8].

The preoperative teaching will also depend on an assessment of the patient's learning style and coping patterns. The hemorrhaging patient needs calm, direct, short explanations. Postoperatively, this patient will need more explanation, reinforcing of information, and clarification of expectations. The patient in a stabilized condition is often more responsive if his anxiety is not too high.

Postoperatively the nurse also needs to recall the effects of long-term liver disease on the cardiorespiratory system. Also the patient with liver damage needs careful dietary counseling.

The nurse should observe and record the post-shunt patient's ability to utilize dietary protein. It is a challenge to encourage adequate intake of food. Small meals attractively served is one method. If the patient is choosing his own menu, the nurse could use this opportunity to assess the patient's educational needs and offer teaching.

Another problem that can occur in the post-shunt phase is hepatic encephalopathy. Long-term nursing care should include particular attention to the evaluation of the patient's functioning within his family and peer group.

Care of the patient with portal hypertension demands a sophisticated level of knowledge and skill of the professional nurse. The pre- and postoperative nursing care must be based on an understanding of pathophysiology and the procedures themselves.

Frequently however the patient recalls small human caring actions taken by nurses. For example treating a chronic alcoholic with respect, the calm assurance when a nurse has handled a sudden bleeding crises or the caring involved in reaching out for the hand of a frightened patient.

By seeking feedback from patients, nurses may learn of those interventions that were most meaningful and helpful and work to implement these approaches in the future.

The patient who undergo liverresektion

Hepatom, primary malignant tumour in the liver, is persistent in Sweden in a frequency of 6.9 (men) – 4,3 (women) per 100.000 inhabitants and year (1980). In other parts of the world the frequency is substantially higher. The only curative treatment is surgical resection of all tumour tissue. Metastatic tumours are 20 times higher in frequency than hepatoms. Quite often it is useful to treat them surgically.

Preoperative care

The preoperative preparations follows the guidelines for major gastrointestinal surgery, so it will not be commented in detail here.

At our department a retrospective study of 10 patients undergoing liver resection due to malignancy has been carried out by two of the staff nurses [9]. They found it to be of vital importance to use a lot of energy in getting the patient calm before surgery. This is accomplished by giving correct information to the patient and family about the postoperative care and by taking time when caring for this type of patient.

Postoperative care

The evening after surgery the patient will be monitored and cared for in the intensive care unit (ICU) and will return to the ward the following morning.

At the ICU the patient will have his vital signs checked as well as CVP, urine output/hour, drainage and pain control. Blood samples will be taken to control the ventilation, hemorrhaging tendencies and liverfunction as well as electrolytes. If the patient can manage, changes of position are done frequently.

When the patient returns to the prepared single-room at the ward the primary nurse is responsible for the nursing care and control of the patient. She makes sure that the things needed for oxygen and suction, as well as mouth care equipment, are ready.

She checks the vital signs four-hourly. Haemoglobin is checked twice a day, other blood samples according to the physicians order. Electrolytes and fluid balance is kept so that glucose in urine is positive, according to medical orders. Urine is collected for control of amount of urea and of creatinine clearance. The patient's weight is taken daily.

The dressing on the op-site is only changed when needed. If needed the area around the drains is cleaned with chlorhexidine-spiritus. If the drainage is heavy, a stoma-bag is put over the drain.

Pain control is carried out so the patient is painfree without a breathing depression which is easy to get with liver-insufficiency. The physiotherapist and the nurse will assist the patient with coughing, breathing and mobilization. The first postoperative day the patient will sit at the edge of the bed. During the next days mobilizing in the room, and in the hall on approximately the fifth postoperative day.

The nurse will also listen to bowel sounds daily, due to the risk of paralysis. When the bowels have moved the patient will start on fluids and solid food after approximately six days.

Joakimsson/Nilsson [9] noted several possible complications for these patients. Loss of appetite, pleural effusion, oedema tendency, possible intoxication from pain medication and depression.

Their conclusion is that through good information the patient will get a feeling of thrust and be able to work towards the same goals as the staff. Possibly this may also reduce some of the depressive and hopeless feelings that many of these patients seem to go through after surgery.

Biliary catheter care

The management of biliary drainage tubes in a patient who has an irresectable tumour, is discussed in three articles written by Bradford [10] from Hammersmith Hospital in London (1981), Miller/Gavant [11] at VA Medical Center in Memphis (1985) and Coleman [12] at John Hopkins University Medical Center in Baltimore (1985).

The design and introduction, at Hammersmith Hospital, of a new closed drainage system, comprising a single-use disposable collecting bag connected via a twist action, self-sealing slit valve, has eliminated bacterial colonisation and enabled significant reduction of associated septic complications. The system allows aseptic flushing of drainage tube, introduction of contrast medium and bile collection for laboratory examination without prejudice to sterility [13].

In order to maintain the patency of the tubes, they are flushed twice a day through the tap with 5 ml of sterile normal saline. To prevent infection occurring in the bilebags, 10 ml of aqueous povidone-iodine is flushed through the tap into the bag. The taps and bile bags are changed twice a week. The entry site of the tube is cleaned and dressed daily. The tube is secured carefully to the patient to prevent pulling and discomfort [10].

Patients managed with this new closed system showed a significant reduction of bacterial colonisation after 20 days drainage, and of bacteraemia during decompression and post-operatively, as well as of positive wound cultures.

Miller/Gavant [11] are describing the use of a palliative percutaneous biliary drainage, where after two or three days, if there are no complications, the catheter stopcock is removed and replaced with a rubber injection site adapter. The drainage bag is discarded and bile will flow internally.

After the catheter first has been placed, the patient is observed for potential complications, such as hemorrhage, sepsis or bile leakage. After the drainage bag is discarded, care will center on ensuring the catheter to remain patent. Once a day, 20 to 30 ml of sterile normal saline or sterile water is flushed through the catheter.

Flushing with 5 ml at a time in a quick, spurting motion breaks up and clears debris and bile accretions in the tube. However, fluid MUST NOT be aspirated during the irrigation. To do so might draw irritating duodenal contents into the biliary tree and lead to an infectious or chemical cholangitis.

Miller/Gavant [11] suggest to clean the skin with saline and cover the coiled catheter and entry site with one or two 4X4 bandages to keep the skin from catching on the clothing.

In Lund we have had fewer complications by cleaning the area around the catheter with chlorhexidinspiritus, covering the skin with a metalline tracheotomy compress and covering the coiled catheter with a sterile gauze swab (7 × 10 cm) with self-adhesive fabric on top. The catheter is flushed twice a day the first 10 days with 10 ml Inspir (acetylcystein), to prevent clotting. The patient also gets acetylcystein per os for the same reason.

Lecates [14] suggests using a skin barrier wafer (e.g., Stomahesive) to treat or prevent blistered, excoriated skin secondary to bile leakage.

In Lund the catheter is often sutured to a skin barrier wafer a little to the side from the punctional site. This is to prevent the catheter from sliding, without too much pain for the patient.

During the daily irrigation the patient and a family member are given instructions on how to care for the catheter at home. Written instructions are helpful to send with the patient when leaving the hospital.

In some cases where a bypass, Roux-En-Y procedure, is necessary it is also necessary to place a U-tube or Silastic stents. Of paramount importance is the security and patency of the stents as well as the color, consistency and amount of drainage. (Within 24 hrs the drainage should be clear bile.) Any bile leakage, leakage of flushing solution at the exit site or absence of bile-flow into the bag should be noted and reported to the surgeon. Gentle flushing with 20 ml sterile normal saline may be ordered to maintain the patency. Aspiration is never done due to the risk of sepsis [12]. The tubes are usually shortened and joined together and the patient and family taught how to care for them at home.

Preparation for home

In general patients with cancer will sooner or later suffer in different ways and might need rehospitalization. To be of maximal assistance to the patient and the family, the nurse must understand the stages of grief, the stage of awareness of the patient and family and, most important, their personal feelings about death. The nurse should assist in deciding if terminal care is to be carried out in the home or in an institution.

Nursing care of the patient with liver-transplantation

Liver transplants are done routinely only at a few medical centers around the world. Approximately 800 transplants had been performed 1985.

Preoperative care

For the patient the procedure in the operating room is vital naturally, but it is not enough to make a liver transplant successful. The pre- and postoperative care is also of great importance.

In 1978 the Nursing Mirror, Great Britain, and The Australian Nurses' Journal both published series of articles on the nursing care of patients having liver transplants.

Law [15] discussed in depth the need for the RN to take a nursing history as part of the nursing assessment. Information is obtained about the patients socio-economic circumstances, his fears and expectations, and his normal pattern of daily living in relation to hygiene, diet, sleeping, elimination, pain and recreational activities.

This information can be used to plan individualized nursing care and make predictions about the patient's learning needs. When taking the nursing history it is also a good time to inform the patient about what to expect and what is expected of him during hospitalization and in the future.

It can also be used as the baseline on which postoperative changes in the patient can be compared. The confidence of the patient is built on him being accepted as an individual, and on the conficence of the nurses in their ability to meet his needs [15].

Lok [16] especially mentions the need to inform the patient and his family about the possibility of death during the operation and that there is no other form of artificial mechanism that can keep the patient alive. He also mentions the need for the patient's next of kin to be prepared for what to expect when the patient arrives back from the theatre.

The preoperative care is the same as that given before general surgery, so here will only be mentioned the need for screening the patient for any signs of preoperative infection. This because of the serious consequences an infection can have after the surgery.

Perioperative care

When the operating room team at The Presbyterian University Hospital of Pittsburgh Medical Center were asked about the most important thing to remember about scrubbing for this procedure the answer was as follows: 'In addition to knowing the procedure step-by-step, all materials must be prepared and ready ahead of time. Organization is crucial because it is an extremely long procedure, with many people involved. You must keep exact counts for the several hundred needles and sponges used.'

Other important things being stressed are that it is crucial to maintain stringent aseptic technique as these patients already have a lowered resistance to infection. It is also important to be well prepared for the possibility of excessive bleeding, and to remember not to waste energy reserves on useless activities since the surgery is very demanding.

Operating room nurses must develop a proper mental attitude and discipline to avoid depression resulting from potential negative outcome of the surgery [17].

Postoperative care

While the operation is in progress, the patient's room is cleaned and prepared. The walls and floor are washed to make it as clean as possible [15]. When the patient returns he is reverse-barrier nursed for 10–14 days.

No matter how the postoperative care is organized, the patient needs intensive care at first. Lok, Mazzola [18] and Law all agree on the need for two RNs to care for the patient constantly for the first couple of days.

The most important measures are to maintain ventilation and monitoring of the patient's general state. Fluid and electrolyte balance and prevention of infection come next. All these actions ought to be well known to the reader, they will not be presented in detail here. The one thing to mention is mouth care, since it is a potential site for infection. The frequency of mouth care often has to be increased to every hour to improve patient comfort.

Pain control is not usually a great problem, but may be needed before physiotherapy. It has also been shown that pain can be influenced by anxiety, and that pain and anxiety can be reduced by giving relevant information. It is therefore of value to the patient to give nursing information also at all stages of care after operation [19].

Prevention of pressure sores, activity and feeding takes place according to the patient's condition. The post-operative recovery should take two or three weeks if there is no rejection crisis or major complications.

Preparation for home

The patient needs to learn how to cope with his own dressings and drugs in preparation for discharge. Knowledge of the signs of rejection and what to do in such a situation is also important. He also needs to re-learn independence of living in between regular hospital outpatient visits.

To assist nurses with improving the knowledge on the critical care nursing of liver transplants, Smith [20] have presented a patient care plan in the american 'Heart & Lung'. The article is followed by an educational program with a special examination.

Smith covers basically the same material as was published 1978, but she adds an interesting fact about how patients realize long before their surgery that another person must die for the transplant to become reality. This morbid waiting period is a time of extreme stress.

She also puts forward the need for a multidisciplinary approach to the care of these patients, beginning early in the preoperative phase if possible. At UCLA Medical Center, a clinical nurse specialist, a clinical social worker, and a psychiatrist join the critical care nursing staff and physicians to form the core group of the in-hospital support system for the patient and family.

Evaluation of nursing care

Nurses should determine things that are important to patients and make provision for them in the plan of care. Emotional support comes when patients feel that the nurse cares for them as human beings, allows them to participate in decisions, knows the therapeutic plan and expectations and spends time with them. A therapeutic atmosphere must be created before patients feel free enough to share their feelings with a team member.

The evaluation of care for the patient with postoperative complications focuses primarily on alleviation of the problem identified. The patient may be in a life-threatening situation that allows little time for the knowledge aspects associated with other phases of care. However, postoperative care assumes much significance to the family members who are waiting to hear the results of the surgery. The presence of a complication strikes fear in the heart and mind of the patient and family alike. This fear if not addressed can adversely affect recovery. For this reason the standards of care developed for postoperative complications need to include the family to a greater extent than other phases of care.

Patients must also understand what they must do, and what others will do, before making any committment to change or adapt their behavior. All nurse-patient interaction should contribute to teaching. The plan for home

430

care must be clear to all, so that patient, family, physicians and nurses all work together.

Finally there is a need for nurses to communicate knowledge concerning care of HPB-patients. Hopefully the amount of published clinical nursing knowledge concerning these patients will increase in forthcoming years.

References

1. Given BA, Simmons SJ: Gastroenterology in clinical nursing, ed 4, St Louis, Mosby, 1984
2. Winifred S: Cholecystectomy and exploration of the common bile duct. Nursing Mirror pp 45–46, July 1976
3. Ulander K: Preoperative information to patients operated with gallbladder resection. Paper given at symposium for HPB-nurses. Lund Univ Hospital, Sweden, 1986
4. Osborne S: Total pancreatectomy and splenectomy for a patient with chronic pancreatitis. Nursing Times pp 1836–1840, Oct 1980
5. Whiteford A: Restless nights. Nursing Mirror pp 48–50, July 1980
6. Levine CD: Preventing complications in the pancreatoduodenectomy patient. Dimensions of critical nursing 2(2): 90–97, March-April 1983
7. Altshuller A, Hilden D: The patient with hypertension. Nursing Clinics of North America 12(2): 317–329, 1977
8. King DE: How to give your portal hypertension patient a fighting chance. RN for managers 46(7): 31–37, July 1983
9. Joakimsson A, Nilsson K: Nursing care planning for patients operated with liver-resection. Paper given at symposium for HPB-nurses. Lund Univ Hospital, Sweden, 1986
10. Bradford F: Malignant strictures of the hepatobiliary system. Nursing times 77(37): 1601–1604, Sept 1981
11. Miller B, Gavant ML: Biliary catheter care. American Journal of Nursing 10: 1115–1117, Oct 1985
12. Coleman JA: Surgical treatment for cholangiocarcinoma. Today's OR Nurse 7(10): 22–27, Oct 1985
13. Jones B: The Hammersmith biliary drainage system improved patient care during preoperative decompression of the obstructed biliary tree. Paper presented at symposium for HPB-nurses. Lund Univ Hosp, Sweden, 1986
14. Lecates E: Bile leakage from biliary cath. American Journal of Nursing 86(1): 28, Jan 1986
15. Law GM: The nursing care of patients having orthotopic liver transplants. Nursing Mirror pp 12–14, Aug 1978
16. Lok P: Nursing management of liver transplant. Australian Nurses Journal 8(4): 38–40, Oct 1978
17. Hepatic surgery saves lives. Today's OR Nurses 7(8): 25–28, 1985
18. Mazzola P: Nursing care of the liver-transplant patient. RN 39(5): 34–37, May 1976
19. Boore J: Prescription for recovery. Royal College of Nursing, Whihtefriars press LTD, London, 1978
20. Smith SL: Liver transplantation – Implications for critical care nursing. Heart & Lung 14(6): 617–628, Nov 1985